St

Challenging Concepts in Oncology

Titles in the Challenging Concepts in series

Anaesthesia (Edited by Dr Phoebe Syme, Dr Robert Jackson, and Professor Tim Cook)

Cardiovascular Medicine (Edited by Dr Aung Myat, Dr Shouvik Haldar, and Professor Simon Redwood)

Emergency Medicine (Edited by Dr Sam Thenabadu, Dr Fleur Cantle, and Dr Chris Lacy)

Infectious Disease and Clinical Microbiology (Edited by Dr Amber Arnold and Professor George Griffin)

Interventional Radiology (Edited by Dr Irfan Ahmed, Dr Miltiadis Krokidis, and Dr Tarun Sabharwal)

Neurology (Edited by Dr Krishna Chinthapalli, Dr Nadia Magdalinou, and Professor Nicholas Wood)

Neurosurgery (Edited by Mr Robin Bhatia and Mr Ian Sabin)

Obstetrics and Gynaecology (Edited by Dr Natasha Hezelgrave, Dr Danielle Abbott, and Professor Andrew Shennan)

Oncology (Edited by Dr Madhumita Bhattacharyya, Dr Sarah Payne, and Professor Iain McNeish)

Oral and Maxillofacial Surgery (Edited by Mr Matthew Idle and Group Captain Andrew Monaghan)

Respiratory Medicine (Edited by Dr Lucy Schomberg and Dr Elizabeth Sage)

Challenging Concepts in Oncology
Cases with Expert Commentary

Edited by

Dr Madhumita Bhattacharyya PhD MRCP
Consultant Medical Oncologist
Berkshire Cancer Centre, Royal Berkshire Hospital NHS Foundation Trust, Reading, UK

Dr Sarah Payne PhD MRCP
Specialist Registrar Clinical Oncology
Guy's and St Thomas' NHS Foundation Trust, London, UK

Professor Iain McNeish PhD FRCP
Professor of Gynaecological Oncology
Institute of Cancer Sciences, University of Glasgow, Glasgow, UK

Series editors

Dr Aung Myat BSc (Hons) MBBS MRCP
BHF Clinical Research Training Fellow, King's College London British Heart Foundation Centre of
Research Excellence, Cardiovascular Division, St Thomas' Hospital, London, UK

Dr Shouvik Haldar MBBS MRCP
Electrophysiology Research Fellow & Cardiology SpR, Heart Rhythm Centre, NIHR Cardiovascular
Biomedical Research Unit, Royal Brompton & Harefield NHS Foundation Trust, Imperial College London,
London, UK

Professor Simon Redwood MD FRCP
Professor of Interventional Cardiology and Honorary Consultant Cardiologist, King's College London
British Heart Foundation Centre of Research Excellence, Cardiovascular Division and Guy's and
St Thomas' NHS Foundation Trust, St Thomas' Hospital, London, UK

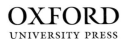

OXFORD
UNIVERSITY PRESS

OXFORD
UNIVERSITY PRESS

Great Clarendon Street, Oxford, OX2 6DP,
United Kingdom

Oxford University Press is a department of the University of Oxford.
It furthers the University's objective of excellence in research, scholarship,
and education by publishing worldwide. Oxford is a registered trade mark of
Oxford University Press in the UK and in certain other countries

Impression: 1

Published in the United States of America by Oxford University Press
198 Madison Avenue, New York, NY 10016, United States of America

British Library Cataloguing in Publication Data
Data available

Library of Congress Control Number: 2014956589

ISBN 978-0-19-968888-3

Printed in Great Britain by
Ashford Colour Press Ltd, Gosport, Hampshire

FOREWORD

All of the professions involved in providing modern care for cancer patients face an information base which is growing in its volume and complexity at a rate which is both gratifying and alarming. The rapid advances in the basic sciences which underpin our understanding of the biology and pathology of cancer are well recognized. These are feeding through steadily to enhance the scientific basis for the evaluation of the diagnosis, stage, prognosis, and risk factors associated with each individual cancer patient. New treatments, which are increasingly deployed on a personalized or stratified basis, are emerging. We have seen a steady growth in the number of targeted therapies for specific tumour types or subtypes. Perhaps the greatest current excitement results from a significant minority of patients who are achieving durable remissions with new biological and immunological therapies. However, not all of the challenges faced by oncologists arise from science at the international forefront or the need to deploy effective, complex, and novel therapies. We also have to deal with increasing numbers of older cancer patients who may have co-morbidities or frailty which make their choice of therapy, in consultation with their clinicians, especially challenging. Communication skills and time for effective consultations that allow for good choices by patients are at a premium. Wide availability of information through the Internet can also add to the quality, but also sometimes to the challenges presented by consultations. The health care is subject to increasing scrutiny of its quality and must be based on evidence which must be evaluated and absorbed by oncologists, in order to deliver excellence. More than 50% of all cancer patients now survive their disease and live for at least 10 years after their diagnosis. No effort can be spared to ensure that all patients have their best chance to benefit from this opportunity.

Against this background, the text in *Challenging Concepts in Oncology* provides oncologists with a valuable opportunity to stay up to date in their subject, both within their areas of special expertise, but also across the wider range of oncology. The text is strongly learning-orientated. By relating each topic to a case history and bringing out 'clinical tips', 'expert comments', and key 'learning points 'in each chapter, the multiple authors are generating a resource which will help oncologists to tackle the many challenges they face. The tips and comments are well chosen to help the busy oncologist update their knowledge and their focus on these important clinical questions. The format is readable, lends itself to the 'occasional 'reading session which, for many oncologists, will be early in the morning, late at night, or on a train. By combining authorship between trainees and the experienced consultants, the editors have ensured a balanced approach which will be valuable for learning and teaching, but also valuable for updates and continuing professional development for established consultants and oncologists of all professions.

Professor Peter Selby
President, Association of Cancer Physicians

PREFACE

Oncology is a rapidly evolving specialty fundamentally supported by peer-reviewed evidence-based trials. Personalized medicine has already taken a significant foothold in cancer pathways and signals an era of very exciting times ahead. Application of translational work to everyday clinical practice is key to ensuring patients receive the best possible care.

With improvements in cancer outcomes, late effects and survivorship are increasingly important, as many cancers become chronic diseases. The provision of acute oncology services in the UK by oncologists is another recent development. This stems from a national initiative influenced by the National Confidential Enquiry into Patient Outcome and Death (NCEPOD) and the National Chemotherapy Advisory Group (NCAG). The recommendations from their reports included the development of dedicated acute oncology services in all trusts involved in reviewing patients presenting with undiagnosed cancer or suspected cancer, complications of chemotherapy, radiotherapy, or with cancer-related complications.

In this book, we have tried to encapsulate the elements of patient-focussed care, principles of acute oncology, and the relevant evidence base. We present 25 clinical cases, written by UK oncology specialty trainees, which have been chosen to provide an overview of the management of the common cancers, with discussion of common complications and acute oncological emergencies. Through the 'learning points', 'clinical tips', 'landmark trials 'and 'expert comments', we have discussed the challenges in diagnosis and evidence for current treatments, including some of the molecular and genetic background to the cancer and its treatments. Additionally, we have sought renowned UK experts in the relevant tumour site to provide a peer review commentary throughout each case. The scenarios have been selected to reflect real-life diagnostic and management challenges that would ordinarily generate debate amongst clinicians. In doing so, we have strived to provide a comprehensive textbook, written in a style which is interesting, informative, and, above all, innovative.

We hope the book will appeal to trainees in both medical and clinical oncology. These subspecialties have separate training programmes, although elements of the curriculum are delivered jointly. We feel our concise textbook, covering common problems, treatments, and latest developments in oncology, will be invaluable for both junior oncology trainees and more senior doctors preparing for their postgraduate examinations.

Challenging Concepts also provides an excellent basis for consultants involved in acute oncology to keep up to date with the latest treatments of a variety of malignancies, as well as their own tumour sites of interest. Allied to this, we hope that this book will be an invaluable reference text for specialist nurses involved in delivering acute oncology services and for the palliative care teams, with whom oncologists work closely.

Management of patients with cancer is multidisciplinary, and the book has been written with this in mind. In addition to the target readership of specialist oncologists, our vision has been to produce a text that will engage and encompass the interest of associated health care professionals (e.g. palliative care specialists, specialist nurses, and radiographers).

We believe the *Challenging Concepts* series platform has allowed us to produce a book that is unique and innovative in this field and will be a worthwhile contribution to the medical literature.

We, the editors, very much hope you enjoy the book.

Sarah Payne
Madhumita Bhattacharyya
Iain McNeish

ACKNOWLEDGEMENTS

We would like to thank all the contributors of the book who have worked very hard together to make it so relevant, inclusive, thorough, and clear.

I would like to say a big thank you to my husband Iain Soulsby and my two wonderful daughters, Emily and Charlotte. Thank you for all your support and patience over the course of this project. Thank you also for ensuring I never ran out of cups of tea.

Sarah Payne

I would like to thank all my family for their support and encouragement, above all, my lovely son Ishaan.

Madhumita Bhattacharyya

With thanks to Geraldine, Angus, and Iona.

Iain McNeish

CONTENTS

EXPERTS

Madhumita Bhattacharyya
Consultant Medical Oncologist
Berkshire Cancer Centre, Royal Berkshire Hospital
NHS Foundation Trust
Reading, UK

Mark Bower
Lead Clinician and Consultant Medical Oncologist
National Centre for HIV Malignancy
Chelsea and Westminster Hospital
London, UK

John Bridgewater
Senior Lecturer and Consultant Medical Oncologist
UCL Cancer Institute
London, UK

John Chester
Professor of Medical Oncology
Institute of Cancer and Genetics
School of Medicine, Cardiff University
Honorary Consultant in Medical Oncology
Velindre Cancer Centre
Cardiff, UK

Pippa Corrie
Consultant Medical Oncologist
Department of Oncology
Cambridge University Hospitals NHS Foundation Trust
Addenbrooke's Hospital
Cambridge, UK

Nicola Dallas
Consultant Clinical Oncologist
Berkshire Cancer Centre, Royal Berkshire Hospital
NHS Foundation Trust
Reading, UK

Angela Darby
Consultant Medical Oncologist
Department of Oncology
York Teaching Hospital NHS Foundation Trust
York, UK

Andrew Davies
Cancer Research UK
Senior Lecturer in Medical Oncology and Honorary
Consultant
University Hospital Southampton
NHS Foundation Trust
Southampton, UK

Mark Harries
Consultant Medical Oncologist
Guy's and St Thomas' NHS Foundation Trust
London, UK

Paul Kooner
Consultant Hepatologist
Bart's Health, NHS Trust
London, UK

Nick Maisey
Consultant Medical Oncologist
Department of Oncology
Guy's and St Thomas' NHS Foundation Trust
London, UK

Iain McNeish
Professor of Gynaecological Oncology
Institute of Cancer Sciences, University of Glasgow
Wolfson Wohl Cancer Research Centre
Glasgow, UK

Clive Mulatero
Consultant Medical Oncologist
St James's Institute of Oncology
Leeds Teaching Hospitals NHS Trust
Leeds, UK

Helen O'Donnell
Consultant Clinical Oncologist
Berkshire Cancer Centre
Royal Berkshire NHS Foundation Trust
Reading, UK

Chris Plummer
Consultant Cardiologist
Department of Cardiology
Freeman Hospital
Newcastle upon Tyne NHS Foundation Trust
Newcastle upon Tyne, UK

David Propper
Consultant Medical Oncologist
Bart's Health NHS Trust
London, UK

Anne Rigg
Consultant Medical Oncologist
Guy's and St Thomas' NHS Foundation Trust
London, UK

Azmat H Sadozye
Consultant Clinical Oncologist
Beatson West of Scotland Cancer Centre
Glasgow, UK

Jonathan Shamash
Consultant Medical Oncologist
Barts Health NHS Trust
London, UK

Amen Sibtain
Consultant Clinical Oncologist
Barts Health NHS Trust
London, UK

Eliot Sims
Consultant Clinical Oncologist
Queens Hospital
Essex, UK

Jeremy Steele
Consultant Medical Oncologist
Barts Health NHS Trust
London, UK

Sandra Strauss
Senior Clinical Research Associate
Research Department of Oncology
University College London Hospitals NHS
Foundation Trust
London, UK

Matthew Wheater
Consultant Medical Oncologist
Department of Medical Oncology
University Hospitals Southampton
Southampton General Hospital
Southampton, UK

CONTRIBUTORS

Bristi Basu
Academic Consultant in Experimental Cancer
Therapeutics
Cancer Research UK
Consultant Medical Oncologist
Cambridge University Hospitals NHS Foundation Trust
Department of Oncology
Addenbrooke's Hospital
Cambridge, UK

Laura Beaton
Specialist Registrar Clinical Oncology
Bart's Health NHS Trust
London, UK

Indrani S Bhattacharya
Specialist Registrar Clinical Oncology
Department of Oncology
Mount Vernon Cancer Centre
London, UK

Jennifer Bradbury
Consultant Medical Oncologist
Department of Oncology
University Hospital Southampton NHS Foundation
Trust
Southampton, UK

Anna C Olsson-Brown
Specialist Registrar Medical Oncology
Clatterbridge Cancer Centre
Wirral, UK

Caroline Chau
Specialist Registrar Medical Oncology
Department of Medical Oncology
University Hospital Southampton NHS Foundation
Trust
Southampton, UK

Meenali Chitnis
Locum Consultant Medical Oncologist
Oxford University Hospital's NHS Trust
Oxford, UK

Shanthini Crusz
Specialist Registrar Medical Oncology
Department of Medical Oncology
Barts Health NHS Trust
London, UK

Gary Doherty
Clinical Lecturer in Oncology
Department of Oncology
Cambridge University Hospitals NHS Foundation Trust
Cambridge, UK

Fatima El-Khouly
Specialist Registrar Medical Oncology
Department of Oncology
University College Hospital
University College London Hospitals NHS Foundation
Trust
London, UK

Sarah Ellis
Specialist Registrar Medical Oncology
Department of Oncology
University Hospital Southampton NHS Foundation Trust
Southampton, UK

Gemma Eminowicz
Specialist Registrar Clinical Oncology
Department of Oncology
Barts Health
London, UK

Khurum Khan
Clinical Research Fellow
GI and Lymphoma Unit
Department of Medicine
The Royal Marsden NHS Foundation Trust
Sutton, UK

Angela Lamarca
Clinical Research Fellow
Department of Medical Oncology
The Christie NHS Foundation Trust
Manchester, UK

Alex Lee
Specialist Registrar Clinical Oncology
The Royal Marsden NHS Foundation Trust
London, UK

Chern Siang Lee
Specialist Registrar Medical Oncology
University Hospital Southampton NHS
Foundation Trust
Southampton, UK

Caroline Manetta
Consultant Clinical Oncologist
Brighton and Sussex University
Hospitals NHS Trust
Brighton, UK

Gargi Patel
Consultant Medical Oncologist
Brighton and Sussex University Hospitals NHS Trust
Brighton, UK

Sarah Payne
Specialist Registrar Clinical Oncology
Guy's and St Thomas' NHS Foundation Trust
London, UK

Imran Petkar
Specialist Registrar Medical Oncology
The Royal Marsden NHS Foundation Trust
London, UK

Marcus Remer
Specialist Registrar Medical Oncology
Department of Medical Oncology
University Hospital Southampton
NHS Foundation Trust
Southampton, UK

Kai-Keen Shiu
Locum Consultant Medical Oncologist
University College London Hospitals NHS
Foundation Trust
London, UK

Kate Smith
Specialist Registrar Medical Oncology
Department of Medical Oncology
Barts Health NHS Trust
London, UK

Kathryn Tarver
Consultant Clinical Oncologist
Queen's Hospital
Essex, UK

Hannah Taylor
Specialist Registrar Medical Oncology
Department of Oncology
University Hospitals Bristol NHS Trust
Bristol Oncology Centre
Bristol, UK

Juan W Valle
Professor of Medical Oncology
Department of Medical Oncology
University of Manchester
The Christie NHS Foundation Trust
Manchester, UK

Swee-Ling Wong
Specialist Registrar Clinical Oncology
Barts Health NHS Trust
London, UK

David K Woolf
Specialist Registrar Clinical Oncology
Department of Academic Oncology
Mount Vernon Cancer Centre
Northwood, UK

ABBREVIATIONS

°	degree
°C	degree Celsius
=	equal to
≥	equal to or greater than
≤	equal to or less than
↓	decreased
↑	increased
>	greater than
<	less than
λ	lambda
%	per cent
±	plus or minus
£	pound sterling
®	registered trademark
Ab	antibody
ABVD	doxorubicin, bleomycin, vinblastine, and dacarbazine
ACE	angiotensin-converting enzyme
ACTH	adrenocorticotrophic hormone
ADL	activity of daily living
AED	anti-epileptic drug
AFP	alpha fetoprotein
AI	aromatase inhibitor
AIDS	acquired immune deficiency syndrome
AJCC	American Joint Committee on Cancer
ALA	5-aminolevulinic acid
ALK	anaplastic lymphoma kinase
ALP	alkaline phosphatase
ALT	alanine aminotransferase
AOS	acute oncology service
AR	androgen receptor
ARDS	adult respiratory distress syndrome
ARSAC	Administration of Radioactive Substances Advisory Committee
ASC	active symptom control
ASCO	American Society of Clinical Oncology
AST	aspartate aminotransferase
AUC	area under the curve
AVP	arginine vasopressin
BAP1	BRCA1-associated protein 1
BCLC	Barcelona-Clinic Liver Cancer
BCT	breast-conserving therapy

bd	*bis die* (twice daily)
BEP	bleomycin, etoposide, cisplatin
BHIVA	British HIV Association
BL	Burkitt's lymphoma
BMI	body mass index
BP	blood pressure
BPH	benign prostate hyperplasia
bpm	beat per minute
BSA	body surface area
BTS	British Thoracic Society
CA19.9	carbohydrate antigen 19-9
CA125	cancer antigen 125
cART	combination antiretroviral therapy
CAV	doxorubicin, cyclophosphamide, vincristine
cc	cubic centimetre
CCC	clear cell carcinoma
ccRCC	clear cell renal cell carcinoma
CCRT	concurrent chemoradiotherapy
CEA	carcinoembryonic antigen
CgA	chromogranin A
CHART	continuous hyperfractionated accelerated radiotherapy
CI	confidence interval
CINV	chemotherapy-induced nausea and vomiting
CK5/6	cytokeratin 5/6
CK7	cytokeratin 7
cm	centimetre
CMF	cyclophosphamide, methotrexate, and 5-fluorouracil
CMV	cytomegalovirus
CNS	central nervous system
CO_2	carbon dioxide
COG	Children's Oncology Group
COX	cyclo-oxygenase
CR	complete remission
CRC	colorectal carcinoma
CRM	circumferential margin
CRP	C-reactive protein
CRT	chemoradiotherapy
CSF	cerebrospinal fluid
CT	computerized tomography

CTCAE	common terminology criteria for adverse events
CT CAP	computerized tomography of the chest, abdomen, and pelvis
CTV	clinical target volume
CTZ	chemoreceptor trigger zone
CUP	carcinoma of unknown primary
CXR	chest X-ray
3D	three-dimensional
DCIS	ductal carcinoma *in situ*
DFS	disease-free survival
dL	decilitre
DLBCL	diffuse large B-cell lymphoma
DNA	deoxyribonucleic acid
DPD	dihydropyrimidine dehydrogenase deficiency
DRE	digital rectal examination
DVT	deep vein thrombosis
EASL	European Association for the Study of the Liver
EBCTCG	Early Breast Cancer Trialists' Collaborative Group
EBRT	external beam radiotherapy
EBUS	endobronchial ultrasound
EBV	Epstein–Barr virus
ECF	epirubicin, cisplatin, and 5-fluorouracil
ECG	electrocardiogram
ECOG	Eastern Cooperative Oncology Group
ECX	epirubicin, cisplatin, and capecitabine
ED	emergency department
ED-SCLC	extensive-disease small cell lung cancer
EEG	electroencephalography
EGCCCG	European Germ Cell Cancer Consensus Group
EGF	epidermal growth factor
EGFR	epidermal growth factor receptor
EIA	enzyme immunoassay
EMA	European Medicines Agency
EMG	electromyography
ENETS	European Neuroendocrine Tumor Society
ENT	ear, nose, and throat
EP	cisplatin and etoposide
EPP	extra-pleural pneumonectomy
ER	oestrogen receptor
ERCP	endoscopic retrograde cholangiopancreatography
ESMO	European Society for Medical Oncology

ESR	erythrocyte sedimentation rate
EUS	endoscopic ultrasound
FBC	full blood count
FDA	Food and Drug Administration
FDG	fluorodeoxyglucose
FEV_1	forced expiratory volume in 1 second
FGFR	fibroblast growth factor receptor
FIGO	*Fédération Internationale de Gynécologie et d'Obstétrique*
FISH	fluorescence *in situ* hybridization
fL	femtolitre
FLIPI	Follicular Lymphoma International Prognostic Index
FNA	fine-needle aspiration
FOLFIRINOX	5-fluorouracil, folinic acid, irinotecan, and oxaliplatin
FSH	follicle-stimulating hormone
FTR	free/total ratio
5-FU	5-fluorouracil
FVC	forced vital capacity
g	gram
GBM	glioblastoma multiforme
GBM-O	glioblastoma with oligodendroglioma component
GBq	giga becquerel
GC	gemcitabine and cisplatin
GCS	Glasgow coma score
G-CSF	granulocyte colony-stimulating factor
GEP	gastroenteropancreatic
GFR	glomerular filtration rate
GI	gastrointestinal
GOJ	gastro-oesophageal junction
GP	general practitioner
G6PD	glucose-6-phosphate dehydrogenase
GTV	gross tumour volume
GU	genitourinary
Gy	gray
HAART	highly active antiretroviral therapy
Hb	haemoglobin
HBV	hepatitis B virus
HCC	hepatocellular carcinoma
HCG	human chorionic gonadotrophin
HCV	hepatitis C virus
HDGC	hereditary diffuse gastric cancer
HDR	high-dose rate
HER2	human epidermal growth factor receptor 2
HGF	hepatocyte growth factor
HGSC	high-grade serous ovarian carcinoma

HHV-8	human herpesvirus-8	kCO	transfer coefficient
HIA	hepatic intra-arterial	kg	kilogram
5-HIAA	5-hydroxyindoleacetic acid	kPa	kilopascal
HIF	hypoxia-inducible factor	KS	Kaposi's sarcoma
hIL-6	human interleukin-6	KSHV	Kaposi's sarcoma-associated
HIV	human immunodeficiency virus		herpesvirus
HNPCC	hereditary non-polyposis colorectal	L	litre
	cancer	LANA-1	latent nuclear antigen-1
HNSCC	head and neck squamous cell	LC	local control
	carcinoma	LCIS	lobular carcinoma *in situ*
HPB	hepatopancreaticobiliary	LCNEC	large cell neuroendocrine carcinoma
HPF	high power field	LDH	lactate dehydrogenase
HPV	human papillomavirus	LDR	low-dose rate
HR	hazard ratio	LD-SCLC	limited-disease small cell lung cancer
HRD	defective homologous recombination	LEMS	Lambert–Eaton myasthenic syndrome
HRT	hormone replacement therapy	LFT	liver function test
Hsp90	heat shock protein 90	LH	luteinizing hormone
HSV	herpes simplex virus	LHRH	luteinizing hormone-releasing hormone
5HT3	5-hydroxytryptamine-3	LMWH	low-molecular-weight heparin
HTLV	human T-lymphotropic virus	LND	lymph node dissection
IASLC	International Association for the Study	LoDLIN	longest diameter of the largest involved
	of Lung Cancer		node
IBS	irritable bowel syndrome	LVEF	left ventricular ejection fraction
ICP	intracranial pressure	LVSI	lymphovascular space invasion
ICU	intensive care unit	m	metre
IDH1	isocitrate dehydrogenase 1	mAb	monoclonal antibody
IFN	interferon	MAC	*Mycobacterium avium* complex
IGCCC	International Germ Cell Consensus	MAP	methotrexate, cisplatin, and
	Classification		Adriamycin®
IGF	insulin-like growth factor	MCD	multicentric Castleman disease
IgG	immunoglobulin G	mCi	millicurie
IHC	immunohistochemistry	mCRC	metastatic colorectal carcinoma
IL	interleukin	M, C & S	microbiology, culture, and sensitivity
IM	intramuscular	MCV	mean corpuscular volume
IMRT	intensity-modulated radiotherapy	MDT	multidisciplinary team
INR	international normalized ratio	MEN	multiple endocrine neoplasia
IPI	International Prognostic Index	MET	mesenchymal–epithelial transition
IPS	International Prognostic Score		factor
irAE	immune-related adverse event	mg	milligram
irCR	immune-related complete response	MGMT	methyl guanine methyl transferase
irPD	immune-related progressive disease	MHRA	Medicines and Healthcare products
irPR	immune-related partial response		Regulation Agency
irRC	immune-related response criteria	MIBC	muscle-invasive bladder cancer
irSD	immune-related stable disease	MIBG	meta-iodobenzylguanidine
ISH	*in situ* hybridization	min	minute
ITT	intention-to-treat	mIU	milli international unit
IU	international unit	mL	millilitre
IV	intravenous	mm	millimitre
K	potassium	mmHg	millimetre of mercury

mmol	millimole	PARP	poly (adenosine diphosphate-ribose) polymerase
mOsm	milliosmole	PBL	plasmablastic lymphoma
MRI	magnetic resonance imaging	PCI	prophylactic cranial irradiation
MSCC	metastatic spinal cord compression	PCL	primary central nervous system lymphoma
MSI	microsatellite instability		
MSKCC	Memorial Sloan Kettering Cancer Center	PCOS	polycystic ovary syndrome CH5; Prostate Cancer Outcomes Study
mTOR	mammalian target of rapamycin	PCP	*Pneumocystis jirovecii* pneumonia
MTP	muramyl tripeptide	PCV	procarbazine, CCNU, and vincristine
MU	million unit	PD-1	programmed death-1
MUGA	multigated acquisition	PDAC	pancreatic ductal adenocarcinoma
MVAC	methotrexate, vinblastine, adriamycin, cisplatin	PDGF	platelet-derived growth factor
		PDGFR	platelet-derived growth factor receptor
Na	sodium	PE	pulmonary embolism
nab	nanoparticle albumin-bound	PEG	percutaneous endoscopic gastrotomy
NANETS	North American NeuroEndocrine Tumor Society	PEI	percutaneous ethanol injection
		PEL	primary effusion lymphoma
NB	*nota bene* (take note)	PET	positron emission tomography
NCAP	computerized tomography scan of the neck, chest, abdomen, and pelvis	PF	performance status
		PFS	progression-free survival
NCCN	National Comprehensive Cancer Network	PICC	peripherally inserted central catheter
		PLD	pegylated liposomal doxorubicin
NCRI	National Cancer Research Institute	Plt	platelet
NET	neuroendocrine tumour	pmol	picomole
ng	nanogram	PNET	pancreatic neuroendocrine tumour
NG	nasogastric	PO	*per os* (taken orally)
NHL	non-Hodgkin's lymphoma	PPE	palmar–plantar erythrodysaesthesia
NHS	National Health Service	PR	progesterone receptor
NICE	National Institute for Health and Care Excellence	PRN	*pro re nata* (as required)
		PS	performance status
NK1	neurokinin 1	PSA	prostate-specific antigen
NMBIC	non-muscle-invasive bladder cancer	PTV	planning target volume
nmol	nanomole	PV	portal vein
NNRTI	non-nucleoside reverse transcriptase inhibitor	qds	*quater die sumendum* (four times daily)
		QoL	quality of life
NRTI	nucleoside reverse transcriptase inhibitor	RAI	radioactive iodine ablation
		RANKL	receptor activator of nuclear factor kappa B ligand
NSAID	non-steroidal anti-inflammatory drug		
		RCC	renal cell carcinoma
NSCLC	non-small cell lung cancer	RCT	randomized controlled trial
NTS	nucleus tractus solitarii	R-CVP	rituximab, cyclophosphamide, vincristine, and prednisolone
NYHA	New York Heart Association		
OAR	organs at risk	RECIST	Response Evaluation Criteria in Solid Tumours
od	*omne in die* (once daily)		
OGD	oesophagogastroduodenoscopy	RFA	radiofrequency ablation
OGJ	oesophagogastric junction	rhTSH	recombinant human thyroid-stimulating hormone
OI	opportunistic infection		
OPG	orthopantomogram		
OS	overall survival	RIG	radiologically inserted gastrostomy

RMI	risk of malignancy index
RNA	ribonucleic acid
RPA	recursive partitioning analysis
RPS	radiation protection supervisor
RR	relative risk
RT-PCR	reverse transcriptase polymerase chain reaction
SALT	speech and language therapy
s/c	subcutaneously
SCC	squamous cell carcinoma
SCLC	small cell lung cancer
SEER	Surveillance, Epidemiology, and End Results
SIADH	syndrome of inappropriate anti-diuretic hormone
SIRT	selective internal radiation therapy
SLE	skeletal-related event
SMA	superior mesenteric artery
SMV	superior mesenteric vein
SPARC	secreted protein acidic and rich in cysteine
SPF	sun protection factor
SRE	skeletal-related event
SVC	superior vena cava
SVCO	superior vena cava obstruction
T3	tri-iodothyronine
T4	thyroxine
TACE	trans-arterial chemo-embolization
TAH-BSO	total abdominal hysterectomy with bilateral salpingo-oophorectomy
TBNA	transbronchial needle aspiration
TBNK	T-cells, B-cells, and natural killer cells
TCC	transitional cell carcinoma
tds	*ter die sumendum* (three times daily)
tFL	transformed follicular lymphoma
Tg	thyroglobulin
TGF	transforming growth factor
TIP	paclitaxel, ifosfamide, cisplatin

TKI	tyrosine kinase inhibitor
TLS	tumour lysis syndrome
TNM	tumour–node–metastasis
TPF	taxane, cisplatin, and 5-FU
TRUS	transrectal ultrasound
TSH	thyroid-stimulating hormone
TTF-1	thyroid transcription factor-1
TURBT	transurethral resection of bladder tumour
TURP	transurethral resection of the prostate
TVUS	transvaginal ultrasound
TYA	teenage young adult
U&Es	urea and electrolytes
UK	United Kingdom
UKI	NETS UK and Ireland Neuroendocrine Tumour Society
ULN	upper limit of normal
US	United States
USS	ultrasound scan
UVA	ultraviolet A
UVB	ultraviolet B
VALSG	Veterans Administration Lung Study Group
VBT	vaginal vault brachytherapy
VEGF	vascular endothelial growth factor
VEGFR	vascular endothelial growth factor receptor
VeIP	cisplatin, ifosfamide, and vinblastine
VHL	von Hippel–Lindau
vIL-6	viral interleukin-6
VIP	etoposide, ifosfamide, and cisplatin; vasoactive intestinal polypeptide
VTE	venous thromboembolism
WBC	white blood count
WCC	white cell count
WHO	World Health Organization
WLE	wide local excision

TABLE 0.1

Challenging Concepts in Oncology Mapped to Clinical Oncology Curriculum 2010

Challenging Concepts in Oncology Chapter:	1. Breast cancer and neutropenic sepsis	2. Non-small cell lung cancer and superior vena cava obstruction	3. Mesothelioma and chemotherapy-induced vomiting	4. Small cell lung cancer (SCLC) and syndrome of inappropriate antidiuretic hormone (SIADH)	5. Endometrial cancer and treatment complications	6. Ovarian cancer and malignant bowel obstruction	7. Oesophageal cancer and dysphagia	8. Gastric cancer and complications of relapsed disease	9. Advanced pancreatic cancer	10. Hepatocellular cancer and venous thromboembolism	11. Colorectal liver metastases	12. Muscle-invasive transitional cell carcinoma of the bladder	13. Metastatic renal cell cancer and hypercalcaemia	14. Metastatic prostate cancer and spinal cord compression	15. Transformed follicular lymphoma	16. Metastatic germ cell cancer	17. Osteosarcoma and the use of high-dose chemotherapy	18. Melanoma and immunotherapy	19. Laryngeal cancer and oral mucositis	20. Glioblastoma multiforme (GMB)	21. Thyroid cancer and radioiodine therapy	22. Neuroendocrine tumours and treatment complications	23. HIV-associated malignancies	24. Late cardiovascular complications of cancer treatment	25. Cancer of unknown primary
10.1 Cytotoxic chemotherapy																									
10.2 Adverse reactions	x		x		x	x				x	x		x	x	x	x	x	x	x	x	x		x		
10.3 Breast cancer	x																								
10.4 Thoracic malignancy		x	x	x																					
10.5 Upper GI cancer							x	x	x	x															
10.6 Lower GI cancer											x														
10.7 Head and neck cancer																			x		x				
10.8 Sarcomas																	x								
10.9 Gynaecological oncology					x	x																			
10.10 Urological malignancy												x	x	x		x									
10.11 Neuro-oncology																				x					
10.12 Skin malignancy																		x							
10.13 Lymphomas															x										
10.14 Paediatric oncology																									

Table 0.2 (*continued*)

10.12 Management of sarcoma						X			
10.13 Management of leukaemia and plasma cell dyscrasia									
10.14 Management of prostate cancer				X					
10.15 Management of immunosuppression-associated malignancies									X
10.16 Management of urothelial cancer		X							
10.17 Management of cervical cancer									
10.18 Management of head and neck cancer							X		
10.19 Management of central nervous system malignancy								X	
10.20 Management of renal cell cancer			X						
10.21 Management of tumours affecting the endocrine organs								X	
10.22 Management of tumours of the thoracic cavity	X								
10.23 Management of teenagers and young adults with cancer					X	X			

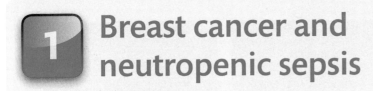

Breast cancer and neutropenic sepsis

Gargi Patel

Ⓒ Expert commentary Anne Rigg

Case history

A 62-year-old retired medical secretary presented to the emergency department (ED) with severe lumbar back pain and constipation for the past few weeks. She had no paraesthesiae, numbness, or weakness, and normal micturition. Eighteen months previously, she had detected a right-sided breast lump, seen on mammography (Figure 1.1), and palpable right axillary lymphadenopathy and was diagnosed with a T2N3M0 grade 3 breast cancer which was oestrogen receptor (ER)- and progesterone receptor (PR)-positive (ER 8/8, PR 8/8) and human epidermal growth factor receptor 2 (HER2)-negative. Following a multidisciplinary meeting and patient consultation, she underwent a wide local excision (WLE) and axillary lymph node dissection (LND); histology showed a 3.3×3.6 cm infiltrating ductal carcinoma. Fourteen out of 18 lymph nodes were involved; margins were clear. She was treated with adjuvant radiotherapy and tamoxifen (20 mg daily) and declined chemotherapy.

She had hypertension controlled with bendroflumethiazide. She was post-menopausal (her periods stopped 2 years prior to diagnosis). She did not smoke and drank alcohol in moderation. Her mother was diagnosed with breast cancer aged 52, whilst going through the menopause, and died of metastatic disease within 2 years.

> **➕ Clinical tip** Diagnosis of breast cancer
>
> 'One-stop' clinics allow triple assessment through clinical, radiological, and histological examination. Common histological groups include infiltrating ductal, lobular, or mixed ductal and lobular carcinoma. Carcinoma *in situ* (ductal or lobular, DCIS or LCIS) is a pre-malignant lesion with different treatment options. Breast cancers may be subtyped by gene expression into luminal A or B, HER2-enriched, and basal subtypes, with implications for prognosis and treatment [1].
>
> Assessment of ER, PR, and HER2 status provides prognostic information and tailoring of treatment.

> **Ⓒ Expert comment**
>
> All new patients with breast cancer will have their case discussed at diagnosis and after surgery to determine further therapies. Multidisciplinary team (MDT) working allows groups of health professionals to debate and decide on recommendations for a patient's care. This ensures that all members of the team are giving the patient accurate and consistent information. It is recommended that the patient's case is re-discussed at each presentation with a new breast cancer event in the metastatic setting to explore the most useful option for the patient at that moment in time.

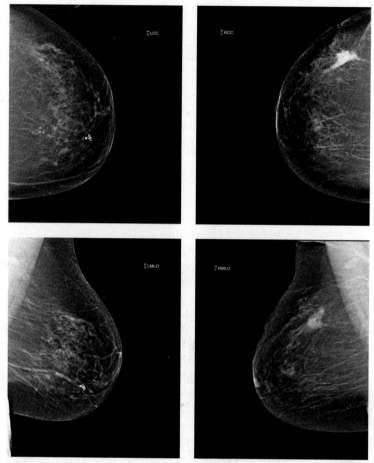

Figure 1.1 Breast cancer diagnosis. Bilateral mammograms of the right and left breasts, demonstrating a spiculated 3 cm mass in the right upper quadrant, suspicious of carcinoma. (R, right; L, left; MLO, medio-lateral oblique view; CC, cranio-caudal view).

> ✪ **Learning point** Risk of relapse
>
> Breast cancer is staged using the TNM system [2]:
>
> - *'early stage'*: stage I, IIA, IIB, or IIIA, node-negative disease
> - *'locally advanced'*: stage IIIA or IIIC with fixed nodal involvement, or T4 disease regardless of nodal status (IIIB)
> - *'metastatic disease'*: stage IV disease (<5% of cases at presentation).
>
> Lymph node involvement is a strong prognostic indicator for relapse. A greater burden of nodal involvement predicts for poorer survival. Patients with locally advanced primary tumours without nodal involvement have a better prognosis than those with locally advanced nodal disease (e.g. clinically fixed axillary lymph nodes or ipsilateral supraclavicular lymph node), as illustrated by 5-year survival rates for stage I, IIA, IIB, IIIA, IIIB, and IV disease: 95%, 85%, 70%, 52%, 48%, and 18%, respectively [2].
>
> Further prognostic factors include tumour size, grade, hormone receptor status, tumour type (inflammatory versus other histological subtypes), lymphovascular invasion, young age (<35 years), or older age (>65 years) [3]. Genomic signatures, which have recently been approved by the Food and Drug Administration (FDA) for recurrence, e.g. MammaPrint, may be used for prognostication but are not widely available [4].

❂ Learning point Adjuvant radiotherapy

Although radical mastectomy is the operation of choice for locally advanced breast cancer, WLE, followed by radiotherapy (breast-conserving therapy, BCT), has been shown to be equivalent for early-stage disease, with fewer morbidities and better cosmesis [5]. Patients typically receive 46–50 Gy over 4–5 weeks, followed by a boost to the lumpectomy site.

With nodal involvement, surgical axillary dissection is normally recommended. The MA.20 trial for node-positive or high-risk node-negative patients demonstrated an improved 5-year disease-free survival (DFS) and a reduction in locoregional relapse (92.4% versus 94.5%), but with higher risks of radiation dermatitis, pneumonitis, and lymphoedema, for patients receiving regional node irradiation. Following mastectomy, radiotherapy is indicated for tumours involving the deep margins or pathologically involved lymph nodes.

❂ Learning point Adjuvant chemotherapy

Adjuvant chemotherapy with cyclophosphamide, methotrexate, and 5-fluorouracil (5-FU) (CMF) demonstrated a survival benefit for patients with high-risk early and locally advanced breast cancer [6]. The introduction of anthracyclines into adjuvant regimens further improved survival rates [7], with a 6.5% reduction in breast cancer mortality and an 8% reduction in the risk of recurrence. Incremental benefits above those observed with CMF were found with higher doses of anthracyclines (i.e. a cumulative dose of >360 mg/m^2 or >240 mg/m^2 for epirubicin or doxorubicin, respectively). The addition of taxane therapy to an anthracycline-based regimen provided a further overall survival (OS) benefit of 2.8% and a 4.5% reduction in the risk of recurrence [7]. The choice of regimen is dependent on patient and tumour characteristics but includes anthracycline- and taxane-based chemotherapy for high-risk patients.

❂ Learning point Adjuvant hormonal therapy

Patients with ER- and/or PR-positive tumours (Allred score of 3 or greater) benefit from treatment with tamoxifen or aromatase inhibitors (AIs). The menopausal status and side effect profiles drive the choice of agent.

Pre- or peri-menopausal status

Tamoxifen, a selective ER modulator, is a competitive antagonist of the ER but demonstrates partial agonist activity. The EBCTG meta-analysis demonstrated a 13% reduction in recurrence (46% versus 33%), and a 15% reduction in risk of breast cancer mortality (33% versus 24%), at 15 years for tamoxifen (20 mg once a day for 5 years), compared to placebo [8].

Post-menopausal status

These patients may be treated with AIs, tamoxifen, or a combination.

For post-menopausal women, treatment with AIs for 5 years is equivalent to a 'switch' regimen (tamoxifen for 2–3 years, followed by anastrozole for 2–3 years, or vice versa) and will be dictated by patient choice and tolerability. For pre- or peri-menopausal patients with high-risk disease, up to 10 years of tamoxifen may be offered, if the initial treatment is well tolerated.

✚ Clinical tip Menopausal status

Chemotherapy treatment may lead to amenorrhoea without true menopause; guidelines for the definition of menopause have been developed by the National Comprehensive Cancer Network (NCCN) [25]:

- >60 years of age
- <60 years of age, with previous bilateral oophorectomy or lack of menstruation for 12 months or more, in the absence of treatment with tamoxifen, chemotherapy, or ovarian suppression.

✚ Clinical tip Aromatase inhibitors (AIs)

AIs, e.g. anastrozole (1 mg once daily, od), letrozole (2.5 mg od), or exemestane (25 mg od), inhibit the peripheral conversion of androgens to oestrogen by aromatase. In patients with minimal residual ovarian function, peripheral inhibition of the aromatization of androgens may lead to the activation of a negative feedback loop stimulation of ovarian function. These drugs are therefore contraindicated in pre- or peri-menopausal patients unless used with ovarian suppression.

✚ Clinical tip Side effects of tamoxifen

Common side effects of tamoxifen include hot flushes, weight gain, mood swings, vaginal discharge, sexual dysfunction, and menstrual irregularities. Less common, but major, side effects include increased risk of venous thrombosis, including stroke and deep vein thrombosis (DVT) (not statistically significant), and endometrial malignancies (4% versus 1% for patients treated with placebo for women aged >55 years). Compared to AIs, tamoxifen has a protective effect on bone mineral density and cardiovascular risk.

⊕ Clinical tip   Side effects of AIs

Common side effects of AIs include hot flushes, vaginal dryness, sexual dysfunction, arthralgia, joint stiffness, and bone pain (may be severe in up to 30% of patients). Major side effects include osteoporosis, fractures, increased cardiovascular, risk and hypercholesterolaemia. Compared to tamoxifen, the risk of venous thrombosis and endometrial cancer is lower.

⊕ Clinical tip   Bone mineral density scans

Post-menopausal patients commencing AIs and pre-menopausal patients who develop premature menopause should have bone mineral density studies performed at the hip and lumbar spines and commence treatment with bisphosphonates, if osteopaenic.

❝ Expert comment

Many breast oncologists use the Adjuvant! Online programme to predict the risk of breast cancer recurrence and death within the next 10 years. This web-based programme is a physician decision making tool and can be useful during consultations to try and quantify an individual patient's risk from breast cancer and the absolute survival benefit that they would get from adjuvant chemotherapy and/or endocrine therapy. It is free for any oncologist to register and use. It would not be recommended that patients use it, without input from a health professional. The risk prediction for this patient at original presentation was that she had a 19% chance of surviving 10 years with surgery only. Endocrine therapy would increase her chances by a further 13%, and chemotherapy by 17%. If she had agreed to both modalities, her risk of death within 10 years would have been 48%. Of note, the programme takes into account co-morbidities, and she would have had a 5% chance of dying of a non-breast cancer condition during the decade.

❝ Expert comment

Tamoxifen is contraindicated if a patient has a past history of venous thromboembolism (VTE). It can only be administered to a patient with a previous VTE event, if the patient agrees to be anticoagulated for the whole duration of time on tamoxifen. For patients who commence tamoxifen, the risk of venous thrombosis is present immediately, and the risk does not increase over time. If the patient has a strong family history of VTE, but no personal history, it can be helpful to check a thrombophilia screen and consult with a specialist in anticoagulation. Conversely, the risk of endometrial malignancy increases, as the duration of exposure to tamoxifen increases.

✔ Evidence base   MA.17 and BIG 1-98 studies: adjuvant hormonal therapy

The MA.17 and BIG 1-98 studies, and an EBCTCG meta-analysis demonstrated a reduction in relapse at 5 years (12% versus 15%, respectively) for patients on an AI, compared to tamoxifen, but no difference in the OS [8–10]. The MA.27 study demonstrated that treatment with different AIs, e.g. exemestane versus anastrozole, was equivalent.

A 'switch' regimen with AI and tamoxifen, switching from one to the other at 2–3 years, did demonstrate a benefit for relapse-free survival (8% versus 11%) and OS (6.5% versus 8%) at 5 years, compared to tamoxifen alone for 5 years [11]. Sequential therapy with 5 years of tamoxifen, followed by 5 years of AI, also demonstrated improved DFS (93% versus 87%), but no definite improvement in the OS, compared to tamoxifen alone for 5 years [10]. Meta-analysis data suggest that the use of an AI alone for 5 years is equivalent to the 'switch' regime for post-menopausal women.

✪ Learning point   Adjuvant trastuzumab

Several large randomized controlled studies have demonstrated the benefit of addition of trastuzumab (Herceptin®) to adjuvant chemotherapy for HER2-positive tumours (score of >2 on immunohistochemistry (IHC) or fluorescence *in situ* hybridization (FISH) positive) of >1 cm [12–14], with improvements in OS and DFS (hazard ratios (HRs) 0.66 and 0.60, respectively). Due to risks of cardiotoxicity, regular monitoring of the left ventricular ejection fraction (LVEF) is required by echocardiogram or multigated acquisition (MUGA); the drug is preferably given with taxanes, as anthracyclines are also cardiotoxic. Trastuzumab is administered for 1 year. The case for HER2-targeted treatment for tumours <1 cm is more controversial.

On examination she had a World Health Organization (WHO) performance status (PS) of 1. Neurological, cardiovascular, respiratory, and abdominal examinations were normal. She had bony tenderness on palpation of the lumbar spine. Breast examination revealed no new lesions.

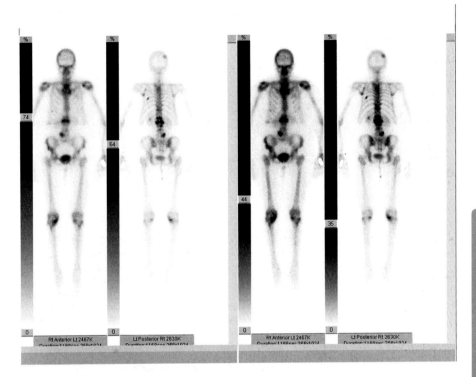

Figure 1.2 Whole-body nuclear medicine bone scan. Bone scan demonstrating several foci of abnormal increased tracer uptake, involving the skull, left scapula, several ribs, the spine, and the pelvis, likely to represent metastatic disease. There is also increased uptake in the region of the left coracoid. Joint-centred uptake is present within both knees, particularly marked within the medial tibial plateau on the right, which may represent degenerative disease.

Blood tests demonstrated hypercalcaemia, with corrected serum calcium of 3.21 mmol/L, but were otherwise normal. Full-staging computerized tomography (CT) did not demonstrate visceral metastases, and no new abnormalities were seen on repeat mammogram. A whole-body bone scan demonstrated multiple bony metastases, including the lumbar spine and pelvis (Figure 1.2). Magnetic resonance imaging (MRI) of the spine did not demonstrate cord compression. She was treated with intravenous (IV) pamidronate (90 mg in 500 mL of 0.9% normal saline over 90 minutes), leading to the normalization of her serum calcium. She continued on 3-weekly pamidronate, alongside anastrozole 1 mg daily and analgesia, and remained on these for a further 3 years.

She subsequently developed weight loss and upper abdominal pain, and restaging CT demonstrated liver metastases and a suspicious lung nodule. She started weekly paclitaxel chemotherapy.

Following cycle 1, she was admitted with a fever of 38.9°C and a neutrophil count of 0.1. She was tachycardic and hypotensive with a blood pressure (BP) of 90/50 mmHg. Peripheral blood cultures and a urine sample were sent for microbiology, prior to commencing IV Tazocin® (piperacillin and tazobactam) and amikacin. She responded well to fluid resuscitation and IV antibiotics, alongside granulocyte colony-stimulating factor (G-CSF, 263 micrograms) for 4 days as an inpatient, until her neutrophils recovered to 1.0×10^9/L. She was then discharged home with a 10-day

❝ Expert comment

The BOLERO-2 study has demonstrated a new standard of care for patients who develop resistance to non-steroidal aromatase inhibitors (NSAIs) [15]. The addition of an mTOR (mammalian target of rapamycin) inhibitor, everolimus, to exemestane was shown to produce an improvement in progression free survival of 6 months (4.1 to 10.6 months), with an objective response rate of 7% versus 0.4%. However, this combination is mainly likely to benefit patients who have previously hormone-sensitive breast cancer, which has become resistant to NSAIs, likely by activation of the PI3kinase/mTOR signalling pathway alongside the ER pathway, and has not shown to be of benefit in first line treatment for patients who are NSAI-naive (HORIZON study) [16].

✪ Learning point Hormonal treatment of relapsed disease

Patients with ER/PR-positive disease with asymptomatic or non-end-organ (e.g. soft tissue) relapse often exhibit an indolent phenotype, responsive to further hormonal therapy. Progression on adjuvant hormonal therapy, or within 12 months of completion, is defined as resistant disease and requires treatment with a different hormonal agent. Rechallenge with previously used hormone treatment is appropriate for relapse >12 months from cessation of that therapy.

course of oral antibiotics. With subsequent chemotherapy cycles, she received G-CSF for 5 days (days 7–12). She completed six cycles of treatment, with a good partial response in her liver lesions. At this stage, her 20-year-old daughter requested referral for genetic counselling.

✪ **Learning point**   Chemotherapy in metastatic breast cancer

Patients with rapidly progressing, visceral, or symptomatic disease demonstrate an aggressive phenotype, with chemotherapy being required to produce rapid response rates. Patients with triple-negative disease or HER2-positive metastatic disease also require chemotherapy.

Combination chemotherapy regimens provide minimal survival benefits at a cost of significant toxicities, when compared to new chemotherapy agents, e.g. capecitabine, docetaxel, vinorelbine, and gemcitabine. Single-agent chemotherapy, ± HER2-targeted agents for HER2-positive disease, forms the mainstay of treatment for metastatic disease, providing equivalent survival rates with better quality of life (QoL). Disease relapse on or within 12 months of chemotherapy is defined as resistance and requires treatment with an alternative chemotherapy agent.

- Taxanes are usually used in the first line, with response rates of 25–35% [17], without cumulative toxicity. Rechallenge within 12 months of treatment may be successful, as paclitaxel and docetaxel do not show complete cross-resistance. Trastuzumab should be prescribed in combination for HER2-positive patients, even if progressing on trastuzumab.
- Anthracyclines may be used with response rates of 35–40% [17] but are limited due to cumulative cardiotoxicity.
- Capecitabine, given orally, may be better tolerated in patients with poor PS and who have received multiple previous lines of treatment, with response rates of 30%. The HER2-targeted drug lapatinib has been approved for use with capecitabine in the metastatic setting, after progression on taxanes and trastuzumab.
- Vinorelbine is also attractive for poor PS patients, with minimal toxicities and response rates of 25–45% for heavily pretreated patients.
- It is always important to consider opportunities for clinical trials in both the metastatic and adjuvant settings.
- ASCO guidelines (2014) now recommend a combination of docetaxel, pertuzumab and trastuzumab in the first line treatment of patients with HER2+ve metastatic disease, due to a 6 month improvement in disease-free survival seen in the CLEOPATRA study. This combination is currently available in the UK by application to the CDF [18, 19].

✪ **Learning point**   Bisphosphonates

Bisphosphonates, e.g. pamidronate, zoledronate, clodronate, and alendronate, have two major roles in breast cancer:

- used with AIs in *early breast cancer* for patients with osteoporosis
- for *metastatic disease* to the bone.

Bisphosphonates cause apoptosis of osteoclasts, reducing bone resorption and slowing the loss of bone mineral density.

Bony metastases may cause significant morbidity, due to pain and skeletal-related events (SREs), e.g. fracture, spinal cord compression, hypercalcaemia, and the need for surgery or radiotherapy to these lesions. Bisphosphonates reduce the risk of SREs by 15%, attenuate bony pain, improve the QoL, and increase the median time to SREs in women with clinically evident bony metastases [20]. No survival benefit has been demonstrated for these drugs; trials are ongoing. There is no evidence to demonstrate the superiority of one type of bisphosphonate over another. The duration of therapy required is unclear, but the risk–benefit ratio seems to be favourable up to at least 2 years, beyond which we have little evidence.

Denosumab, an inhibitor of the receptor activator of nuclear factor kappa B ligand (RANKL), which inhibits osteoclast activity, has been shown to be superior to bisphosphonates, with a greater delay to the first SRE (32.4 months versus 26.4 months), no difference in OS, and similar tolerability [21]. Although this drug is preferred for patients with metastatic breast cancer, drug costs currently restrict clinical use.

❝ Expert comment

Oncology is a relatively young specialty and is heavily evidence-based. Most cancer centres will participate in clinical research trials and will try to have a trial for every clinical scenario. Many patients like to be informed about the option of taking part in a clinical trial, whether it is to study a new intervention or more focussed on observation. All staff involved in clinical trials need to have up-to-date training in Good Clinical Practice based on the Declaration of Helsinki. Centres that have a high commitment to clinical trials produce better outcomes for patients. All of the treatment recommendations for this patient were based on the published results of previous clinical trials in breast cancer.

➕ Clinical tip Side effects of bisphosphonates

Side effects of bisphosphonates are uncommon but include acute renal injury, electrolyte imbalance with hypocalcaemia, ocular inflammation, and osteonecrosis of the jaw. Patients are recommended to undergo full dental assessment, prior to commencing bisphosphonate therapy.

❝ Expert comment

Denosumab is a monoclonal antibody (mAb) against RANKL and inhibits osteoclast activity. In clinical trials, it has been shown to be even more potent than zoledronic acid at preventing skeletal events from bone metastases. As it is administered subcutaneously (s/c), it lends itself to being given in a community setting and may enable patients to have fewer hospital visits and will help those that have poor venous access. In addition, it does not lead to renal impairment so does not require patients to have the renal function monitored. It can cause significant hypocalcaemia, especially in the first 6 months of treatment, so it is essential that patients take calcium and vitamin D supplements.

✪ Learning point Familial breast cancer and *BRCA*

Familial breast cancer is defined as a history of breast cancer in one or more first-degree relatives. Approximately 10% of the population have a positive family history of breast cancer, with an associated lifetime risk of 10–13% of developing breast cancer. A positive family history of breast cancer may be due to inherited (germline) mutations, rather than acquired (somatic) mutations, few of which have been identified.

The major germline mutation characterized in breast cancer is the breast cancer susceptibility gene (*BRCA*) mutation. *BRCA* is a tumour suppressor gene, essential for the production of proteins which repair DNA double-stranded breaks. Mutation is inherited in a dominant manner from either parent and leads to the loss of function of one of a pair of diploid genes, leaving one functional copy. Mutation in both copies, either germline or somatic, results in the loss of heterozygosity and a high propensity to errors in DNA repair. Mutations in *BRCA1* and/or *BRCA2* vary widely, as may genetic penetrance and phenotype, according to the type of mutation, resulting in a range of no increased risk to a lifetime risk of over 50% for breast cancer [22].

BRCA1 mutations are associated with a higher risk of breast cancer at a younger age, compared to *BRCA2* mutations. The risk of ovarian, Fallopian tube, and peritoneal cancers is also increased in *BRCA1* and *BRCA2* mutation carriers. *BRCA1* mutations are further associated with an increased risk of cervical, uterine, pancreatic, gastric, and prostate cancers, and *BRCA2* mutations are associated with biliary, prostate, pancreatic, and gastric cancers, and melanoma.

❝ Expert comment

Breast cancer patients can be referred to a clinical geneticist to discuss whether they might carry a germline mutation in *BRCA1*, *BRCA2*, or *p53*. Patients developing breast cancer under the age of 45 should be considered for genetic referral, especially if the cancer is triple receptor-negative (ER-, PR-, and HER2-negative). Family history should also be considered as an important risk factor for carrying a gene mutation which predisposed to breast cancer. Most genetic clinics will use an algorithm to assess the likelihood of the patient having a known gene mutation and will recommend testing for those with an intermediate or high probability of there being a mutation. The testing is performed from an ordinary blood sample. It is essential that the patient is counselled properly, prior to the test being performed, as there are numerous consequences to discovering a genetic mutation for both the patient and family members. In the first instance, the test is usually performed for the person who has actually had cancer; then, if a mutation is identified, the test can be offered to unaffected adult blood relatives.

> ⊕ **Clinical tip** Management of *BRCA* patients
>
> Early identification and surveillance is recommended, with clinical examination at least annually from the age of 25, annual mammography and breast MRI from the age of 25, and twice-yearly ovarian screening with transvaginal ultrasound and serum CA125 levels from the age of 35. Risk-reducing mastectomy reduces the risk of breast cancer by over 90% and should be considered for women with a *BRCA1* or *BRCA2* mutation. Similarly, salpingo-oophorectomy should be considered for women with these mutations who have completed their families.

> ✪ **Learning point (Acute oncology)** Neutropenic sepsis (acute oncology)
>
> Neutropenic sepsis is a medical emergency and is defined as neutropenia (neutrophil count < 0.5 or $< 1.0 \times 10^9$/L and expected to fall) with a fever (core temperature of $>37.5°C$).
>
> Neutropenic fever may rapidly progress to systemic sepsis syndrome, and even death, if not treated urgently within an hour of presentation with broad-spectrum IV antibiotics. Fever may not be present, but other warning symptoms are rigors, general deterioration in condition, and confusion, especially in the elderly. Use of anti-pyretics, e.g. paracetamol or non-steroidal anti-inflammatory drugs (NSAIDs), and immunosuppressants, e.g. steroids, can mask a fever and the signs of sepsis until a late stage.
>
> **Pathogenesis**
>
> Cytotoxic therapy may lead to compromised integrity and immunity of mucosal surfaces in the oropharynx, gut, and lung. Translocation of commensal bacteria, which are predominantly Gram-negative organisms, may lead to systemic infection and sepsis.
>
> **Investigations**
>
> - Full history, including dates and type of chemotherapy, drug history, and history of allergies.
> - Clinical examination.
> - Microbiological investigations:
>   - ○ urine, blood cultures (peripheral and indwelling central venous catheters)
>   - ○ swabs, sputum sample, diarrhoea, if appropriate.
> - Chest X-ray (CXR).
>
> **Management**
>
> - Treatment with broad-spectrum IV antibiotics should be commenced within 1 hour of presentation with a clinical suspicion of neutropenic sepsis.
> - Monitor fluid balance and urine output.
> - Consider the use of G-CSF.
> - If further spikes in temperature after 48 hours from the initiation of first-line antibiotics, further cultures must be taken and antibiotics switched to second line, as per local protocol.
> - Further spikes in temperature, 48 hours after the initiation of second-line antibiotics, usually require the addition of IV anti-fungal and/or anti-viral treatment and discussion with the microbiology team.
>
> Patients are usually discharged from hospital, once they have been free of fever for 24 hours and the neutrophil counts are $>1.0 \times 10^9$/L, with a course of appropriate oral antibiotics.

> ⊕ **Clinical tip** Neutropenic sepsis
>
> Aggressive fluid resuscitation should be commenced, alongside broad-spectrum first-line antibiotics, in haemodynamically unstable patients. Urinary catheterization is usually necessary to monitor the hourly urine output, and an arterial blood gas should be taken for measurement of serum pH and lactate levels. If patients do not stabilize with fluid resuscitation, they should be referred early for intensive care input, for potential treatment with inotropes.

Discussion

In summary, this is a case of a patient with breast cancer who developed bony metastases and hypercalcaemia, after inadequate adjuvant treatment. She had high-risk, locally advanced stage IIIA (T2N2aM0) disease, with a large (over 2 cm) primary tumour, and was heavily node-positive. She should have received adjuvant chemotherapy, with a combination of anthracycline and taxane. It could be argued that adjuvant tamoxifen only was also suboptimal for this post-menopausal patient. Her clinical outcome could have been improved by the switch to an AI at 2 years, had she not developed metastatic disease.

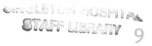

She was fully investigated to exclude cord compression and commenced treatment with bisphosphonates for the prevention of further SREs and to control hypercalcaemia which was probably contributing to constipation. Her disease exhibited the typically indolent phenotype associated with breast cancer with bony metastases alone.

On re-presentation with symptomatic visceral disease, she was treated with chemotherapy, in order to obtain a more rapid response rate. Weekly paclitaxel is associated with an OS advantage, compared to 3-weekly docetaxel, but with higher toxicities, especially neuropathy. A further option would have been anthracycline-based chemotherapy, as she had not received this previously and had no cardiac morbidity.

She was appropriately treated for neutropenic sepsis. Although G-CSF was given alongside broad-spectrum antibiotics, the evidence to support its use is controversial. Although several trials have demonstrated reduced duration of neutropenia and length of hospital stay, a meta-analysis has found no survival benefit [23]. However, the benefit of using G-CSF as secondary prophylaxis, after the development of neutropenic sepsis, has been shown to reduce the risk of further neutropenic fever by 50% [24].

A final word from the expert

This case is a good example of the complex journey that a woman with breast cancer can experience. Ideally, this woman should have had adjuvant chemotherapy at the time of her initial diagnosis with breast cancer, as this would have significantly reduced her risk of developing distant metastases. As has been shown, there can be long periods of time where ER-positive breast cancer bony metastases can be controlled with hormonal therapy and bisphosphonates or denosumab. When a patient develops visceral metastases, the preferred course of action would be to use chemotherapy instead, as, although more toxic, it can produce a response in the tumour faster. Chemotherapy can be associated with significant toxicity, and it is essential that the patient is counselled appropriately about the intention of the treatment and understands the procedure for contacting the oncology team for help. Multidisciplinary working between oncology, surgery, radiology, pathology, and palliative care is essential to maintain the highest standards of care for all patients with breast cancer throughout their journey.

References

1. Perou CM, Sorlie T, Eisen MB et al. Molecular portraits of human breast tumours. *Nature* 2000; **406**(6797): 747–52.
2. Newman LA. Epidemiology of locally advanced breast cancer. *Seminars in Radiation Oncology* 2009; **19**(4): 195–203.
3. Rosen PP, Groshen S, Kinne DW, Norton L. Factors influencing prognosis in node-negative breast carcinoma: analysis of 767 T1N0M0/T2N0M0 patients with long-term follow-up. *Journal of Clinical Oncology* 1993; **11**(11): 2090–100.
4. van't Veer LJ, Dai H, van de Vijver MJ et al. Gene expression profiling predicts clinical outcome of breast cancer. *Nature* 2002; **415**(6871): 530–6.
5. [No authors listed]. Effects of radiotherapy and surgery in early breast cancer. An overview of the randomized trials. Early Breast Cancer Trialists' Collaborative Group. *The New England Journal of Medicine* 1995; **333**(22): 1444–55.
6. Bonadonna G, Rossi A, Valagussa P. Adjuvant CMF chemotherapy in operable breast cancer: ten years later. *The Lancet* 1985; **1**(8435): 976–7.
7. Peto R, Davies C, Godwin J et al. Comparisons between different polychemotherapy regimens for early breast cancer: meta-analyses of long-term outcome among 100,000 women in 123 randomised trials. *The Lancet* 2012; **379**(9814): 432–44.

8. Davies C, Godwin J, Gray R *et al.* Relevance of breast cancer hormone receptors and other factors to the efficacy of adjuvant tamoxifen: patient-level meta-analysis of randomised trials. *The Lancet* 2011; **378**(9793): 771–84.

9. Thurlimann B, Keshaviah A, Coates AS *et al.* A comparison of letrozole and tamoxifen in postmenopausal women with early breast cancer. *The New England Journal of Medicine* 2005; **353**(26): 2747–57.

10. Goss PE, Ingle JN, Martino S *et al.* A randomized trial of letrozole in postmenopausal women after five years of tamoxifen therapy for early-stage breast cancer. *The New England Journal of Medicine* 2003; **349**(19): 1793–802.

11. Coombes RC, Kilburn LS, Snowdon CF *et al.* Survival and safety of exemestane versus tamoxifen after 2–3 years' tamoxifen treatment (Intergroup Exemestane Study): a randomised controlled trial. *The Lancet* 2007; **369**(9561): 559–70.

12. Romond EH, Perez EA, Bryant J *et al.* Trastuzumab plus adjuvant chemotherapy for operable HER2-positive breast cancer. *The New England Journal of Medicine* 2005; **353**(16): 1673–84.

13. Piccart-Gebhart MJ, Procter M, Leyland-Jones B *et al.* Trastuzumab after adjuvant chemotherapy in HER2-positive breast cancer. *The New England Journal of Medicine* 2005; **353**(16): 1659–72.

14. Slamon D, Eiermann W, Robert N *et al.* Adjuvant trastuzumab in HER2-positive breast cancer. *The New England Journal of Medicine* 2011; **365**(14): 1273–83.

15. Baselga J, Campone M, Piccart M *et al.* (2012) Everolimus in postmenopausal hormone-receptor-positive advanced breast cancer. *The New England Journal of Medicine* 366:520–529.

16. Wolff AC, Lazar AA, Bondarenko I, et al. (2013) Randomized phase III placebo-controlled trial of letrozole plus oral temsirolimus as first-line endocrine therapy in postmenopausal women with locally advanced or metastatic breast cancer. *Journal of Clinical Oncology* 31:195–202.

17. Paridaens R, Biganzoli L, Bruning P *et al.* Paclitaxel versus doxorubicin as first-line single-agent chemotherapy for metastatic breast cancer: a European Organization for Research and Treatment of Cancer Randomized Study with cross-over. *Journal of Clinical Oncology* 2000; **18**(4): 724–33.

18. Giordano SH, Temin S, Kirshner JJ *et al.* Systemic therapy for patients with advanced human epidermal growth factor receptor 2–positive breast cancer: American Society of Clinical Oncology Clinical Practice Guideline. *Journal of Clinical Oncology* 2014 **32**(19):2100–8.

19. Swain SM, Kim SB, Cortés J *et al.* Pertuzumab, trastuzumab, and docetaxel for HER2-positive metastatic breast cancer (CLEOPATRA study): overall survival results from a randomised, double-blind, placebo-controlled, phase 3 study. *Lancet Oncology* 2013; **14**(6): 461–71.

20. Wong MH, Stockler MR, Pavlakis N. Bisphosphonates and other bone agents for breast cancer. *Cochrane Database of Systematic Review* S 2012; **2**: C D003474.

21. Stopeck AT, Lipton A, Body JJ *et al.* Denosumab compared with zoledronic acid for the treatment of bone metastases in patients with advanced breast cancer: a randomized, double-blind study. *Journal of Clinical Oncology* 2010; **28**(35): 5132–9.

22. Chen S, Parmigiani G. Meta-analysis of BRCA1 and BRCA2 penetrance. *Journal of Clinical Oncology* 2007; **25**(11): 1329–33.

23. Berghmans T, Paesmans M, Lafitte JJ *et al.* Therapeutic use of granulocyte and granulocyte-macrophage colony-stimulating factors in febrile neutropenic cancer patients. A systematic review of the literature with meta-analysis. *Supportive Care in Cancer* 2002; **10**(3): 181–8.

24. Crawford J, Ozer H, Stoller R *et al.* Reduction by granulocyte colony-stimulating factor of fever and neutropenia induced by chemotherapy in patients with small-cell lung cancer. *The New England Journal of Medicine* 1991; **325**(3): 164–70.

25. National Comprehensive Cancer Network. *NCCN Clinical Practice Guidelines in Oncology* (NCCN Guidelines), Breast Cancer, Version 2.2013. Available at: <http://www.nccn.org/professionals/physician_gls/PDF/breast.pdf>

2 Non-small cell lung cancer and superior vena cava obstruction

Laura Beaton and Swee-Ling Wong

⊕ Expert commentary Clive Mulatero

Case history

A 64-year-old woman presented to her general practitioner (GP) with a 3-month history of cough, increasing shortness of breath on exertion, and small-volume haemoptysis. Her only significant past medical history was that of mild asthma, for which she was taking Symbicort®. She was a never-smoker and worked as a teacher. Of note, her father had died of lung cancer at the age of 75. At presentation she was performance status (PS) 1.

Despite a course of antibiotics and steroids, her cough and haemoptysis did not settle, and a routine CXR was organized. This showed a spiculated opacity in the left upper lobe, and she was referred for an urgent appointment with the respiratory team, given the concern of an underlying malignancy.

A CT scan of the chest and abdomen showed a 4.5 cm left upper lobe mass and an enlarged left hilar lymph node. There was no evidence of other enlarged lymph nodes or sites of distant disease. Spirometry was organized by the respiratory team, and, despite her background of mild asthma, her lung function was good. It was felt that the left upper lobe lesion was amenable to a bronchoscopic biopsy, and this was performed the following week. The patient's case was presented at the next lung MDT meeting. Histology revealed a moderately differentiated non-small cell carcinoma that was thyroid transcription factor-1 (TTF-1)-positive and consistent with an adenocarcinoma of lung origin (Table 2.1). On CT imaging, her disease was staged as T2aN1M0 (stage IIA).

⊕ Expert comment

The management of each individual NSCLC patient differs on the basis of morphological, immunohistochemical, and genetic features of their tumours. It has become clinically important to distinguish between squamous and non-squamous tumours, as well as those with actionable somatic mutations. Tumours may contain a mixture of squamous and non-squamous NSCLC phenotypes and, if so, are managed, using algorithms for the non-squamous component. Occasionally, tumours may contain mixed SCLC and NSCLC features. In these circumstances, most clinicians would manage the patient, using an SCLC treatment pathway. Whilst large cell neuroendocrine carcinoma (LCNEC) is classified as an NSCLC variant, according to WHO [2], it is currently managed similarly to SCLC, given its high-grade neuroendocrine features and clinical course. Carcinoid tumours are low-grade neuroendocrine malignancies and are managed in the same way as carcinoids that arise from other anatomical sites such as the intestine.

Table 2.1 Histology of non-small cell lung cancer (NSCLC)

Histological subtype	Immunohistochemical profile	Additional notes
Adenocarcinoma	TTF-1, CK7, napsin A	Seen in smokers and non-smokers, especially women Usually peripheral Tendency to spread to lymph nodes and brain TTF-1 helps distinguish between lung primary and metastatic adenocarcinoma CK20 positivity suggests gastrointestinal (GI) adenocarcinoma origin
Squamous cell	p63, CK5/6	Central tumours Associated with smoking Decreasing incidence No markers to distinguish between lung primary and metastatic SCC
Large cell, including neuroendocrine tumours (NETs)	NCAM (CD6), synaptophysin, and chromogranin	High tendency to spread to lymph nodes Markers may be negative in poorly differentiated NETs
Carcinoid		Usually small, endobronchial, and patients are young Unrelated to smoking Typical (70–90%)—rarely metastasizes and not associated with smoking Atypical (10–30%)—frequently metastasizes, and this appears to be associated with smoking

Source: data from Brambilla *et al.,* The new World Health Organization classification of lung tumours, *European Respiratory Journal,* Volume 18, Number 6, Copyright © 2001 ERS Journals Ltd.

<table>
<tr><td>

➕ Clinical tip

NSCLC is any type of epithelial lung cancer, other than small cell lung cancer (SCLC). The commonest subtypes are adenocarcinoma, large cell carcinomas, and squamous cell carcinomas (SCC).

</td></tr>
</table>

Table 2.2 Survival rates of NSCLC by stage

Stage	TNM	5-year OS (%) [3]
IA	T1a–1bN0M0	58–73
IB	T2aN0M0	43–58
IIA	T1a–T2aN1M0 T2bN0M0	36–46
IIB	T2bN1M0 T3N0M0	25–36
IIIA	T3N1M0 T1a–T3N2M0 T4N0M0	19–24
IIIB	T4N2M0 T1a–T4N3M0	7–9
IV	Any T, any N, M1a–b	2–13

Source: data from Office of National Statistics, *Cancer Survival in England: Patients Diagnosed 2005–2009 and Followed up to 2010,* © Crown Copyright 2011, reproduced under the Open Government Licence 2.0.

The MDT concluded that the patient was fit enough to be considered for radical treatment with surgery, and a positron emission tomography (PET) scan was arranged to exclude any distant disease or any regional nodal spread not visible on the CT scan. This test confirmed the staging to be T2aN1M0, and she was referred to a cardiothoracic surgeon to discuss the option of radical surgery. However, following this consultation, the patient decided against surgery. Given that her disease was encompassable in a radical radiotherapy field, she was therefore referred to an oncologist for discussion of radical concurrent chemoradiotherapy (CRT) [1]. After careful discussion of the practicalities of the treatment and its potential side effects, the patient consented to proceed to CRT. Although aware of the curative intent of the proposed treatment, the patient was also aware of the risk of recurrence.

> **⊘ Evidence base** Cochrane review of concurrent radiotherapy [1]
>
> - *Nineteen randomized studies (2728 participants) of concurrent CRT versus radiotherapy alone.*
>   - CRT significantly:
>   - reduced overall risk of death (HR 0.71, 95% CI 0.64–0.80; $n=1607$)
>   - reduced overall progression-free survival (PFS) at any site (HR 0.69, 95% CI 0.58–0.81; $n=1145$)
>   - increased the risk of acute oesophagitis, neutropenia, and anaemia.
> - *Six trials (1024 patients) of concurrent versus sequential CRT.*
>   - Concurrent CRT showed:
>   - significant benefit in OS (HR 0.74, 95% CI 0.62–0.89; $n=702$)
>   - 10% absolute survival benefit at 2 years
>   - increased risk of severe oesophagitis (RR 4.96, 95% CI 2.17–11.37; $n=947$).
> - Chemotherapy combinations used include:
>   - carboplatin/cisplatin±etoposide, vinorelbine, or paclitaxel.
>   - *No significant difference in PFS or locoregional control.*
>   - *Analysis favours concurrent CRT over sequential CRT.*
>
> *Source*: data from O'Rouke *et al.*, Concurrent chemoradiotherapy in non-small cell lung cancer, *The Cochrane Collaboration*, Issue 6, Copyright © 2010 The Cochrane Collaboration.

> **✪ Learning point** Staging and initial work-up
>
> Investigation for patients suspected of lung cancer should be tailored, according to whether the patient is to be treated with radical or palliative intent.
>
> One of the challenges in diagnosis lies in the technical difficulty of lymph node staging, as this is crucial in determining the most appropriate management option, if radical treatment is being considered. Mediastinal lymph node staging may be performed using endobronchial ultrasound (EBUS)-guided transbronchial needle aspiration (TBNA), endoscopic ultrasound (EUS)-guided fine-needle aspiration (FNA), or surgically with a mediastinoscopy and/or anterior mediastinotomy, depending upon the anatomical location of the nodes. Surgical staging is more accurate and allows more extensive exploration of the lymph node stations, but it is more invasive with higher risk, carrying a morbidity risk of 3% and mortality risk of 0.08% (Figure 2.1).

> **⑥ Expert comment**
>
> It is important for the management of both radically treatable and advanced NSCLC to obtain histological confirmation at diagnosis. The most appropriate means of obtaining tissue for pathological and genetic characterization of NSCLC vary, according to the site of individual tumour deposits, patient fitness, and the intent of treatment. Tissue yields vary by modality, and the more technically demanding techniques tend to produce a lower yield of tissue. The clinician must therefore balance the risk to the individual patient from the procedure chosen against the risk of obtaining insufficient tissue, to accurately guide management when determining the mode of biopsy and number of biopsy needle passes to take.
>
> It is considered optimal practice to obtain sufficient diagnostic tissue through biopsy or cytology of the lesion that will yield pathological confirmation at the highest stage possible, if this is technically feasible, in order to assist therapeutic decision making.

The patient proceeded to treatment with concurrent chemotherapy and radiotherapy. The first cycle of chemotherapy consisted of cisplatin 80 mg/m^2 IV administered on day 1 and vinorelbine 30 mg/m^2 IV on days 1 and 8 of a 21-day cycle. A total of four cycles of chemotherapy were given. The second and subsequent cycles were administered with cisplatin 75 mg/m^2 IV and vinorelbine 15 mg/m^2 IV on days 1 and 8. Radiotherapy commenced with cycle 2, and she was treated with 64 Gy in 32 fractions over 6.5 weeks.

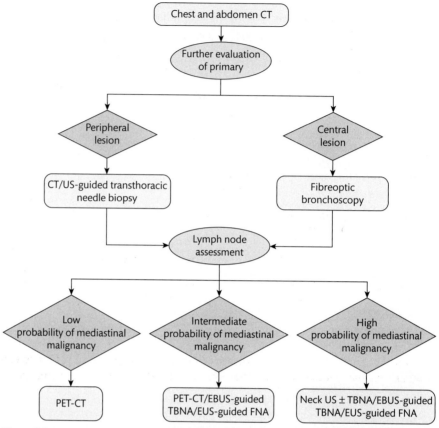

Figure 2.1 Investigation pathway for NSCLC [4]

Source: data from National Institute for Health and Clinical Excellence (NICE), Clinical Guidance 121, *Lung cancer: The diagnosis and treatment of lung cancer,* April 2011, Copyright © NICE 2011, available from <http://www.nice.org.uk/nicemedia/live/13465/54202/54202.pdf>.

✅ **Evidence base** Randomised multicentre trial: CHART (continuous hyperfractionated accelerated radiotherapy) vs. conventional radiotherapy in NSCLC [6]

- Total of 563 patients.
- 54 Gy in 36 fractions, given three times a day (tds) over 12 consecutive days, versus conventional radiotherapy of 60 Gy in 30 fractions, given over 6 weeks in a 3:2 ratio.
- Overall 24% reduction in relative risk of death.
- Absolute improvement in 2-year survival of 9%, from 20% to 29% ($p = 0.004$, 95% CI 0.63–0.92).
- Largest benefit in SCCs: 34% reduction in relative risk of death (an absolute improvement at 2 years of 14%, from 19% to 33%).
- Short-term toxicity was worse in CHART group: severe dysphagia in CHART was 19% versus 3% in the conventional radiotherapy group.
- No difference in long-term morbidity between the groups.
- Criticism of study: control arm used 60 Gy in 30 fractions, instead of 66 Gy in 33 fractions.

Source: data from *Radiotherapy Oncology*, Volume 52, Issue 2, Saunders M, *et al.*, Continuous, hyperfractionated, accelerated radiotherapy (CHART) versus conventional radiotherapy in non-small cell lung cancer: mature data from the randomised multicentre trial: CHART Steering committee, pp. 137–48, Copyright © 1999 Elsevier Inc. All rights reserved.

⭐ **Learning point** Management of early-stage NSCLC (Stages I, II, and III disease)

Early-stage disease (stages I and II) is optimally managed with surgery, if the patient is fit enough.

Although there is some evidence suggesting a role for neoadjuvant chemotherapy, this is not currently approved by National Institute for Health and Care Excellence (NICE) and does not reflect current clinical practice. Adjuvant radiotherapy is recommended, if there are positive margins (both microscopic and macroscopic) following surgery, and considered for pathological N2 disease.

Adjuvant platinum-based combination chemotherapy is offered to patients with T1–3, N1–2, M0 and considered in T2–3, N0, M0 with tumours >4 cm in diameter. The *Lung Adjuvant Cisplatin Evaluation (LACE) meta-analysis* [5] showed a 5-year absolute benefit of 5.4% from chemotherapy in patients with stages II and III disease. However, toxicity was significant, and patients therefore should be of good PS.

Radical radiotherapy is a potential alternative option for patients with stages I–II disease who are not candidates for radical surgery, or for patients with stage III who cannot tolerate combination CRT. The disease must be safely encompassed in a radical radiotherapy volume and should follow ideally the *CHART regime* [6]. If this is not available, a radical dose regimen, such as 64–66 Gy in 32–33 fractions over 6.5 weeks, or 55 Gy in 20 fractions over 4 weeks, should be offered.

CRT was the treatment chosen by the patient in this case. Whilst this is not the first-choice treatment for patients with good PS and stage II disease, it can be offered as a reasonable alternative, if surgery is declined, as CRT is superior to radiotherapy alone [1]. CRT is usually offered to patients with stage II disease who are not appropriate surgical candidates, and can be considered in selected patients with stage IIIB disease, and is the treatment of choice for those with stage IIIA disease.

💬 **Expert comment**

Chemotherapy drugs can potentiate the effect of radiotherapy, acting as radiosensitizers, and it is important that the chemotherapy regimen and doses administered alongside radical radiotherapy are both evidence-based and regularly reviewed during the radiotherapy course.

Adjuvant chemotherapy currently has no place, following CRT, for radically treatable NSCLC. A placebo-controlled randomized trial of adjuvant erlotinib (RADIANT) recruiting all NSCLC subtypes has reported no improvement in disease free or overall survival (ref). The value of adjuvant epidermal growth factor receptor (EGFR) inhibition in EGFR mutation positive patients is still uncertain [25].

After completion of treatment, the patient was closely followed up by both the respiratory and oncology teams, and routine imaging showed no evidence of recurrence.

⭐ **Learning point (Acute Oncology)** Diagnosis of SVCO

- SVCO results from compression of the SVC.
- Nearly always occurs because of a malignancy.
- Can be caused by invasion, external compression, or by thrombus.
- Is a clinical diagnosis in the first instance.
- Dyspnoea is the commonest presenting symptom.
- Other symptoms include:
  - facial swelling
  - headache/head fullness
  - cough
  - chest pain
  - dysphagia
  - hoarseness
  - orthopnoea
  - distorted vision.
- Characteristic signs include:
  - thoracic vein distension
  - neck vein distension
  - tachypnoea
  - facial/conjunctival oedema
  - plethora
  - cyanosis
  - arm oedema
  - confusion/coma (due to cerebral oedema).
- Symptoms and signs are often worse in the mornings and can increase on bending forwards.

However, just over 2 years following her radical treatment, the patient presented with a 2-month history of increasing shortness of breath, a new cough, and generalized lethargy. On examination, she looked plethoric and had slight facial swelling. Her neck and chest veins were not distended, but she appeared short of breath at rest. There was clinical suspicion of superior vena cava obstruction (SVCO) with disease recurrence as the most likely aetiology. An urgent CT scan of the chest and abdomen was performed which showed a new large right-sided mediastinal mass with obstruction of the superior vena cava (SVC). Unfortunately, multiple liver metastases were also detected. An endovascular SVC stent was therefore inserted to offer rapid symptomatic benefit.

✪ **Learning point (Acute Oncology) Causes of SVCO [7–9]**

- *Malignant (60–85%)*:
  ○ bronchogenic tumours:
    - NSCLC—50% of all cases
    - SCLC—25% of all cases.
  ○ non-Hodgkin's lymphoma (NHL):
    - 10% of all cases.
  ○ rare malignant causes:
    - Hodgkin's lymphoma
    - thymoma
    - primary mediastinal germ cell tumours
    - mesothelioma
    - primary leiomyosarcomas of mediastinal vessels
    - plasmacytomas.
- *Non-malignant (15–40%)*:
  ○ thrombosis
  ○ mediastinal fibrosis
  ○ histoplasmosis
  ○ tuberculosis
  ○ benign mediastinal tumours
  ○ post-radiation fibrosis

⊕ **Clinical tip Initial management of SVCO**

- SVCO is no longer considered as a medical emergency [7].
- Treatment can usually wait, until a histological diagnosis is made, dependent on the severity of symptoms at presentation.
- Investigations include:
  ○ observations, including pulse oximetry
  ○ bloods:
    - full blood count (FBC), urea and electrolytes (U&Es), liver function tests (LFTs), clotting (in case of interventional procedure)
    - human chorionic gonadotrophin (HCG), alpha fetoprotein (AFP), lactate dehydrogenase (LDH) (if a new diagnosis to exclude germ cell tumour)
  ○ imaging:
    - CXR
    - CT of the chest.
- Treatment may be either symptomatic or aimed at the underlying cause.
- Traditionally, systemic corticosteroids and either external beam radiotherapy (EBRT) (for NSCLC) or chemotherapy (for SCLC) were used.
- Symptomatic relief rates of SVCO are similar for chemotherapy and radiotherapy in both cell types [1]:
  ○ 76.9% and 77.6%, respectively, for SCLC
  ○ 59.0% and 63.0%, respectively, for NSCLC.

(Continue)

- Complete relief of symptoms usually occurs within 2 weeks with radiotherapy.
- Clinical response to chemotherapy in SCLC usually more rapid.
- Relapse rates from chemotherapy and radiotherapy:
  o 17% in SCLC
  o 19% in NSCLC.
- Stenting now appears to be the most effective and rapid treatment for the relief of symptoms, with relief in 95% of patients [7]:
  o relapse rate of 11%
- NICE guidelines now state that stent insertion should be considered for the immediate relief of severe symptoms of SVCO [4].
- Corticosteroids can be helpful in resolving symptoms when SVCO is caused by steroid-responsive malignancies (i.e. lymphoma, thymoma) but can affect interpretation of the biopsy, particularly in high-grade lymphoma. Their role, however, in NSCLC has never been studied. In practice, steroids are generally prescribed, but the use of high doses should be of limited duration.

❻ Expert comment

The balance of risk of the procedure against the likelihood of relieving symptoms should guide the management of SVCO in lung cancer patients. Response rates to SCLC chemotherapy are generally excellent and those responses are rapid, so primary treatment with chemotherapy may be considered appropriate. However, NSCLC has a lower chance of response and responses are slower, so initial stent insertion may be preferred in symptomatic patients.

At relapse of NSCLC, repeat biopsy is appropriate, if practicable for patients with NSCLC, as clonal evolution causing the development of resistance or transformation of the recurrent disease to a different phenotype from the original primary may occur.

One week later, the patient's facial swelling had settled; her breathing had started to improve, and her PS had improved from 2 to 1. Further treatment options were discussed with her at an outpatient visit. Her original histopathology was sent for EGFR testing and showed an EGFR mutation in exon 19. The benefit of first-line EGFR tyrosine kinase inhibitors (TKIs) in metastatic NSCLC was discussed, and she was consented for erlotinib (see OPTIMAL trial) [10]. She began taking erlotinib at a dose of 150 mg once daily orally and was reviewed 2 weeks later to assess for acute toxicity.

She underwent a repeat CXR after a month of therapy to assess response, which showed a slight improvement in the size of her mediastinal mass. She continued taking erlotinib, and interval imaging at 3 months showed an ongoing response, with a reduction in the size of both the right-sided mediastinal mass and liver lesions. Her breathing continued to improve; her energy levels had increased, and she was even now considering going back to work.

✪ Learning point EGFR mutations and TKIs

- *EGFR*
  o A receptor tyrosine kinase that plays an important role in tumour cell survival.
  o Activated phosphorylated EGFR results in the phosphorylation of downstream proteins that cause cell proliferation, invasion, metastasis, and inhibition of apoptosis.
- *EGFR mutations.*
  o Most frequently seen in:
    – non-smokers
    – non-SCCs (mostly adenocarcinomas)
    – females
    – Asians (seen in 50% of Asians with NSCLC, compared to 10% of Caucasians with NSCLC)

(Continue)

o Two commonest sensitizing mutations occurring in the EGFR-TK domain are exon 19 deletion (45% and L858R point mutation in exon 21 (45%).
o The remaining 10% of mutations involve exons 18 and 20 [11].
o A range of activating and de novo resistance mutations of the EGFR gene are now recognized [12,13].
o EGFR mutation is predictive for response and prognostic for survival.
o All never-smokers should be considered for testing and all non-SCCs:
  – 1 in 1000 of lung SCCs carry the EGFR mutation, but it is still reasonable to test for the mutation in these patients.

Three EGFR TKIs are currently licensed in the United Kingdom (UK) for the management of EGFR mutation-positive NSCLC. A subtle, but distinct, difference between efficacy and toxicity for each of these agents has been demonstrated through clinical trials [10,14,15]. These differences influence clinicians' current choice for individual patients.

* *Gefitinib (IRESSA®).*
  o Potent selective small molecule inhibitor of the EGFR tyrosine kinase, thereby inhibiting EGFR autophosphorylation.
  o Option in first line treatment for patients with sensitising mutations [14]
* *Erlotinib (TARCEVA®).*
  o Potent selective small molecule inhibitor of the EGFR tyrosine kinase, thereby inhibiting EGFR autophosphorylation.
* Option in first line treatment for patients with sensitising mutations [10]
  o second- or third-line systemic treatment, following failure of at least one prior chemotherapy regime (see *BR21 trial*) [15]
  o response rate of 8.9%, compared to placebo
  o median duration of response of 7.9 months, compared with 3.7 months
  o OS advantage of 2 months, compared to placebo.
* *Afatinib (GILOTRIF®).*
  o Selective inhibitor of EGFR, human epidermal growth factor receptor 2 (HER2), and ErbB4 and has wide-spectrum preclinical activity against EGFR mutations.
  o Option in first line treatment for patients with sensitising mutations but not yet NICE approved [16]

⊘ Evidence base OPTIMAL: erlotinib versus chemotherapy in first-line treatment of EGFR-mutated NSCLC [10]

* Phase III trial in China.
* A total of 165 patients with EGFR-mutated NSCLC:
  o randomized in a 1:1 ratio to receive erlotinib (150 mg/day), until disease progression or unacceptable adverse side effects, or up to four cycles of gemcitabine and carboplatin
  o median PFS was 13.1 months (erlotinib group) versus 4.6 months (chemotherapy group) (HR 0.16, 95% CI 0.10–0.26; p <0.0001)
  o erlotinib had fewer associated grade 3 or 4 toxic effects.

Source: data from *The Lancet Oncology*, Volume 12, Issue 8, Zhou C *et al.*, Erlotinib versus chemotherapy as first-line treatment for patients with advanced EGFR mutation-positive non-small-cell lung cancer (OPTIMAL, CTONG 0803): a multicentre, open label, randomised phase 3 study, pp. 735–4, Copyright © 2012.

⊘ Evidence base IPASS: gefitinib versus chemotherapy in lung adenocarcinoma [14]

* Phase III study conducted in East Asia.
* Patients randomized to gefitinib or carboplatin and paclitaxel.
* Superior PFS of 9.5 months, compared to 6.3 months in the chemotherapy group.
* For EGFR wild-type patients, PFS was longer when treated with carboplatin and paclitaxel.
* Greatest benefit in non-smokers or former light smokers with EGFR mutation-positive adenocarcinoma.

Source: data from Mok TS *et al.*, Gefitinib or Carboplatin–Paclitaxel in Pulmonary Adenocarcinoma, *New England Medical Journal*, Volume 361, Number 10, pp. 47–57, Copyright © 2009 Massachusetts Medical Society. All rights reserved.

✓ Evidence base LUX-Lung 3 study: afatinib versus chemotherapy in NSCLC [16]

- Phase III study.
- A total of 1269 patients with EGFR-mutated NSCLC.
- Randomized to afatinib versus cisplatin and pemetrexed.
- Median PFS was 11.1 months (afatinib group) versus 6.9 months (chemotherapy group).
- Median PFS higher at 13.6 months (afatinib group) in patients with exon 19 deletions and L858R mutations.

Source: data from Sequist L *et al.*, Phase III Study of Afatinib or Cisplatin Plus Pemetrexed in Patients with Metastatic Lung Adenocarcinoma with EGFR Mutations, *Journal of Clinical Oncology*, Volume 31, Number 27, pp. 3327–3334, Copyright © 2013 by the American Society of Clinical Oncology.

⊕ Clinical tip Practicalities of EGFR TKIs

- Taken orally.
- Side effects include [17,18]:
  - diarrhoea
    - onset can be within 12 days
  - rash (Figure 2.2)
    - onset can be within 8 days
    - typically occurs on sun exposed sites (e.g. face and upper body)
    - erythematous papulopustular rash
  - anorexia
  - nausea
  - vomiting
  - GI bleeding and perforation (rarely)
  - keratitis.
- If severe adverse reactions, consider dose interruption or dose reduction, if possible.
- Use with caution in hepatic impairment—dose reduction or interruption should be considered.
- Metabolism is primarily by liver microsomal CYP3A4 enzyme:
  - inducers increase drug metabolism, resulting in reduced levels of TKI
  - inhibitors decrease drug metabolism, resulting in increased levels of TKI.
- Cigarette smoking reduces EGFR TKI exposure; therefore, patients should be advised to quit.

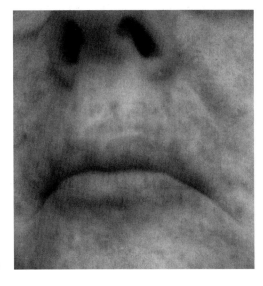

Figure 2.2 EGFR TKI related rash

❝ Expert comment

Relative to traditional chemotherapy, the daily oral administration schedule for EGFR TKIs results in less acute severe cyclical toxicities, but more chronic milder ones that can nonetheless have a significant detrimental impact upon patients' QoL. New consensus toxicity management algorithms should be consulted to guide management of these toxicities [17,18].

The role of EGFR inhibitors in patients who do not carry an activating EGFR mutation has recently been questioned by the TAILOR trial [19].

✪ Learning point Treatment of locally advanced or metastatic disease

Palliative systemic therapy is generally indicated for patients who present with advanced or metastatic disease and for those who have relapsed with advanced disease following prior definitive treatment. A number of factors influence the choice of therapy, including the presence or absence of symptoms, PS, co-morbidities, tumour histology, *EGFR* mutation status, and patient preference.

The discovery of EGFR mutations and the advent of TKIs have changed the face of the management of advanced lung cancer. The landmark *IPASS* study [14] established gefitinib as the first-line treatment in EGFR mutation-positive patients with locally advanced and metastatic NSCLC. Since then, the *OPTIMAL* trial [10] has established erlotinib, and the *LUX-Lung 3* trial [16] afinitinb, as alternatives.

For those without a sensitizing EGFR mutation, chemotherapy is considered standard of care for those with good PS.

Chemotherapy with doublet combinations of platinums (cisplatin or carboplatin) with gemcitabine, vinorelbine, or taxanes are well-established reference regimes. They have been shown to offer a survival benefit and can improve the QoL. The *BTOG2 trial* [20] established an equivalence of cisplatin (at $80 \, mg/m^2$) and carboplatin, in terms of response rates and OS, and thus carboplatin can be used when cisplatin is contraindicated. Furthermore, Scagliotti *et al.* [21] showed that pemetrexed was advantageous over other doublet agents for patients with non-squamous histology. Treatment with docetaxel (at $75 \, mg/m^2$) in the second line, following progression after platinum-based chemotherapy, prolongs PFS over best supportive care alone [22].

For elderly patients (over 70 years), those who are of borderline PS, or those for whom a platinum agent is not suitable, then the *ELVIS trial* [23] showed that the single agent vinorelbine provides a reasonable alternative.

✔ Evidence base : Phase III study Cisplatin plus Pemetrexed vs Cisplatin plus Gemcitabine in NSCLC [21] Pemetrexed in non-squamous NSCLC [21]

- Differential response in accordance to the different histological subtypes.
- Patients with adenocarcinoma and large cell carcinoma did better on cisplatin and pemetrexed.
  - Improved OS: 12.6 months versus 10.9 months, $p = 0.0$.
  - Better tolerated—lower rates of neutropenia, anaemia, and thrombocytopenia.
- Patients with squamous cell carcinoma (SCC) did better on gemcitabine and cisplatin.
  - Improved OS: 10.8 months versus 9.4 months.
  - Chemoresistance of SCCs to pemetrexed may be due to overexpression of thymidylate synthase.

Source: data from Scagliotti GV *et al.*, Phase III Study Comparing Cisplatin Plus Gemcitabine With Cisplatin Plus Pemetrexed in Chemotherapy-Naïve Patients With Advanced Stage Non-Small Cell Lung Cancer, *Journal of Clinical Oncology*, Volume 26, Number 21, pp. 3543–3551, Copyright © 2013 by the American Society of Clinical Oncology.

Discussion

This case underlines the challenges in the investigation and management of early NSCLC and the complexities of late-stage disease, especially when complicated by SVCO. Furthermore, it highlights the advances made in the management of meta-static disease, given the availability of EGFR testing and the number of TKIs now in clinical use (Figure 2.3). There are a number of potential management options for NSCLC (Table 2.3), but the choice of modality is ultimately determined by each patient performance status and disease stage.

Table 2.3 Treatment options for NSCLC [4]

Stage	Surgery	Radical radiotherapy	CRT	Systemic therapy
I	++	+	X	X
II	++	+	+	X
IIIA	+	+	++	+
IIIB	X	+	+	++
IV	X	X	X	++

++, first choice for eligible patients; +, suitable for some patients; X, not recommended.

Source: data from National Institute for Health and Clinical Excellence (NICE), Clinical Guidance 121, *Lung cancer: the diagnosis and treatment of lung cancer*, April 2011, Copyright © NICE 2011, available from <http://www.nice.org.uk/nicemedia/live/13465/54202/54202.pdf>.

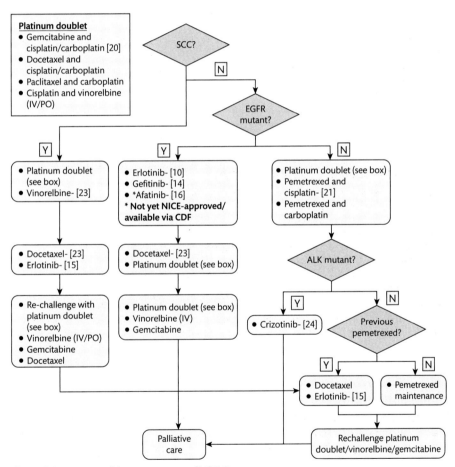

Figure 2.3 Overview of the management of NSCLC.

Source: data from National Institute for Health and Clinical Exce.llence (NICE), Clinical Guidance 121, *Lung Cancer: The diagnosis and treatment of lung cancer*, April 2011, Copyright © NICE 2011, available from <http://www.nice.org.uk/nicemedia/live/13465/54202/54202.pdf>

> ✅ **Evidence base** Crizotinib versus chemotherapy in anaplastic lymphoma kinase (ALK)-positive NSCLC [24]
>
> - ALK rearrangements are present in approximately 5% of patients with NSCLC.
> - Crizotinib is an oral small molecule TKI, targeting ALK, MET, and ROS1 tyrosine kinases.
> - Phase III trial comparing crizotinib with chemotherapy.
> - 347 patients with locally advanced or metastatic ALK-positive lung cancer, who received one prior platinum-based regimen were randomized to crizotinib (250 mg) twice daily (bd) or pemetrexed (500 mg/m^2) or docetaxel (75 mg/m^2) every 3 weeks.
> - Cross-over was allowed.
> - Median PFS was 7.7 months (crizotinib group) versus 3.0 months (chemotherapy group).
> - Response rates were 65% (crizotinib group) versus 20% (chemotherapy group).
> - Interim analysis of OS showed no significant improvement with crizotinib over chemotherapy.
>
> *Source:* data from Shaw AT *et al.*, Crizotinib versus Chemotherapy in Advanced ALK-Positive Lung Cancer, *New England Medical Journal*, Volume 368, Number 25, pp. 2385–94, Copyright © 2013 Massachusetts Medical Society. All rights reserved.

A final word from the expert

Given the large number of carcinogens present in tobacco, it is not surprising that wide variations are seen in the presentation and clinical course for patients with NSCLC.

As technologies evolve and our understanding of the cancer genome increases, an incredible genetic complexity of NSCLC tumours is becoming apparent.

It is increasingly understood that morphologically similar NSCLC tumours harbour distinct differences in their genetic and gene expression characteristics that can now be differentiated. This has resulted in a shift away from a 'one size fits all' approach to the management of NSCLC, with treatment guided by the specific abnormalities of individual tumours through increasingly complex algorithms.

New treatments for 'actionable' targets, such as crizotinib, an ALK TKI inhibitor that is beneficial in *ALK* gene-translocated tumours, are being developed for the observed range of low-prevalence genetic abnormalities in NSCLC. Clinical trials of targeted treatments in selected populations such as PROFILE 1007 [24] increasingly show significant improvements in response rate and PFS. However care in interpretation of negative OS data is warranted as many patients cross over to receive the targeted therapy at some point after progression if they draw the study control arm treatment (112 of 174 patients in the PROFILE 1007 study).

As more becomes known about the differences between individual patients' tumours, the natural history of clonal evolution of tumours within patients, and the mechanisms of resistance to targeted treatment, the future care for NSCLC patients is likely to become increasingly personalized.

References

1. O'Rourke N, Roqué I, Figuls M, Farré Bernadó N, Macbeth F. Concurrent chemoradiotherapy in non-small cell lung cancer. *Cochrane Database of Systematic Reviews* 2010; **6**: CD002140.

2. Brambilla E, Travis WD, Colby TV, Corrin B, Shimosato Y. The new World Health Organization classification of lung tumours. *European Respiratory Journal* 2001; **18**(6): 1059–68.

3. Office for National Statistics. *Cancer survival in England: patients diagnosed 2005-2009 and followed up to 2010.* 2011. Available at: <http://www.ons.gov.uk/ons/dcp171778_240942.pdf>.

4. National Institute for Health and Care Excellence. *Lung cancer: the diagnosis and treatment of lung cancer. Clinical guidance 121.* 2011. Available at: <http://www.nice.org.uk/guidance/cg121>.

5. Pignon JP, Tribodet H, Scagliotti GV *et al.* Lung adjuvant cisplatin evaluation: a pooled analysis by the LACE Collaborative Group. *Journal of Clinical Oncology* 2008; **26**(21): 3552–9.

6. Saunders M, Dische S, Barrett A, Harvey A, Griffiths G, Palmar M. Continuous, hyper-fractionated, accelerated radiotherapy (CHART) versus conventional radiotherapy in non-small cell lung cancer: mature data from the randomised multicentre trial. CHART Steering Committee. *Radiotherapy Oncology* 1999; **52**(2): 137–48.

7. Rowell NP, Gleeson FV. Steroids, radiotherapy, chemotherapy and stents for superior vena caval obstruction in carcinoma of the bronchus. *Cochrane Database of Systematic Reviews* 2001; **4**: CD001316.

8. Zelen M. Keynote address on biostatistics and data retrieval. *Cancer Chemotherapy Reports 3* 1973; **4**(2): 31–42.

9. Rice TW, Rodriguez RM, Light RW. The superior vena cava syndrome: clinical characteristics and evolving etiology. *Medicine (Baltimore)* 2006; **85**(1): 37–42.

10. Zhou C, Yi-Long W, Chen G *et al.* Erlotinib versus chemotherapy as first-line treatment for patients with advanced EGFR mutation-positive non-small-cell lung cancer (OPTIMAL, CTONG 0803): a multicentre, open label, randomised phase 3 study. *The Lancet Oncology* 2011; **12**(8): 735–42.

11. Sharma SV, Bell DW, Settleman J, Haber DA. Epidermal growth factor receptor mutations in lung cancer. *Nature Reviews Cancer* 2007; **7**(3): 169–81.

12. Ohashi K, Maruvka YE, Michor F, Pao W. Epidermal growth factor receptor tyrosine kinase inhibitor-resistant disease. *Journal of Clinical Oncology* 2013; **31**(8): 1070–80.

13. Riely GJ, Politi KA, Miller VA, Pao W. Update on epidermal growth factor receptor mutations in non-small cell lung cancer. *Clinical Cancer Research* 2006; **12**(24): 7232–41.

14. Mok TS, Wu Y-L, Thongprasert S *et al.* Gefitinib or carboplatin-paclitaxel in pulmonary adenocarcinoma. *The New England Journal of Medicine* 2009; **361**(10): 947–57.

15. Shepherd FA, Rodrigues Pereira J, Ciuleanu T *et al.* Erlotinib in previously treated non-small-cell lung cancer. *New England Journal of Medicine* 2005; **353**(2): 123–32.

16. Sequist L, Yang J, Yamamoto N *et al.* Phase III study of afatinib or cisplatin plus pemetrexed in patients with metastatic lung adenocarcinoma with EGFR mutations. *Journal of Clinical Oncology* 2013; **31**(27): 3327–34.

17. Lacouture ME, Schadendorf D, Chu CY *et al.* Dermatologic adverse events associated with afatinib: an oral ErbB family blocker. *Expert Review of Anticancer Therapy* 2013; **13**(6): 721–8.

18. Hirsh V. Managing treatment-related adverse events associated with EGFR tyrosine kinase inhibitors in advanced non-small cell lung cancer. *Current Oncology* 2011; **18**(3): 126–38.

19. Garassino MC, Martelli O, Broggini M *et al.* Erlotinib versus docetaxel as second-line treatment of patients with advanced non-small-cell lung cancer and wild-type EGFR tumours (TAILOR): a randomised controlled trial. *The Lancet Oncology* 2013; **14**(10): 989–8.

20. Ferry D, Billingham LJ, Jarrett HW, Dunlop D *et al.* S85 British Thoracic Oncology Group Trial, BTOG2: Randomised phase III clinical trial of gemcitabine combined with cisplatin 50 mg/m^2 (GC50) vs cisplatin 80 mg/m^2 (GC80) vs carboplatin AUC 6 (GCb6) in advanced NSCLC. *Thorax* 2011; **66**: A41.

21. Scagliotti GV, Parikh P, von Pawel J *et al.* Phase III study comparing cisplatin plus gemcitabine with cisplatin plus pemetrexed in chemotherapy-naïve patients with advanced stage non-small cell lung cancer. *Journal of Clinical Oncology* 2008; **26**(21): 3543–51.

22. Shepherd FA, Dancey J, Ramlau R, *et al.* Prospective trial of docetaxel versus best supportive care in patients with non-small-cell lung cancer previously treated with platinum-based chemotherapy. *Journal of Clinical Oncology* 2000; **18**: 2095–103.

23. Gridelli C. The ELVIS trial: a phase III study of single-agent vinorelbine as first-line treatment in elderly patients with advanced non-small cell lung cancer. Elderly Lung Cancer Vinorelbine Italian Study. *The Oncologist* 2001; **6** (Supp): 4–7.

24. Shaw AT, Kim DW, Nakagawa K *et al.* Crizotinib versus chemotherapy in advanced ALK-positive lung cancer. *The New England Journal of Medicine* 2013; **368**(25): 2385–94

25. Kelly K, Nasser K, Wilifried Ernst Erich Eberhardt *et al.* A randomized, double-blind phase 3 trial of adjuvant erlotinib (E) versus placebo (P) following complete tumor resection with or without adjuvant chemotherapy in patients (pts) with stage IB-IIIA EGFR positive (IHC/FISH) non-small cell lung cancer (NSCLC): RADIANT results. *Journal of Clinical Oncology* 2014; **32**:5s (suppl; abstr 7501).

3 Mesothelioma and chemotherapy-induced vomiting

Sarah Payne

Expert commentary Jeremy Steele

Case history

A 65-year-old builder attended his GP with a 2-month history of progressive shortness of breath, fatigue, and weight loss of 1 stone. The patient had been a 20-pack-year smoker, until a year prior to presentation, and acknowledged previous asbestos exposure. The gentleman was performance status (PS) 1. Clinical examination revealed reduced air entry of the left lung and dullness to percussion of the left lung base. A CXR demonstrated pleural plaques bilaterally and left-sided pleural thickening, with a small associated pleural effusion. There were no intra-pulmonary masses or cardiac abnormalities. These findings were seen more clearly on the staging CT scan (Figure 3.1).

✚ Clinical tip Malignant pleural effusions

Firstly, it is important to confirm that a pleural effusion is malignant. In 75% of cases, this will be related to lung, breast, or ovarian cancer, or lymphoma [1]. Only half of effusions in cancer patients are malignant. Non-malignant causes include infection, pulmonary embolism (PE), cardiac failure, and impaired pleural lymphatic drainage from a mediastinal tumour. Cytology is positive in about 60% of cases. Cytology, plus a pleural biopsy, increases the chance of detecting a malignancy to 80–90% [2]. A histological sample is ideally required to make a definitive diagnosis.

✚ Clinical tip Management of malignant pleural effusions

Management of a malignant pleural effusion depends on:

- symptoms
- performance status (PS)
- primary tumour
- likely response to treatment, and
- degree of lung expansion following pleural fluid aspiration [1].

Current British Thoracic Society (BTS) guidelines (2010) initially recommend [1]:

- observation if the patient is asymptomatic and the tumour type is known
- ultrasound-guided aspiration for symptomatic patients of no more than 1.5 L

Repeat pleural aspiration is only recommended for palliation of patients with a very short life expectancy (<1 month) [1]. Without treatment of the primary tumour, a malignant pleural effusion will usually recur within a month. Pleurodesis should therefore be discussed. Options include small-bore intercostal tube insertion, with chemical pleurodesis (tetracycline, doxycycline, and bleomycin) and operative talc poudrage. The latter is preferable for patients with good PS and has a success rate of 77–100% [1]. Failure is usually secondary to the tumour bulk preventing lung re-expansion.

Chronic indwelling catheters may offer a solution for recurrent pleural effusions [3]. Pleurectomy has been described but is not superior to pleurodesis or the use of a long-term catheter [1].

❝ Expert comment

Histological diagnosis is very important in the case of malignant mesothelioma because of the medicolegal implications of a diagnosis. Histological confirmation is best achieved with a CT-guided pleural biopsy or a thoracoscopic biopsy performed under general anaesthesia. The Abrams' pleural biopsy needle approach is no longer recommended for routine use, in view of the excessive false negative rate and the discomfort caused by the technique.

❝ Expert comment

Radiotherapy to drain sites to treat tumour seedlings is controversial. There are no randomized trials which support its use. Data assessing the incidence of associated morbidity from tract metastases suggest that rates are relatively low. Instead of prophylactic irradiation, patients are currently clinically monitored and only treated if they develop symptomatic deposits.

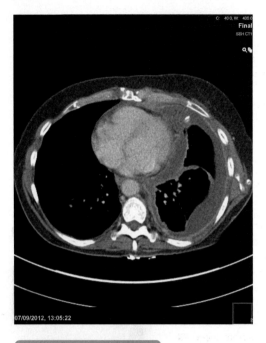

Figure 3.1 CT scan showing left-sided mesothelioma. The CT scan shows marked circumferential pleural thickening in the left hemithorax. The thickening looks malignant because of the uneven margins, extensive mediastinal component, and contraction of the hemithorax. There is an associated encased unilateral pleural effusion.

⑥ Expert comment

There is no single immunohistochemical marker that confirms mesothelioma. Diagnosis is best made by an expert histopathologist who will use a panel of markers. Typically, cytokeratin 5/6 and calretinin are positive. A more recently deployed antibody is WT-1, which is usually positive, and is helpful in supporting the diagnosis of malignant mesothelioma.

⑥ Expert comment

Asbestos is a naturally occurring mineral that has been used in shipbuilding, construction, and manufacturing for thousands of years. Chrysotile ('white' asbestos), amosite ('brown' asbestos), and crocidolite ('blue' asbestos) are the three commonest types. Exposure to the latter two is commonly linked with mesothelioma, although exposure to all types can be harmful. Most subforms of asbestos are contaminated with small amounts of other types; thus, there is no 'safe' asbestos.

The case was discussed in the respiratory multidisciplinary meeting. A decision was made to perform a thoracotomy to obtain tissue for histology. Pathological review of the pleural biopsy confirmed the diagnosis of an epithelioid malignant mesothelioma, based on haematoxylin and eosin staining and the outcome of a panel of immunohistochemical stains (positivity for calretinin, N-cadherin, thrombomodulin, WT-1, and cytokeratin 5/6, and negativity for TTF-1, carcinoembryonic antigen (CEA), and E-cadherin).

✪ Learning point Mesothelioma aetiology

Malignant mesothelioma is a tumour that arises from the mesothelial surfaces of the pleural and peritoneal cavities, tunica vaginalis, or pericardium. Ninety per cent are pleural in origin. It is caused by asbestos exposure, and long-term survival is rare.

Radiation exposure has also been implicated as a causative agent [4]. Autosomal dominant familial forms have been reported in Turkey [5]. Incidence is between 2 and 30 per 100 000 population worldwide but is on the increase, despite a ban on asbestos use in the Western world in the 1970s [6,7].

Malignant pleural mesothelioma usually affects men (ratio of men to women 5:1), and patients are predominantly over 70 years of age [8]. The time lag to developing a tumour is approximately 30–50 years [9]. Median survival after diagnosis is 4.5–17 months, depending on the histological type, tumour stage, PS, and treatment, as well as other factors such as gender and age [10–13].

There are three main histological subtypes of mesothelioma:

● epithelial (60%)
● sarcomatous (20%)
● mixed (20%).

Epithelial tumours are the commonest and associated with the best prognosis.

😊 **Learning point** Peritoneal mesothelioma

Peritoneal mesothelioma affects approximately 10% of patients with malignant mesothelioma. It usually presents as advanced disease but rarely spreads outside the peritoneal cavity. Patients usually complain of vague symptoms, including weight loss, abdominal pain, or abdominal bloating because of ascites, or, less frequently, night sweats and hypercoagulability [15,16].

CT findings are non-specific but aid in diagnosis, staging, and guiding biopsy of peritoneal masses. There are three types:

- dry: one solitary mass or multiple masses, with no associated ascites
- wet: ascites and widespread small nodules and plaques, but no masses
- mixed

Cytological analysis is of low diagnostic potential. Histological review is needed for definitive diagnosis, using a panel of immunohistochemical markers.

Where feasible, radical surgery to remove the entire tumour is preferable. Hyperthermic intraoperative or early post-operative intraperitoneal chemotherapy and immunotherapy are additional strategies being explored for radical disease management [17].

Systemic palliative chemotherapy should be considered for patients with inoperable disease. Given the rarity of the tumour type, there are no randomized controlled studies, so the management strategies employed for advanced pleural mesothelioma are often applied.

The patient was deemed inoperable and offered palliative chemotherapy with pemetrexed and cisplatin. One week prior to starting treatment, the patient received an injection of vitamin B12 and folic acid tablets.

😊 **Learning point** Criteria for operability of malignant pleural mesothelioma

Extra-pleural pneumonectomy (EPP) offers radical treatment of patients with mesothelioma of the thoracic wall alone and includes resection of the hemidiaphragm and the pericardium en bloc. It can be considered for patients with good PS and adequate cardiopulmonary function. Operative mortality is high (6–30%) [18,19]. The procedure may increase DFS but has no impact on OS [18].

A pleurectomy is a less invasive operation, which may be indicated for elderly patients with an intracavity mesothelioma. This involves an open thoracotomy, removal of the parietal pleura, the pleura over the mediastinum, pericardium, and diaphragm, and stripping of the visceral pleura for decortication. Post-operative radiotherapy should be considered, given the greater chance of local recurrence, compared to EPP. Operative mortality is significantly less than that of an EPP [20].

Standard treatment for all but localized pleural disease is rarely curative [21–23]. A parietal pleurectomy may also be considered as a palliative procedure to help alleviate symptoms of shortness of breath and pain in patients with more advanced disease [24].

💬 **Expert comment**

The MARS trial questioned the benefit of EPP. This was a multicentre randomized controlled trial (RCT) designed to review trimodal therapy for locally advanced malignant mesothelioma. Due to slow accrual, only the pilot phase of the trial was completed. All patients underwent induction platinum-based chemotherapy. Following clinical review, of the 112 patients who registered for the study, 50 patients were subsequently randomized to EPP, followed by post-operative hemithorax irradiation, or to no EPP. EPP was only completed satisfactorily in 16, out of a possible 24, patients. The procedure was associated with a high morbidity and mortality rate, with an HR for OS between EPP and no EPP groups of 1.90 (95% CI 0.92–3.93; exact $p = 0.082$) [25]. Median survival for the EPP group was 14.4 months versus 19.5 months for the no EPP group [25]. No significant differences were seen in QoL data between the groups, but the numbers involved were small. Because the trial was terminated at completion of the pilot phase, it was statistically underpowered, and the survival data have to be viewed with caution. Nevertheless, this remains the only randomized data on EPP, and the results suggest that EPP should only be undertaken after a full and open discussion of the risks of the operation between the surgeon and patient.

💬 **Expert comment**

Germline mutations of BRCA1-associated protein 1 (BAP1) have recently been discovered in two families with a high incidence of mesothelioma [14]. Truncating and aberrant BAP1 expression has also been found in cases of malignant mesothelioma without germline mutations [14]. Screening for this mutation may help identify individuals at high risk of developing mesothelioma in the future.

> ★ **Learning point** Summary of the role of radiotherapy in the management of malignant pleural mesothelioma
>
> **Adjuvant radiotherapy**
>
> Adjuvant hemithoracic radiotherapy after EPP improves local control but does not enhance OS [26,27].
>
> **Curative radiotherapy**
>
> The role of curative hemithoracic radiotherapy is limited by the large target volume of tissue involved and may be associated high toxicity and morbidity (i.e. fatal pneumonitis) [28].
>
> **Palliative radiotherapy**
>
> Radiotherapy can be used to manage pain associated with an invasive tumour, although the benefit is often short-lived [29,30].

The first cycle of chemotherapy was delivered without immediate complication. Unfortunately, on day 3, the gentleman was admitted with severe nausea and vomiting, despite concordance with empirical anti-emetics dispensed on day 1. The patient was initially managed with IV fluids and IV anti-emetics, with careful monitoring of the fluid balance and electrolytes. His anti-emetic schedule was modified for the next cycle of treatment, according to the hospital protocol.

> ★ **Learning point** Management of chemotherapy-induced vomiting
>
> Chemotherapy-induced nausea and vomiting (CINV) is a common side effect. There are several subtypes:
>
> - *acute:* <24 hours of chemotherapy
> - *delayed:* 24 hours to 5 days after treatment
> - *breakthrough:* occurring despite prophylatic treatment
> - *anticipatory:* triggered by taste, odour, memories, visions, or anxiety related to chemotherapy
> - *refractory:* occurring during subsequent cycles when anti-emetics have failed in earlier cycles
>
> **Aetiology**
>
> The exact mechanism for CINV is unclear but is thought to include direct stimulation by emetic toxins, such as chemotherapy, of the:
>
> - chemoreceptor trigger zone (CTZ) in the medulla oblongata, and
> - enterochromaffin cells in the GI tract
>
> Activated chemoreceptors in these areas relay information about emetic agents to the nucleus tractus solitarii (NTS). The neurotransmitters involved include serotonin, dopamine, histamine, and substance P. Nerve impulses are then sent to the vomiting centre in the medulla, which initiates vomiting once a certain threshold is reached (Figure 3.2).
>
> **Classification of agents**
>
> The risk of CINV varies, depending on the chemotherapy regimen (drugs, dose, and schedule), as well as external factors, including:
>
> - younger age
> - female sex, and
> - high pretreatment expectation of severe nausea.
>
> Chemotherapy agents are often divided into four categories, based on their emetogenicity:
>
> - highly emetic: >90% risk of emesis
> - moderately emetic: >30–90% risk of emesis
> - low emetogenicity: 10–30% risk of emesis
> - minimally emetic: <10% risk of emesis.   (Continued)

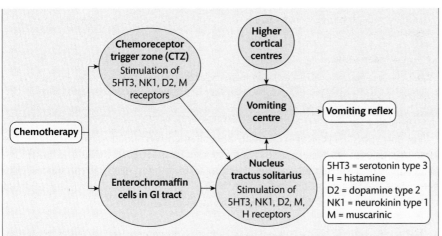

Figure 3.2 Diagram depicting a simplified pathway of the vomiting reflex following administration of chemotherapy.

Examples of these are given in Table 3.1.

Table 3.1 Examples of chemotherapy drugs with different levels of emetogenicity

Level of emetogenicity	Examples of chemotherapy agents
Minimally emetic	• Vinorelbine • Bleomycin • Vincristine • Fludarabine
Low emetogenicity	• Paclitaxel • Docetaxel
Moderate emetogenicity	• Carboplatin • Cyclophosphamide (<1500 mg/m²) • Doxorubicin • Oxaliplatin • Ifosfamide • Irinotecan
High emetogenicity	• Cisplatin • Cyclophosphamide (>1500 mg/m²)

Anti-emetic choices

For combination treatments, the emetic level is determined by the most emetic agent. The three categories of drugs with the highest therapeutic index for the management CINV include:

- 5-HT$_3$ receptor antagonists (e.g. ondansetron, granisetron)
- NK$_1$ receptor antagonists (e.g. aprepitant), and
- glucocorticoids.

Poor control of emesis

Despite anti-emetic prophylaxis, some patients experience significant CINV. Before changing the anti-emetic regimen, it is important to exclude other causes for emesis. These include:

- opiate analgesics
- antibiotics (e.g. erythromycin)
- sepsis

(Continued)

- central nervous system (CNS) metastases
- GI obstruction
- hypercalcaemia
- abdominopelvic radiotherapy.

Assuming these factors have been excluded, then check the patient has received the appropriate anti-emetics. If this is the case, then the patient's anti-emetic therapy should be escalated to one appropriate for a higher-risk group.

For the second cycle of treatment, anti-emetics were altered, according to the hospital protocol, and the dose of chemotherapy was reduced by 20% to minimize the chance of a subsequent severe reaction to treatment. The patient successfully completed four cycles of chemotherapy, with an outcome scan confirming a partial response, consistent with reported improvement in symptoms.

Discussion

Diagnosis of malignant pleural mesothelioma

The case highlights a common presentation of malignant pleural mesothelioma and the challenges associated with diagnosis and management. Diagnosis of malignant mesothelioma can be challenging because:
- it is a rare cancer
- often only a limited amount of tissue is available for histological evaluation
- the histological appearance can vary greatly within one patient, and
- many other tumours can mimic mesothelioma (e.g. lung adenocarcinoma, sarcoma of the chest wall, and carcinosarcoma of the female genital organs).

Malignant mesothelioma is not a particularly chemosensitive disease; however, there is an established role of using chemotherapy in managing the disease.

Neoadjuvant chemotherapy

Very few patients are candidates for radical surgery. Small studies considering platinum doublets in single-arm trials have demonstrated a median survival of 19–25 months [31–35]. Patients who demonstrate a complete response or partial response to treatment have a trend to prolonged OS [35]. Efficacy overall remains controversial, and neoadjuvant chemotherapy is not delivered routinely.

Adjuvant chemotherapy

Adjuvant chemotherapy after EPP is difficult to administer, because of toxicities, and has only been assessed in a handful of trials. To date, the addition of chemotherapy after radical surgery has not been shown to increase survival [26]. The three prognostic variables that are associated with improved survival are [36]:

- epithelial cell type
- negative resection margins, and
- extra-pleural nodes.

Intracavity chemotherapy

Intracavity chemotherapy has been shown to cause tumour shrinkage and control of effusions [26,37]. Its role is currently being defined.

Palliative chemotherapy

Before 2003, few chemotherapy agents in the treatment of malignant mesothelioma had response rates higher than 20% [38]. The Medical Research Council conducted a randomized phase III trial, comparing active symptom control (ASC) and two different chemotherapy regimens (mitomycin, vinblastine, and cisplatin; or weekly vinorelbine), and reported that chemotherapy did not improve survival [39]. The results from the single-agent arm did demonstrate a trend to improved survival, although this did not reach statistical significance, likely because the study was underpowered [39]. This suggests that certain chemotherapy can improve outcome.

A review of 119 trials of chemotherapy for unresectable malignant pleural mesothelioma (eight randomized and 111 non-comparative) concluded that combination chemotherapy had higher response rates, compared to single agents [40]. Additionally, platinum-based regimens were superior to those without platinum, achieving response rates of up to 32% [40].

First-line pemetrexed/cisplatin chemotherapy has been shown to improve survival and symptom control, compared to cisplatin alone, in an RCT by Vogelzang *et al.* [41]. Carboplatin can be substituted for cisplatin in elderly patients and offers an effective alternative [42]. Single-agent pemetrexed yields response rates of approximately 10% [42] and is the agent currently recommended by NICE for the treatment of malignant mesothelioma in patients with inoperable disease who are PS 0 or 1. Other anti-folates have been investigated, but they are less commonly used than pemetrexed [43].

⊘ **Evidence base** MSO1: Active symptom control (ASC) with or without chemotherapy in the treatment of patients with malignant pleural mesothelioma [39]

A total of 409 patients were randomly assigned to:

- ASC alone (treatment included steroids, analgesia, bronchodilators, palliative radiotherapy)
- ASC plus MVP (four cycles of mitomycin 6 mg/m^2, vinblastine 6 mg/m^2, and cisplatin 50 mg/m^2 every 3 weeks)
- ASC plus vinorelbine (one injection of vinorelbine 30 mg/m^2 every week for 12 weeks).

Because of slow accrual, the two chemotherapy groups were combined.

- There was a small, non-significant survival benefit for ASC plus chemotherapy (HR 0.89; $p=0.29$).
- Median survival was 7.6 months for ASC versus 8.5 months for ASC plus chemotherapy.
- Subgroup analysis showed a survival advantage for ASC plus vinorelbine versus ASC alone (HR 0.80; $p=0.08$), with a median survival of 9.5 months.
- There was no difference in QoL measures.

Source: data from *The Lancet*, Volume 371, Issue 9625, Muers MF *et al.*, Active symptom control with or without chemotherapy in the treatment of patients with malignant pleural mesothelioma (MS01): a multicentre randomised trial, pp. 1685–94, Copyright © 2008 Elsevier Ltd All rights reserved.

⊘ **Evidence base** Pemetrexed–cisplatin compared to cisplatin alone [41]

- Randomized phase III trial.
- 3-weekly pemetrexed (500 mg/m^2) and cisplatin (75 mg/m^2) ($n=226$) versus 3-weekly single-agent cisplatin (75 mg/m^2) ($n=222$).
- Median OS was significantly increased in the combination arm (12.1 months versus 9.3 months; $p=0.020$, HR 0.77).
- Median time to progression was significantly increased with pemetrexed–cisplatin (5.7 months versus 3.9 months; $p=0.001$).
- Folic acid and vitamin B12 injections in the pemetrexed arm reduced the frequency of grades 3–4 events.

Source: data from Vogelzang NJ *et al.*, Phase III study of pemetrexed in combination with cisplatin versus cisplatin alone in patients with malignant pleural mesothelioma, *Journal of Clinical Oncology*, Volume 21, Number 14, pp. 2636–44, Copyright © 2003 by American Society of Clinical Oncology.

> **✔ Evidence base** EORTC-08983: cisplatin–raltitrexed, compared to cisplatin alone, in first-line treatment [43]
>
> - Randomized phase III trial, 250 patients.
> - Cisplatin (80 mg/m^2) alone or combined with raltitrexed (3 mg/m^2) every 3 weeks.
> - Response rate for single-agent cisplatin 13.6% versus 23.6% for combination treatment ($n=213$) ($p=0.056$).
> - No difference in QoL.
> - Median OS for single-agent cisplatin was 8.8 months versus 11.4 months for combination treatment ($p=0.048$).
> - The main grade 3 or 4 toxicities were neutropenia and emesis, which were reported twice as often in the combination arm.
>
> *Source:* data from van Meerbeeck JP et al., Randomized phase III study of cisplatin with or without raltitrexed in patients with malignant pleural mesothelioma: an intergroup study of the European Organisation for Research and Treatment of Cancer Lung Cancer Group and the National Cancer Institute of Canada, *Journal of Clinical Oncology*, Volume 23, Number 28, pp. 6881–9, Copyright © 2005 by American Society of Clinical Oncology.

Phase II trials have looked at the role of gemcitabine and vinorelbine, either as single agents or in combination with a platinum agent. These studies have not demonstrated superiority to pemetrexed and cisplatin [23]. They may, however, have a role in the second-line setting.

Treatment response

Treatment response can be difficult to assess in mesothelioma, given the complexity of measuring an asymmetric tumour rind. The modified Response Evaluation Criteria in Solid Tumours (RECIST) can be used [44].

Recurrent disease

Where possible, patients with recurrent mesothelioma should be considered for a clinical trial (phase I or II) evaluating new biologicals, chemotherapeutic agents, or physical approaches.

Biological therapy

Given the poor response to chemotherapy, there is a need to consider alternative approaches to managing malignant mesothelioma. Unfortunately, to date, there are no specific targets that have been demonstrated to result in an improved outcome. For example, despite overexpression of EGFR, there is no evidence that dedicated inhibitors demonstrate any efficacy [45,46]. Some targeted therapies to date seem promising, notably anti-angiogenic agents and histone deacetylase inhibitors.

A final word from the expert

Malignant mesothelioma remains an important cancer in industrialized countries. The annual incidence continues to rise. Unfortunately, asbestos is being increasingly used in the developing world, thereby making an epidemic of malignant mesothelioma likely in the middle of the twenty-first century, with a peak predicted for 2020 in the UK and Ireland. Treatment options are limited, but recent insights have increased our understanding of the biology, and there is an increased interest in developing targeted treatments in the future.

References

1. Roberts ME, Neville E, Berrisford RG, Antunes G, Ali NJ; BTS Pleural Disease Guideline Group. Management of a malignant pleural effusion: British Thoracic Society Pleural Disease Guideline 2010. *Thorax* 2010; **65**(Suppl 2): ii32–40.

2. Fenton KN, Richardson JD. Diagnosis and management of malignant pleural effusions. *American Journal of Surgery* 1995; **170**(1): 69–74.

3. Putnam JB, Jr., Walsh GL, Swisher SG *et al.* Outpatient management of malignant pleural effusion by a chronic indwelling pleural catheter. *The Annals of Thoracic Surgery* **69**(2) 2000 369–75

4. Robinson BW, Lake RA. Advances in malignant mesothelioma. *The New England Journal of Medicine* 2005; **353**(15) 1591–603.

5. Dogan AU, Baris YI, Dogan M *et al.* Genetic predisposition to fiber carcinogenesis causes a mesothelioma epidemic in Turkey. *Cancer Research* 2006; **66**(10): 5063–8.

6. Weill H, Hughes J, Churg A. Changing trends in US mesothelioma incidence. *Occupational and Environmental Medicine* 2005; **62**(4): 270.

7. Price B. Analysis of current trends in United States mesothelioma incidence. *American Journal of Epidemiology* 1997; **145**(3): 211–18.

8. Larson T, Melnikova N, Davis SI, Jamison P. Incidence and descriptive epidemiology of mesothelioma in the United States, 1999-2002. *International Journal of Occupational and Environmental Health* 2007; **13**(4): 398–403.

9. Bianchi C, Bianchi T, Malignant mesothelioma: global incidence and relationship with asbestos. *Industrial Health* 2007; **45**(3): 379–87

10. Okada M, Mimura T, Ohbayashi C, Sakuma T, Soejima T, Tsubota N. Radical surgery for malignant pleural mesothelioma: results and prognosis. *Interactive CardioVascular and Thoracic Surgery* 2008; **7**(1): 102–6.

11. Borasio P, Berruti A, Bille A *et al.* Malignant pleural mesothelioma: clinicopathologic and survival characteristics in a consecutive series of 394 patients. *European Journal of Cardiothoracic Surgery* 2008; **33**(2):307–13.

12. Ceresoli GL, Locati LD, Ferreri AJ *et al.* Therapeutic outcome according to histologic subtype in 121 patients with malignant pleural mesothelioma. *Lung Cancer* 2001; **34**(2): 279–87.

13. Roe OD, Creaney J, Lundgren S *et al.* Mesothelin-related predictive and prognostic factors in malignant mesothelioma: a nested case-control study. *Lung Cancer* 2008; **61**(2): 235–43.

14. Testa JR, Cheung M, Pei J *et al.* Germline BAP1 mutations predispose to malignant mesothelioma. *Nature Genetics* 2011; **43**(10) 1022–5.

15. Baker PM, Clement PB, Young RH. Malignant peritoneal mesothelioma in women: a study of 75 cases with emphasis on their morphologic spectrum and differential diagnosis. *American Journal of Clinical Pathology* 2005; **123**(5): 724–37.

16. Le DT, Deavers M, Hunt K, Malpica A, Verschraegen CF. Cisplatin and irinotecan (CPT-11) for peritoneal mesothelioma. *Cancer Investigation* 2003 **21**(5): 682–9.

17. Bridda A, Padoan I, Mencarelli R, Frego M. Peritoneal mesothelioma: a review. *Medscape General Medicine* 2007; **9**(2): 32.

18. Rusch VW, Piantadosi S, Holmes EC. The role of extrapleural pneumonectomy in malignant pleural mesothelioma. A Lung Cancer Study Group trial. *Journal of Thoracic and Cardiovascular Surgery* 1991; **102**(1): 1–9.

19. Sugarbaker DJ, Mentzer SJ, DeCamp M, Lynch TJ. Jr, Strauss GM. Extrapleural pneumonectomy in the setting of a multimodality approach to malignant mesothelioma. *Chest* 1993; **103**(4 Suppl): 377S–81S

20. Tsao AS, Wistuba I, Roth JA, Kindler HL, Malignant pleural mesothelioma. *Journal of Clinical Oncology* 2009; **27**(12): 2081–90.

21. Sugarbaker DJ, Strauss GM, Lynch TJ *et al.* Node status has prognostic significance in the multimodality therapy of diffuse, malignant mesothelioma. *Journal of Clinical Oncology* 1993; **11**(6): 1172–8.

4

Small cell lung cancer (SCLC) and syndrome of inappropriate antidiurectic hormone (SIADH)

Alex Lee

Expert commentary Angela Darby

Case study

A 65-year-old man presented to his GP with a 2-month history of cough and intermittent haemoptysis. He reported a 5 kg weight loss, persistent malaise, and fatigue, as well as a subtle increase in exertional dyspnoea. He had no diagnosed cardiac or respiratory conditions and no personal history of cancer. He was a current smoker, having smoked approximately 20 cigarettes a day since the age of 16. On examination of the chest, transmitted sounds were heard in the mid and lower zones of the right chest. Abdominal and neurological examinations were unremarkable.

> **⊙ Learning point** Diagnosis of small cell lung cancer (SCLC)
>
> SCLC often presents with a distinct clinical picture:
>
> - rapid onset of symptoms, with a typical duration of only 2–3 months before presentation
> - intra-thoracic disease may cause cough, wheeze, haemoptysis, and dyspnoea
> - locally invasive or metastatic disease may cause superior vena cava obstruction (SVCO), recurrent laryngeal nerve palsy, chest wall or bone pain, and symptomatic brain metastases
> - systemic paraneoplastic effects include cachexia, anorexia, symptoms of paraneoplastic endocrine, neurological, or dermatological syndromes.

> **⊕ Expert comment**
>
> As SCLC grows and metastasizes rapidly, patients frequently deteriorate during the course of investigations. Every effort must be made to gain an early histological diagnosis and prompt review by an oncologist. The majority of patients will respond to chemotherapy, making it appropriate to consider treatment, even in patients with poor performance status (PS).

The GP made an urgent referral to the respiratory medicine team at the local hospital who arranged for immediate haemato-biochemistry screening, which was within the normal range, and chest imaging. The CXR showed a right hilar opacification, and the contrast chest CT showed a 42 mm spiculated right middle lobe pulmonary nodule, arising from the right hilum, and two smaller (10 mm and 18 mm) satellite lesions within the same lobe. Multiple enlarged ipsilateral hilar and paratracheal lymph nodes, the largest measuring 32 mm, were also seen.

A staging CT scan of the abdomen and pelvis did not reveal any abnormalities, and a bronchoscopy showed nodular mucosal thickening in the posterior wall of the lateral bronchioles of the right middle lobe. Histopathology of the biopsy revealed small epithelial cells with scant cytoplasm and poorly defined cell borders. Immunohistochemical staining was positive for synaptophysin, CK7, and TTF-1.

➕ **Clinical tip** Classification of SCLC [1]

The WHO classifies SCLC morphologically as 'a malignant epithelial tumour consisting of small cells with scant cytoplasm, ill-defined cell borders, finely granular nuclear chromatin, and absent or inconspicuous cytoplasm. The cells are round, oval and spindle-shaped. Nuclear moulding is prominent. Necrosis is typically extensive and the mitotic count is high' [1].

➕ **Clinical tip** Pathological diagnosis of SCLC

Pathological diagnosis should be sought in all cases of suspected SCLC (Figure 4.1). Flexible bronchoscopy, endoscopic ultrasound (EUS), mediastinoscopy, transthoracic needle biopsy, or thoracoscopy can be used to seek biopsies of primary thoracic disease—biopsy of metastatic or lymph node disease is adequate for diagnosis.

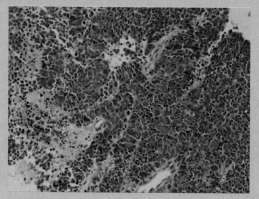

Figure 4.1 Characteristic haematoxylin and eosin-stained sample of SCLC. Slide showing disordered proliferation of cells, large nuclei, and little cytoplasm, characteristic of SCLC.

➕ **Clinical tip** Immunohistochemical profiling

Immunohistochemical profiling is useful in confirming histopathological diagnosis. Over 90% of SCLCs are positive for neuroendocrine markers such as chromogranin and synaptophysin. CD56 (N-CAM) and TTF-1 are often positive, with cytokeratin profiling distinguishing SCLC from other morphologically small, round cancer cells such as lymphoma.

The patient's case was referred to the lung cancer MDT who agreed with the diagnosis of SCLC with provisional staging T3N2M0; stage IIIa. A PET-CT scan, CT head, and pulmonary function testing were requested to complete baseline assessments (Box 4.1).

Box 4.1 Further staging investigations

Fluorodeoxyglucose (FDG)-PET-CT: significant FDG uptake in all right middle lobe lesions, with similar FDG avidity seen in enlarged hilar and mediastinal lymph nodes. No FDG-avid lesions seen elsewhere in the body.

CT head: no evidence of metastatic cerebral disease.

Pulmonary function tests: FEV1 1.98 L/min (61% expected), FVC 3.80 L/min (86% expected), FEV1/FVC 52%, kCO 1.23 mmol/min/kPa/L.

The patient met with the oncology team who recommended concomitant chemo-radiotherapy (CRT), followed by prophylactic cranial irradiation (PCI).

ⓖ Expert comment

PET scans are increasingly performed as part of the staging of patients with SCLC. Many patients with a radiological diagnosis of lung cancer that may be suitable for radical treatment have a PET scan, before histology is available with tissue subsequently obtained at endobroncial ultrasound (EBUS). PET is also increasingly used for potential candidates for chemoradiation, as PET may lead to upstaging/downstaging of patients and to alteration of radiation fields resulting from the detection of additional sites of nodal metastasis. However, it should be noted that the sensitivity, specificity, and positive or negative predictive value of PET and its additional value to accuracy of standard staging are uncertain [2]. Figure 4.2 shows upstaging of SCLC on PET imaging in two separate cases.

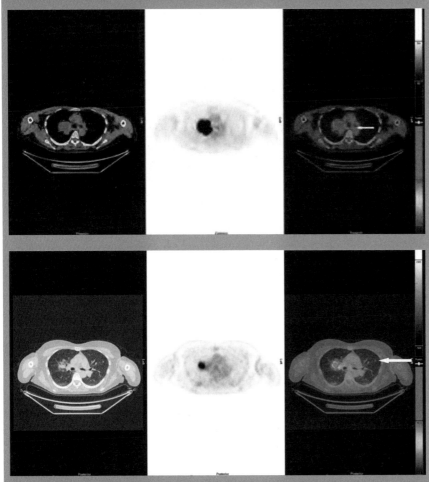

Figure 4.2 Two cases of PET imaging in SCLC which demonstrate upstaging of the disease, compared to the assessments based on conventional CT imaging alone. Each figure includes axial slices with low-dose CT (left), PET (middle), and fused (right) images. The PET and fused images are displayed to a maximum SUV of 10 (colour scale on far right of figure, CT Hounsfield units displayed in grey).

Case 1. Low-grade uptake is seen in a left paratracheal node, suggesting possible involvement of the contralateral mediastinum. Sampling of the nodes, using EBUS, revealed involvement of nodes by SCLC.
Case 2. The PET scan in this case additionally highlighted some small lung nodules, including the nodule arrowed in the left upper lobe, which were suspicious for lung metastases.

> ⊕ **Learning point** SCLC staging
>
> Disease extent is the strongest prognostic factor in SCLC. The Veterans Administration Lung Study Group (VALSG) proposed a binary staging system in 1957, dividing SCLC into either limited (LD-SCLC) or extensive (ED-SCLC) disease, on the basis of whether all disease could be encapsulated in a single radiotherapy port, i.e. LD-SCLC is restricted to one hemithorax, including involved ipsilateral hilar, mediastinal, and supraclavicular lymph nodes; ED-SCLC is all other extent of disease, including malignant pleural or pericardial effusion [3].
>
> The dichotomous VALSG staging remains in wide use, with a 1987 revision by the International Association for the Study of Lung Cancer (IASLC) expanding LD-SCLC to include contralateral mediastinal and supraclavicular nodes and ipsilateral pleural effusion [4].
>
> The IASLC has recently proposed the application of its seventh edition of TNM staging for lung cancer to SCLC, on the basis of ongoing analysis of the 12 000+ cases of SCLC within its database [5]. This analysis has shown that subdivision of LD-SCLC by T and N stages is prognostically informative, that N2 or 3 nodal involvement confers worse survival, compared to N0/1, and that LD-SCLC with cytologically proven malignant ipsilateral pleural effusion falls into an intermediate prognosis between LD-SCLC without pleural involvement and ED-SCLC.
>
> IASLC TNM stage can be translated easily into VALSG staging, with LD-SCLC equating to ≤ stage IIIB and ED-SCLC to ≥ stage IIIB.

> ⊕ **Learning point** Treatment of limited-stage SCLC
>
> **Surgery**
>
> A small proportion of SCLC patients who present with early disease (T1/2, N0/1) may benefit from radical surgical resection. Early randomized trials did not indicate superiority of surgery over radiotherapy [1, 6]. More recent surgical series report high local control rates, with 5-year survival of over 50% for selected patients with stages I–III disease [7]. Surgery should be followed by adjuvant chemotherapy and PCI. pN1 and unexpected pN2 disease should be considered for post-operative thoracic radiotherapy [8].
>
> **CRT**
>
> Thoracic radiotherapy, with concurrent cisplatin–etoposide chemotherapy, is the current standard of care for limited-stage SCLC.

> ✔ **Evidence base** Meta-analyses of the addition of radiotherapy to chemotherapy
>
> Two meta-analyses, published in 1992, have demonstrated a small, but significant (approximately 5%), survival benefit from the addition of thoracic radiotherapy to chemotherapy in the treatment of LD-SCLC [9, 10].
>
> Pignon *et al.* [9]:
> - a total of 2140 patients from 13 randomized trials (individual patient data):
>   - RR of death 0.86 (95% CI 0.78–0.94; $p = 0.001$), in favour of combination CRT versus chemotherapy alone
>   - 3-year survival 14.3% versus 8.9%.
>
> Warde and Payne [10]:
> - a total of 2011 patients from 11 randomized trials (individual and abstracted data):
>   - odds ratio for 2-year survival 1.53 (95% CI 1.30–1.76; $p < 0.001$), in favour of combination therapy
>   - 2-year survival improved by 5.4%
>   - local control odds ratio 3.02 (95% CI 2.8–3.2; $p < 0.001$)
>
> - Warde and Payne report a small, but significant, increase in treatment-related death with combination treatment (3.3% versus 1.4%).
>
> (continued)

Of note:

- overlap of nine trials between two meta-analyses
- no platinum-based chemotherapy used. Mostly cyclophosphamide and/or doxorubicin-based combinations
- variety in radiotherapy doses, mostly 40–50 Gy in 15–25 fractions. PCI administered in approximately two-thirds of trials
- timing of radiotherapy ranged from concomitant, starting on day 1 of chemotherapy, to sequential starting from day >200
- concomitant CRT is superior to sequential administration, in terms of locoregional control and survival, although it is associated with greater acute toxicity [11]. In patients with good PS and non-bulky disease, starting concomitant radiotherapy, alongside either the first or second cycle of chemotherapy, is advised.

✅ **Evidence base** Systematic review of the timing of radiotherapy in combined chemotherapy regimens

- Systematic review of 1524 patients from seven randomized trials comparing early and late start of radiotherapy as part of combined CRT for LD-SCLC [12].
- Early radiotherapy defined as within 9 weeks of the first cycle and before the third cycle of chemotherapy; late radiotherapy defined as after 9 weeks of the first cycle and after beginning the third cycle of chemotherapy.
- OS at 2 years RR 1.17 (95% CI 1.02–1.35; $p = 0.03$), in favour of early radiotherapy.
- Benefit of early radiotherapy was greatest when hyperfractionated radiotherapy and platinum-based chemotherapy used.

The optimal radiotherapy dose and fractionation remain under investigation. Retrospective reviews suggest a dose–response relationship, with up to78% local control rates at 3 years with doses >50 Gy [13].

Optimal definition of radiotherapy target volumes minimizes toxicity to normal tissues. However, the omission of elective irradiation of radiologically uninvolved mediastinal nodes resulted in unexpectedly high mediastinal relapse rates in one prospective phase II study [14]. As such, elective nodal irradiation remains recommended. The use of FDG-PET to assess nodal involvement in this context appears promising, with only 3% nodal failure in one prospective series where only FDG-positive mediastinal lymph nodes were irradiated [15].

PCI

In the absence of disease progression, all patients should be considered for PCI following surgery or CRT for LD-SCLC.

Follow-up

In patients who achieve long-term survival following SCLC, second primary cancer rates approach 10% per year. All patients embarking on treatment for SCLC should be ardently encouraged and supported in smoking cessation, as ongoing smoking increases early and late toxicities of radiotherapy and chemotherapy, worsens cancer-related symptoms, and negatively impacts survival. Radically treated patients should have long-term follow-up, with surveillance for disease relapse and new primary tumours. New lung masses should be biopsied, as *de novo* lung cancers of both small cell and non-small cell subtypes are common.

Within 2 weeks of the first cycle of cisplatin and etoposide (IV cisplatin 75 mg/m^2 on day 1, oral etoposide 100 mg/m^2 once daily on days 1–3), the patient noted a significant improvement in his symptoms. Concomitant thoracic radiotherapy was commenced on day 1 in cycle 2 of chemotherapy. The patient went on to receive 64 Gy in 30 once-daily fractions on consecutive weekdays. A total of four 21-day cycles of chemotherapy were administered. Treatment toxicities included grade 2 fatigue, grade 2 oesophagitis, grade 2 alopecia, grade 1 nausea, and grade 1 peripheral sensory neuropathy. No grade 3 or 4 toxicities were experienced, including haematological toxicities.

> **✪ Expert comment**
>
> Platinum and etoposide are standard first-line chemotherapy. Etoposide is active in IV and oral formulations, with advantages to each route of administration. As the bioavailability of oral etoposide can be unpredictable, I would use IV etoposide for patients having radical treatment. Oral etoposide is useful when it is appropriate to minimize hospital attendances, such as days 2 and 3, when treating extensive-stage disease.

An end-of-treatment CT showed a complete radiological response. The patient went on to receive PCI (25 Gy over ten fractions). The patient was able to return to work, 2 months after completion of his treatment.

> **✪ Learning point** PCI
>
> Metastatic brain disease is common in SCLC and is present at diagnosis in approximately 20% of patients. Intracranial relapse occurs in over 50% of patients and is the sole site of recurrence in up to a third. Whole-brain radiotherapy to treat brain-only relapse is associated with response rates of < 50% and a median survival of 4–5 months [16]. PCI aims to prevent this from developing.
>
> PCI after first-line systemic treatment has been shown to be beneficial in both LD- and ED-SCLC when patients achieve a response to induction therapy. A standard dose of 20–25 Gy in 5–10 fractions is recommended to be delivered within 6 weeks of completion of systemic therapy. Concomitant chemotherapy and PCI is not recommended. PCI improves 3-year survival by 5% and reduces rates of brain metastasis after 3 years by 25% [17].

> **✔ Evidence base** Meta-analysis of PCI delivered to patients with LD- or ED-SCLC in remission after induction therapy [17]
>
> - A 2000 Cochrane review of seven randomized phase III trials ($n = 987$).
> - PCI dosing from 8 Gy in one fraction to 40 Gy in 20 fractions.
> - Significant survival benefit with PCI: RR of death 0.84 (95% CI 0.73–0.97; $p < 0.01$); absolute risk of death at 3 years 15.3% versus 20.7%.
> - Significant reduction in rate of brain metastasis: RR of brain metastasis 0.46 (95% CI 0.38–0.57; $p < 0.001$); absolute cumulative risk of brain metastasis at 3 years 33.3% versus 58.6%.
> - Larger radiotherapy doses significantly decreased the risk of brain metastasis; no significant effect on survival.
> - Earlier administration of PCI significantly reduced the rate of brain metastasis.
>
> *Source*: data from Prophylactic Cranial Irradiation Overview Collaborative Group, Cranial irradiation for preventing brain metastases of small cell lung cancer in patients in complete remission, *The Cochrane Library*, Issue 4, 2000, Copyright © 1999 The Cochrane Collaboration.

> **✔ Evidence base** PCI in extensive-stage SCLC [18]
>
> - EORTC randomized phase III study of PCI versus no PCI after response to first-line chemotherapy [18].
> - 25% reduction in the rate of brain metastasis at 1 year (14.6% versus 40.4%; HR 0.27, 95% CI 0.16–0.44; $p < 0.001$).
> - Improved median PFS in the PCI group (14.7 weeks versus 12.0 weeks; HR 0.76, 95% CI 0.59–0.96; $p = 0.02$).
> - 1-year survival rate 27.1% versus 13.3%, in favour of PCI.
> - Significantly increased hair loss and fatigue in the PCI group. Trend towards increased anorexia, nausea and vomiting, and leg weakness in the PCI group.
> - No significant difference in cognitive or global health scores between groups (NB < 50% compliance with QoL follow-up).
>
> *Source*: data from Slotman B *et al.*, Prophylactic cranial irradiation in extensive small-cell lung cancer, *New England Journal of Medicine*, Volume 357, Number 7, pp. 664–72, Copyright © 2007 Massachusetts Medical Society. All rights reserved.

Five months later, the patient experienced a 2-week history of fatigue and malaise. On review, the patient appeared generally unwell with impaired PS (PS = 2). Urgent blood tests were arranged (Table 4.1). These supported a biochemical diagnosis of syndrome of inappropriate anti-diuretic hormone (SIADH). This raised concerns for recurrent disease.

Table 4.1 Urgent blood test results

Haematology	Biochemistry	
Hb 9.4 g/L	Na 122 mmol/L	Serum osmolality 269 mOsm/L
WBC 13.2 × 10^9/L	K 3.6 mmol/L	Urinary osmolality 412 mOsm/L
Neutrophils 12.2 × 10^9/L	Urea 7.2 mmol/L	Urinary Na 55 mmol/L
Lymphocytes 0.4 × 10^9/L	Creatinine 101 μmol/L	Serum total cholesterol 6.2mmol/L
Platelets 547 × 10^9/L	LDH 299	Serum triglycerides 1.6 mmol/L
	CRP 29	TSH 2.8 mIU/L
		Free T4 15 pmol/L

✪ Learning point SIADH

SIADH affects around 15% of SCLC patients. Symptoms include headache, lethargy and nausea, seizure, or coma [19]. Low serum sodium is a negative prognostic factor in SCLC, with failure to correct hyponatraemia predicting poor outcome [20]. SIADH is characterized by hypo-osmotic hyponatraemia, resulting from inappropriate renal retention of water in response to excess levels of the physiological anti-diuretic hormone arginine vasopressin (AVP). This may occur due to ectopic extrapituitary secretion occurring as a paraneoplastic phenomenon of some malignancies (e.g. SCLC, haematological and head and neck cancers) or in infective or inflammatory pulmonary conditions. Alternatively, excess pituitary secretion of AVP can occur following intracranial trauma or in response to a range of drugs that include platinum agents, vinca alkaloids, or anticonvulsants.

Diagnosis

A diagnosis of SIADH is made on establishing all of the following criteria:

- low serum sodium and osmolality (exclude pseudo-hyponatraemia due to hyperglycaemia or hyperlipidaemia)
- failure of appropriate urinary dilution, i.e. normal or high urinary osmolality
- normal or high urinary sodium (usually >40 mmol/L)
- absence of clinical volume depletion
- absence of other causes of hyponatraemia, including:
  o adrenal insufficiency
  o hypothyroidism
  o congestive heart failure or cirrhosis
  o renal salt wasting.

Treatment

Paraneoplastic SIADH in SCLC often resolves with tumour response to first-line chemotherapy. However, significant symptomatic hyponatraemia may preclude safe administration of chemotherapy or radiotherapy. Alternatively, SIADH may accompany relapsed or refractory disease where a response to further anti-cancer treatment is less likely. In these scenarios, specific management of SIADH may be required. This includes:

1. fluid restriction (500 mL below the patient's average daily urine output)—may see improvement in days
2. stopping drugs which may contribute to low sodium
3. when the above are ineffective or impractical, consider:
  a. demeclocycline—inhibits AVP effect on renal tubules. Use limited by renal toxicity and limited efficacy
  b. tolvaptan—specific V2 receptor antagonist. Rapid and safe correction of hyponatraemia, although sodium levels fall on discontinuation [21]. Patients should be allowed free water intake to prevent overly rapid sodium rise.

The use of fluid restriction and potentially nephrotoxic drugs may prove problematic if cisplatin is used, as it necessitates large-volume IV hydration to prevent platinum-induced renal damage. Cisplatin can also induce SIADH and a salt-wasting renal tubulopathy.

> **⊕ Clinical tip** Paraneoplastic syndromes
>
> SCLC is the cancer most commonly associated with paraneoplastic syndromes (Table 4.2). Many of these can be broadly classified into: (1) endocrine syndromes resulting from the ectopic production and secretion of hormones by cancer cells, and (2) neurological syndromes caused by immune cross-reactivity between antigens found in both tumour cells and components of the nervous system. The emergence of a paraneoplastic syndrome is unrelated to the cancer stage and may form the initial presentation of SCLC. The synchronous presence of >1 paraneoplastic syndrome is exceedingly rare.

Table 4.2 Paraneoplastic syndromes associated with SCLC other than SIADH [22, 23, 24]

Syndrome	Prevalence (% of SCLC)	Cause	Presentation	Diagnosis	Treatment	Prognosis
Cushing's syndrome	5%	Ectopic adrenocorticotrophic hormone (ACTH) secretion	Weakness; lethargy; hypertension; ataxia; altered mental state; weight gain; cushingoid facies; glucose intolerance; proximal myopathy; acne; abdominal striae; hyperpigmentation	Hypokalaemia; hypernatraemia; high serum and urinary cortisol; normal/high midnight ACTH that is not suppressed with dexamethasone	Adrenal suppression (ketoconazole, mitotane, mifepristone, adrenalectomy); antihypertensives; diuretics	Low rate of improvement with chemotherapy. Presence of Cushing's is a poor prognostic factor
Lambert–Eaton myasthenic syndrome (LEMS)	3%; 50% of LEMS secondary to SCLC	Auto-antibodies against pre-synaptic voltage-gated calcium channels	Muscle weakness (predominantly in hip girdle); hyporeflexia; eye and bulbar movement disorders; improvement of weakness and reflexes with repeat muscle use; autonomic dysfunction	Electromyography (EMG) shows low-amplitude compound muscle action potentials, incremental response with high-rate stimulation	3,4-diaminopyridine; IV immunoglobulin	50% of cases refractory to chemotherapy
Limbic encephalitis and encephalomyelitis	< 1%; 40–75% of cases secondary to SCLC	Auto-antibodies against Hu family of neuronal proteins, leading to temporal lobe-predominant neuronal destruction	Rapidly progressive short-term memory loss; personality change; psychiatric disturbance; seizure	Electroencephalography (EEG)—focal temporal lobe epileptic/slow activity; MRI—temporal lobe hyperintensity on T2 or FLAIR sequence; cerebrospinal fluid (CSF)—raised WBC and protein, IgG oligoclonal bands	IV immunoglobulin; high-dose corticosteroid; plasmapheresis; cyclophosphamide; rituximab. Little evidence of efficacy of any of the above	Neurological impairment irreversible. Poor prognosis
Paraneoplastic cerebellar degeneration	< 1%	Auto-antibodies against neuronal epitopes (Hu, Yo, CRMP5, Ma, Tr, Ri, VGCC, mGluR1)	Ataxia; dysarthria; inability to walk, stand, or sit; abnormalities of ocular movement	MRI—appearances of cerebellar atrophy in later stages of syndrome	As per limbic encephalitis	Neurological impairment irreversible

Table 4.2 Paraneoplastic syndromes associated with SCLC [22, 23, 24] (continued)

Syndrome	Prevalence (% of SCLC)	Cause	Presentation	Diagnosis	Treatment	Prognosis
Opsonoclonus–myoclonus	< 1% SCLC most commonly associated cancer in adults (neuroblastoma in children)	Auto-antibodies against neurons (no defined specific antigen)	Involuntary, irregular, continual, chaotic conjugated eye movements; saccadic head movement; limb myoclonus; ataxia	Clinical—no recognized characteristic imaging or CSF findings	Immunosuppression and immunomodulation— corticosteroid, IV immunoglobulin, cyclophosphamide, rituximab	Approximately 50% respond to chemotherapy
Dermatomyositis	Rare in SCLC. Underlying cancer found in 15–40% of cases, most commonly ovarian or NSCLC	Not fully understood— immune-mediated proximal muscle and vascular injury, with likely humoral and cell-mediated autoimmune aetiology	Heliotropic rash; Gottron's papules; shawl sign; proximal muscle pain and weakness	Elevated creatinine kinase, liver transaminases, LDH; muscle biopsy— perifascicular atrophy, infarcts, perivascular and septal inflammation; EMG—fibrillations, positive sharp waves	Corticosteroid, further immunomodulation, e.g. azathioprine, methotrexate, ciclosporin, cyclophosphamide, IV immunoglobulin	Commonly improves with cancer response to chemotherapy; muscle impairment may persist

Source: data from Heinemann S *et al.,* Paraneoplastic syndromes in lung cancer, *Cancer Therapy,* Volume 6, pp. 687–98, Copyright © 2008; *Mayo Clinic proceedings,* Volume 85, Issue 9, Pelosof LC and Gerber DE, Paraneoplastic syndromes: an approach to diagnosis and treatment, *Mayo Clinic Proceedings,* pp. 838–54, Copyright © 2010 Mayo Foundation for Medical Education and Research; and *Seminars in Oncology,* Volume 33, Issue 3, Darnell RB and Posner JB, Paraneoplastic syndromes affecting the nervous system, pp. 270–98, Copyright © 2006 Elsevier Inc.

A CT restaging scan showed widespread recurrent disease involving both lungs, mediastinal and supraclavicular lymph nodes, the liver, and adrenal glands. Following correction of hyponatraemia and medical stabilization, second-line treatment options were discussed with the patient.

The patient commenced second-line oral topotecan (2.3 mg/m² once daily on days 1–5 of a 21-day cycle) and was referred to the local palliative care team. Prior to cycle 2, the patient's PS had improved to 1, and the serum biochemistry normalized. Restaging CT after two cycles revealed a partial response. The patient went on to receive four cycles of chemotherapy. An end-of-treatment CT scan revealed several new areas of liver disease, with interval progression of some lung lesions and mediastinal lymphadenopathy. At this point, the patient expressed a wish not to pursue further anti-cancer treatment and was followed up by his local palliative care team.

> **✪ Learning point** Management of relapsed SCLC
>
> Despite high rates of response to first-line chemotherapy, the duration of response is often disappointing, with average PFS approximately 4 months in ED-SCLC and 12 months in LD-SCLC. Median survival after relapse is 2–3 months, without second-line treatment. Response rates of up to 40% can be seen with second-line treatment, although these are typically short-lived, with median survival rarely >6 months.
>
> Second-line treatments are stratified, according to the response to first-line therapy:
>
> ● patients with PFS > 90 days are classed as 'sensitive'
> ● patients with PFS < 90 days are classed as 'resistant'
> ● patients with no response to first-line treatment are classed as 'refractory'.
>
> Sensitive patients can be rechallenged with first-line combination chemotherapy. Single-agent topotecan is the only licensed second-line agent for relapsed or refractory SCLC. Both oral and IV topotecan preparations have been shown to be equivalent in randomized studies [25].

✪ Expert comment Second-line chemotherapy in SCLC

It was correct to commence second-line chemotherapy after a treatment-free interval of approximately 6 months. With lower response rates, it is vital to recognize the palliative aim of this treatment and introduce palliative care alongside chemotherapy, to monitor the toxicity of treatment closely, and only continue if evidence of clinical benefit.

✔ Evidence base Oral topotecan as second-line treatment of extensive-stage SCLC [26]

Phase III trial comparing supportive care (SC) alone with supportive care plus oral topotecan in patients with relapsed SCLC.

- Randomized study of SC versus SC + oral topotecan (2.3 mg/m^2 on days 1–5 of 21-day cycle).
- A total of 141 patients stratified by sensitivity to first-line chemotherapy.
- Patients with symptomatic brain metastases excluded.
- Median OS significantly longer with topotecan (25.9 weeks versus 13.9 weeks; $p = 0.01$):
  o survival benefit maintained in chemoresistant and PS >1 subgroups.
- Topotecan response rates: 7% partial response; 44% stable disease at >56 days.
- Significantly slower deterioration in QoL in the topotecan group.

In the rare scenario of the fit SCLC patient being considered for third-line therapy, an anthracycline-based regimen or clinical trial can be considered.

Progress in the development of novel targeted therapies for SCLC has been slow, with a lack of predictive biomarkers of response a significant hurdle. Anti-angiogenic mAbs and TKIs, immune checkpoint inhibitors, and cancer vaccines have been investigated, with little success.

Source: data from O'Brien ME *et al.*, Phase III trial comparing supportive care alone with supportive care with oral topotecan in patients with relapsed small-cell lung cancer, *Journal of Clinical Oncology*, Volume 24, Number 24, pp. 5441–7, Copyright © 2006 by American Society of Clinical Oncology.

✔ Evidence base Cochrane review of platinum-containing chemotherapy compared with non-platinum-containing regimens [28]

- A total of 5530 patients (including both LD- and ED-SCLC) from 29 randomized trials, examining the use of platinum-containing and non-platinum-containing schedules in separate arms.
- Platinum arms: 80% cisplatin, 20% carboplatin.
- Commonest non-platinum agents: etoposide 83%; cyclophosphamide 76%; vincristine 62%; doxorubicin 62%.
- Radiotherapy (thoracic and/or PCI) used in 76%.
- No significant difference between the platinum and non-platinum groups in survival at 6, 12, and 24 months.
- Greater rates of complete response in platinum group (RR 1.33; 95% CI 1.13–1.56), but no significant difference in overall response rates.
- No difference in toxic death between the two groups, but higher rates of nausea and vomiting in platinum group (RR 1.51; 95% CI 1.20–1.90).

The substitution of cisplatin with carboplatin is widely accepted in the treatment of extensive disease.

Source: data from Amarasena IU *et al.*, Platinum versus non-platinum chemotherapy regimens for small cell lung cancer, *The Cochrane Library*, Issue 4, 2008, Copyright © 2009 The Cochrane Collaboration.

✪ Learning point Treatment of extensive-stage SCLC

Chemotherapy

Chemotherapy is the treatment of choice for ED-SCLC. The disease is very sensitive to first-line treatment, resulting in rapid reversal of symptoms, thus justifying treatment of selected patients with impaired PS. Trials have also demonstrated a significant improvement in OS [27]. Combination of cisplatin and etoposide (EP) is the current first-line standard, although superiority over anthracycline-based regimens, such as CAV (doxorubicin, cyclophosphamide, vincristine), has not been consistently demonstrated in phase III trials.

> **✔ Evidence base** Meta-analysis comparing first-line cisplatin and carboplatin-based chemotherapies [29]
>
> - A total of 663 patients from four randomized trials.
> - ED-SCLC in 68.3% of patients.
> - No significant difference between cisplatin (P) and carboplatin (C) group in:
>   - median OS—9.6 months (P) versus 9.4 months (C)
>   - median PFS—5.5 months (P) versus 5.3 months (C)
>   - overall response rate—67.1% (P) versus 66.0% (C).
> - More haematological toxicity with carboplatin; more non-haematological toxicity with cisplatin.
>
> The use of single-agent chemotherapy, such as oral etoposide, in frail or elderly patients has been shown to be inferior to combination regimens [30].
>
> **Maintenance chemotherapy**
>
> Trials examining the role of maintenance chemotherapy, investigating both the continuation of first-line regimen beyond six cycles or a switch to a non-cross-resistant maintenance regimen, have failed to show any impact upon survival whilst causing excess toxicity.
>
> **Thoracic radiotherapy**
>
> The benefit of thoracic radiotherapy in ED-SCLC is still to be defined. A randomized study showed patients who achieved complete response or partial response after three cycles of cisplatin and etoposide had significantly improved survival when randomized to concurrent hyperfractionated thoracic irradiation, delivered alongside two final cycles of chemotherapy [31].
>
> Source: data from Rossi A *et al.*, Carboplatin- or cisplatin-based chemotherapy in first-line treatment of small-cell lung cancer: the COCIS meta-analysis of individual patient data, *Journal of Clinical Oncology*, Volume 30, Number 4, pp. 1692–8, Copyright © 2012 by American Society of Clinical Oncology.

Discussion

SCLC accounts for approximately 20% of all lung cancers worldwide, with a UK incidence of around 12 cases per 100 000 per year. It is a classical smoking-related lung cancer, with cases in never-smokers exceedingly rare. Due to changes in smoking habits, SCLC incidence has fallen in the industrialized world over the past 30 years, although the proportion of female cases is increasing.

This case represents a typical history of SCLC, with rapid clinical onset and progression of symptoms that respond early and markedly to first-line treatment. As described, early metastasis is common, despite radical treatment, with preferential spread to bone, brain, liver, and adrenals. Responses to second-line therapy are seen but rarely endure more than a few months.

A final word from the expert

SCLC remains a challenging disease, being highly chemotherapy- and radiation-sensitive at presentation but rapidly developing chemoresistance. Whilst clinical trials including patients with limited-stage disease achieve median survivals of 18–24 months, there has been no consistent survival benefit from increased dose intensity, increased dose density, administration of additional drugs, or the use of maintenance chemotherapy. However, small improvements in survival are seen with optimizing radiotherapy, and PCI, and participation in clinical trials will hope to improve outcomes for future patients.

References

1. Sobin LH. The international histological classification of tumours. *Bulletin of the World Health Organization* 1981; **59**(6): 813–19.

2. Bradley JD, Dehdashti F, Mintun MA, Govindan R, Trinkaus K, Siegel BA. Positron emission tomography in limited-stage small-cell lung cancer: a prospective study. *Journal of Clinical Oncology* 2004; **22**(16): 3248–54.

3. Zelen M. Keynote address on biostatistics and data retrieval. *Cancer Chemotherapy Reports Part 3* 1973; **4**(2): 31–42.

4. Mountain CF. A new international staging system for lung cancer. *Chest* 1986; **89** (4 Suppl): 225S–33S.

5. Vallieres E, Shepherd FA, Crowley J *et al.* The IASLC Lung Cancer Staging Project: proposals regarding the relevance of TNM in the pathologic staging of small cell lung cancer in the forthcoming (seventh) edition of the TNM classification for lung cancer. *Journal of Thoracic Oncology* 2009; **4**(9): 1049–59.

6. Lad T, Piantadosi S, Thomas P, Payne D, Ruckdeschel J, Giaccone G. A prospective randomized trial to determine the benefit of surgical resection of residual disease following response of small cell lung cancer to combination chemotherapy. *Chest* 1994; **106**(6 Suppl): 320S–3S.

7. Puglisi M, Dolly S, Faria A, Myerson JS, Popat S, O'Brien ME. Treatment options for small cell lung cancer—do we have more choice? *British Journal of Cancer* 2010; **102**(4): 629–38.

8. Stahel R, Thatcher N, Fruh M *et al.* 1st ESMO Consensus Conference in lung cancer; Lugano 2010: small-cell lung cancer. *Annals of Oncology* 2011; **22**(9): 1973–80.

9. Pignon JP, Arriagada R, Ihde DC *et al.* A meta-analysis of thoracic radiotherapy for small-cell lung cancer. *The New England Journal of Medicine* 1992; **327**(23): 1618–24.

10. Warde P, Payne D. Does thoracic irradiation improve survival and local control in limited-stage small-cell carcinoma of the lung? A meta-analysis. *Journal of Clinical Oncology* 1992; **10**(6): 890–5.

11. Takada M, Fukuoka M, Kawahara M *et al.* Phase III study of concurrent versus sequential thoracic radiotherapy in combination with cisplatin and etoposide for limited-stage small-cell lung cancer: results of the Japan Clinical Oncology Group Study 9104. *Journal of Clinical Oncology* 2002; **20**(14): 3054–60.

12. Fried DB, Morris DE, Poole C *et al.* Systematic review evaluating the timing of thoracic radiation therapy in combined modality therapy for limited-stage small-cell lung cancer. *Journal of Clinical Oncology* 2004; **22**(23): 4837–45.

13. Roof KS, Fidias P, Lynch TJ, Ancukiewicz M, Choi NC. Radiation dose escalation in limited-stage small-cell lung cancer. *International Journal of Radiation Oncology, Biology, Physic* S2003; **57**(3): 701–8.

14. De Ruysscher D, Bremer RH, Koppe F et al. Omission of elective node irradiation on basis of CT-scans in patients with limited disease small cell lung cancer: a phase II trial. *Radiotherapy and Oncology* 2006; **80**(3): 307–12.

15. van Loon J, De Ruysscher D, Wanders R *et al.* Selective nodal irradiation on basis of (18)FDG-PET scans in limited-disease small-cell lung cancer: a prospective study. *International Journal of Radiation Oncology *Biology* Physics* 2010; **77**(2): 329–36.

16. Postmus PE, Haaxma-Reiche H, Gregor A *et al.* Brain-only metastases of small cell lung cancer; efficacy of whole brain radiotherapy. An EORTC phase II study. *Radiotherapy and Oncology* 1998; **46**(1): 29–32.

17. Prophylactic Cranial Irradiation Overview Collaborative Group. Cranial irradiation for preventing brain metastases of small cell lung cancer in patients in complete remission. *Cochrane Database of Systematic Review* S2000; **4**: CD002805.

18. Slotman B, Faivre-Finn C, Kramer G, *et al.* Prophylactic cranial irradiation in extensive small-cell lung cancer. *The New England Journal of Medicine* 2007; **357**(7): 664–72.

19. Sorensen JB, Andersen MK, Hansen HH. Syndrome of inappropriate secretion of antidiuretic hormone (SIADH) in malignant disease. *Journal of Internal Medicine* 1995; **238**(2): 97–110.

20. Castillo JJ, Vincent M, Justice E. Diagnosis and management of hyponatremia in cancer patients. *The Oncologist* 2012; **17**(6): 756–65.

21. Schrier RW, Gross P, Gheorghiade M *et al.* Tolvaptan, a selective oral vasopressin V2-receptor antagonist, for hyponatremia. *The New England Journal of Medicine* 2006; **355**(20): 2099–112.

22. Heinemman S, Zabel P, Hauber H. Paraneoplastic syndromes in lung cancer. *Cancer Therapy* 2008; **6**: 687–98.

23. Pelosof LC, Gerber DE. Paraneoplastic syndromes: an approach to diagnosis and treatment. *Mayo Clinic Proceedings* 2010; **85**(9): 838–54.

24. Darnell RB, Posner JB. Paraneoplastic syndromes affecting the nervous system. *Seminars in Oncology* 2006; **33**(3): 270–98.

25. Eckardt JR, von Pawel J, Pujol JL *et al.* Phase III study of oral compared with intravenous topotecan as second-line therapy in small-cell lung cancer. *Journal of Clinical Oncology* 2007; **25**(15): 2086–92.

26. O'Brien ME, Ciuleanu TE, Tsekov H *et al.* Phase III trial comparing supportive care alone with supportive care with oral topotecan in patients with relapsed small-cell lung cancer. *Journal of Clinical Oncology* 2006; **24**(34): 5441–7.

27. Pelayo Alvarez M, Gallego Rubio O, Bonfill Cosp X, Agra Varela Y. Chemotherapy versus best supportive care for extensive small cell lung cancer. *Cochrane Database of Systematic Reviews* 2009; **4**: CD001990.

28. Amarasena IU, Walters JA, Wood-Baker R, Fong K. Platinum versus non-platinum chemotherapy regimens for small cell lung cancer. *Cochrane Database of Systematic Reviews* 2008; **4**: CD006849.

29. Rossi A, Di Maio M, Chiodini P *et al.* Carboplatin- or cisplatin-based chemotherapy in first-line treatment of small-cell lung cancer: the COCIS meta-analysis of individual patient data. *Journal of Clinical Oncology* 2012; **30**(14): 1692–8.

30. Rossi A, Maione P, Colantuoni G *et al.* Treatment of small cell lung cancer in the elderly. *The Oncologist* 2005; **10**(6): 399–411.

31. Jeremic B, Shibamoto Y, Nikolic N *et al.* Role of radiation therapy in the combined-modality treatment of patients with extensive disease small-cell lung cancer: a randomized study. *Journal of Clinical Oncology* 1999; **17**(7): 2092–9.

> **⊕ Clinical tip** Presentation of gynaecological malignancy
>
> The presentation of gynaecological malignancy depends on the site involved and the stage. Some classically present at an early stage (e.g. endometrial cancer), whilst others typically present late (e.g. ovarian cancer). Symptoms can be due to local disease or distant spread.
>
> - Asymptomatic: incidental or screening-detected (e.g. cervical cancer).
> - Local symptoms:
>   - mass: vaginal or vulval lesion, inguinal lymphadenopathy
>   - vaginal bleeding: post-menopausal bleeding, intermenstrual or post-coital bleeding, menorrhagia
>   - vaginal discharge or itch
>   - pain: dyspareunia, pelvic or back pain due to tumour or lymphadenopathy
>   - abdominal symptoms: pain, bloating, change in bowel habit due to pressure effect or direct invasion of tumour, peritoneal deposits or ascites
>   - other: bladder symptoms from pressure or direct invasion, renal failure from ureteric obstruction, lower limb oedema or venous thromboembolic disease from pelvic lymphadenopathy or tumour.
> - Distant metastases: fatigue, anorexia, cachexia, shortness of breath, bone pain, nausea, jaundice, paraneoplastic syndrome.

> **✪ Learning point** Risk factors for endometrial carcinoma [1]
>
> | Factors increasing risk | Factors reducing risk |
> | --- | --- |
> | - Age | - Grand multiparity |
> | - Obesity | - Late menarche |
> | - Diabetes, metabolic syndrome | - Combined oral contraceptive pill |
> | - Early menarche | - Use of intrauterine device |
> | - Nulliparity (especially infertility) | - Smoking |
> | - Atypical endometrial hyperplasia | - Diet—isoflavones (soya), coffee |
> | - Polycystic ovary syndrome (PCOS) | |
> | - Breast cancer | |
> | - Long-term unopposed oestrogens | |
> | - Tamoxifen | |
> | - Family history—first-degree relative, hereditary non-polyposis colorectal cancer (HNPCC) | |
>
> Source: data from *The Lancet*, Volume 366, Issue 9484, Amant F *et al.*, Endometrial cancer, pp. 491–505, Copyright © 2005 Elsevier Ltd.

Obesity is a key risk factor. A body mass index (BMI) >25 doubles the risk of endometrial cancer, and almost 50% of women presenting with endometrial cancer are obese. Diabetes is linked to obesity but is also a risk factor in women with a normal BMI.

Breast cancer shares many of the same risk factors as endometrial cancer. In addition, tamoxifen is a well-recognized risk factor for benign and malignant endometrial disease. The impact of AIs on the risk of endometrial cancer is unclear [1].

The exact risk with PCOS is not fully understood. PCOS leads to anovulation and so higher levels of unopposed oestrogen. Obesity and hyperinsulinaemia are risk factors common to both PCOS and endometrial cancer.

HNPCC is an autosomal dominant syndrome of mismatch repair, leading to an increased risk of colonic and endometrial cancers, as well as gastric, pancreatic, and small bowel cancers. Women with HNPCC have a 40–60% lifetime risk of endometrial cancer and typically develop it at a younger age.

Women with a uterus should only be prescribed HRT with combined oestrogen and progesterone, as unopposed oestrogens increase the risk of endometrial cancer.

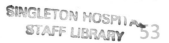

> ⊕ **Clinical tip** Diagnostic work-up of endometrial carcinoma
>
> TVUS is often the initial investigation for women with post-menopausal bleeding. Endometrial thickness in post-menopausal women (not on HRT) should be <5 mm. TVUS in pre-menopausal women is less helpful, as endometrial thickness varies with the menstrual cycle. Outpatient pipelle biopsy is possible in most women and has a sensitivity of 81% and a specificity of >98% for endometrial cancer [2]. If not tolerated or not possible, patients require hysteroscopy and biopsy. Pre-menopausal women presenting with vaginal bleeding need a pregnancy test.
>
> MRI of the pelvis is key to staging the local extent of disease. Most women will also have a staging CT of the chest, abdomen, and pelvis (CT CAP). Although the yield in early-stage disease is low, CT is helpful in assessing nodal disease. Bone scan is not routine but is used if clinical symptoms or signs raise concern of bone metastases. CA125 is not a helpful diagnostic tool but may be raised. There is no routine role for PET currently.

> ⑥ **Expert comment**
>
> For low-grade endometrial cancer (grades 1/2), there is no consensus in the UK regarding the role of routine MRI, much less CT CAP. In grade 3 or other high-risk histologies, MRI is recommended. CT is usually reserved for those patients where MRI, or symptoms, indicate the possibility of more advanced disease.

> ✪ **Learning point** Staging of carcinoma of the endometrium—*Fédération Internationale de Gynécologie et d'Obstétrique* (FIGO)
>
> Staging of gynaecological cancers uses the FIGO system [3]. It was revised in 2009; Table 5.1 shows the current staging. Most of the landmark trials in endometrial cancer were based on the previous 1988 FIGO staging system. This has implications when interpreting the studies. The FIGO classification for endometrial cancer is based on surgical staging. The regional lymph nodes are the pelvic, common iliac, external iliac, parametrial, and sacral nodes. Uterine sarcomas have a separate FIGO classification and are managed differently.
>
> **Table 5.1 FIGO staging of endometrial cancer**
>
> | | |
> |---|---|
> | Stage I* | Tumour confined to the corpus uteri |
> | IA* | No or less than half myometrial invasion |
> | IB* | Invasion equal to or more than half of the myometrium |
> | Stage II* | Tumour invades the cervical stroma but does not extend beyond the uterus** |
> | Stage III* | Local and/or regional spread of the tumour |
> | IIIA* | Tumour invades the serosa of the corpus uteri and/or adnexae# |
> | IIIB* | Vaginal and/or parametrial involvement# |
> | IIIC* | Metastases to pelvic and/or para-aortic lymph nodes# |
> | IIIC1* | Positive pelvic nodes |
> | IIIC2* | Positive para-aortic lymph nodes with or without positive pelvic lymph nodes |
> | Stage IV* | Tumour invades the bladder and/or bowel mucosa, and/or distant metastases |
> | IVA* | Tumour invasion of the bladder and/or bowel mucosa |
> | IVB* | Distant metastases, including intra-abdominal metastases and/or inguinal lymph nodes |
>
> * Either G1, G2, or G3.
> ** Endocervical glandular involvement only should be considered as stage I and no longer as stage II.
> # Positive cytology has to be reported separately without changing the stage.
> Reprinted from *International Journal of Gynecology and Obstetrics*, Volume 105, Number 2, Pecotelli S. *et al.*, Revised FIGO staging for carcinoma of the vulva, cervix and endometrium, pp. 103–104, Copyright © 2009, with permission from Elsevier, <http://www.sciencedirect.com/science/journal/00207292>.

Preoperative routine blood tests and CT were normal. She underwent a total abdominal hysterectomy with bilateral salpingo-oophorectomy (TAH-BSO) and peritoneal washings. The histology showed a grade 2 endometrioid adenocarcinoma invading more than half of the myometrium. The tumour was 3 mm from the serosal margin. Vascular invasion was present. Unexpectedly, there was a 10 mm deposit in the right ovary. There was no cervical invasion, and peritoneal cytology was negative, FIGO stage IIIA.

✚ Clinical tip Endometrial cancer risk stratification

Endometrial cancer can be divided into early, locally advanced, and metastatic. It is also grouped into low risk, intermediate/high-intermediate risk, and high risk. This is useful when considering the potential benefit of adjuvant therapy. The exact definition of risk categories varies across the trials. Risk factors include:

- stage III and above
- deep myometrial invasion
- grade 3
- clear cell or serous subtype
- lymphovascular invasion
- age >60–65 years.

❝ Expert comment

Risk categories started being used widely after the publication of PORTEC 1 trial. This randomized trial, comparing adjuvant radiotherapy versus observation in stage I endometrial cancer, found three independent risk factors for relapse: age >60, grade 3, and depth of myometrial invasion >50%. Two out of these three risk factors meant a risk of recurrence between 15% and 20%. Lymphovascular space invasion (LVSI) is a separate risk factor that is now recognized to indicate an increased risk of nodal metastasis and distant recurrence.

★ Learning point Management of early endometrial cancer

Early endometrial cancer (FIGO stage 1) is defined as cancer that has not spread outside the uterus. Approximately 75% of patients present with stage I disease. Most of these cancers are low risk. Stage IB and grade 3 tumours are considered high risk, as they have a higher incidence of pelvic and distant metastases and so are managed more aggressively. Clear cell and serous histology tumours have a similar prognosis to grade 3 disease and are also considered high risk.

The primary treatment is surgery with TAH-BSO (uterus, Fallopian tubes, and ovaries removed) and peritoneal washings. Positive peritoneal cytology should be reported but does not change the stage. Patients not fit for surgery due to co-morbidities or PS can be treated definitively by radiotherapy alone (combined EBRT and brachytherapy, or brachytherapy alone).

There are two key areas of controversy for early-stage endometrial cancer: the role of pelvic lymphadenectomy and the use of post-operative radiotherapy.

★ Learning point Pelvic Lymphadenectomy for early-stage endometrial cancer

The role of pelvic (and para-aortic) lymphadenectomy, in addition to hysterectomy, has been a key area of debate. Pelvic lymphadenectomy provides accurate staging of lymph nodes. It may also have a therapeutic role, but this is not certain. There is an increased risk of complications, including lymphoedema, lymphocysts, deep vein thrombosis (DVT), and small bowel obstruction. Operation times are longer. These risks are higher if para-aortic, as well as pelvic, lymph nodes are removed.

For patients with stage I disease, the risk of occult lymph node involvement is low at 7%. Patients with a high (>15%) risk of microscopic lymph node involvement are more likely to have therapeutic benefit from lymphadenectomy, if such a benefit exists.

The landmark trial for lymphadenectomy in stage I disease is the ASTEC study. There was no disease free survival (DFS) or overall survival (OS) benefit for any stage I patients [4]. Some centres continue to offer pelvic lymphadenectomy for all but stage 1 grade 1 disease because of the staging information gained.

❝ Expert comment

There have been several valid criticisms of the MRC ASTEC trial which means that questions are far from answered, and, in fact, a new trial is being considered to try and address this all important question.

✔ Evidence base MRC ASTEC trial: efficacy of systematic pelvic lymphadenectomy in endometrial cancer [4]

- Surgery with lymphadenectomy versus standard surgery alone in stage I patients.
- Randomized, international, multicentre trial.
- Surgery (TAH-BSO, peritoneal washings, palpation of para-aortic lymph nodes) with pelvic lymphadenectomy (iliac and obturator lymph nodes) ($n=704$) versus standard surgery alone ($n=704$) in stage I patients.
- Pre-defined subgroup analysis by risk group and surgical centre.
- Separate randomization for patients with intermediate- or high-risk disease into the ASTEC radiotherapy trial.
- Median follow-up of 37 months.
- 1% difference in OS (95% CI –4 to 6). HR for OS 1.04 (0.74–1.45; $p=0.83$).
- HR for recurrence-free survival 1.25 (0.93–1.66; $p=0.14$).
- No significant difference by subgroup analysis.
- No therapeutic benefit from pelvic lymphadenectomy in early endometrial cancer.

Source: data from *The Lancet*, Volume 373, Issue 9658, ASTEC Study Group *et al.*, Efficacy of systematic pelvic lymphadenectomy in endometrial cancer (MRC ASTEC trial): a randomised study, pp. 125–136, Copyright © 2009 Elsevier Ltd.

⊗ **Learning point** Adjuvant radiotherapy for early-stage disease

Adjuvant radiotherapy can be external beam radiotherapy (EBRT) to the pelvis and/or vaginal vault brachytherapy (VBT). Pelvic EBRT covers the obturator, external iliac, internal iliac, and common iliac lymph node chains up to the level of the aortic bifurcation. The primary role is to reduce the risk of lymph node metastases. The potential benefit of EBRT therefore depends on how high the risk is of lymph node involvement. For stage I, grades 1 and 2 disease, the risk of occult lymph node spread is 7%. This risk is outweighed by the potential toxicity associated with pelvic radiotherapy [5]. The role of VBT is to reduce local recurrence at the vaginal vault, as this is the commonest site of first relapse.

The role of radiotherapy for stage I disease has been evaluated in eight randomised controlled trials (RCTs) included in a Cochrane review [6]. Radiotherapy reduces the risk of local recurrence but does not improve OS or endometrial cancer-specific survival for stage I disease. However, there is limited evidence in the high-risk group, so these women may still gain from EBRT [6]. Brachytherapy reduces the risk of local recurrence but does not improve OS in low-risk women. The benefit of brachytherapy alone in intermediate- and high-risk women is not clear, due to a lack of data. However, as EBRT has not shown a survival benefit, brachytherapy is unlikely to do so. Nevertheless, as intermediate- and high-risk disease have a high rate of local recurrence (13–23.1%), most advocate radiotherapy in these groups [7,8] The move in many centres has been towards offering more brachytherapy, and less EBRT, in an effort to reduce toxicity. This is supported by data from PORTEC 2 study [10]. EBRT is indicated in stage IB, grade3 tumours, and tumours with a clear cell and serous histology. Table 5.2 gives an outline of the use of radiotherapy in stage I disease.

Table 5.2 Adjuvant radiotherapy for early-stage endometrial cancer

FIGO stage	Grade	Risk group	Adjuvant treatment options
1A (endometrium or less than half of myometrium invaded)	1	Low	None
	2	Low	None
	3	Intermediate	EBRT or VBT alone
1B (half or more of myometrium invaded)	1	Intermediate	VBT alone
	2	Intermediate	VBT alone
	3	High	EBRT

✓ **Evidence base** Cochrane review of adjuvant radiotherapy for stage I endometrial cancer

The Cochrane Collaboration carried out a review of adjuvant radiotherapy for stage I disease. Eight studies met their criteria for review, including the key studies ASTEC/EN.5, GOG 99, PORTEC 1, and PORTEC 2. The trials used the 1988 FIGO staging system and varied in their use of lymphadenectomy. They used different combinations of radiotherapy—EBRT alone, brachytherapy alone, and EBRT plus brachytherapy. In some trials, brachytherapy was allowed in both treatment arms (Figure 5.2). The Cochrane review concluded that radiotherapy reduces the risk of local recurrence but does not improve OS or endometrial cancer-specific survival for stage I disease [6].

(continued)

❝ **Expert comment**

Although the American Patterns of Care Study showed that, in patients with deeply penetrating stage I tumours (>50% myometrial invasion), whether grade 1 or 3, there was a survival advantage for EBRT.

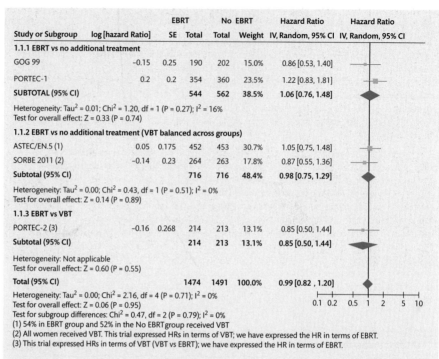

Study or Subgroup	log [hazard Ratio]	EBRT SE	EBRT Total	No EBRT Total	Weight	Hazard Ratio IV, Random, 95% CI	Hazard Ratio IV, Random, 95% CI
1.1.1 EBRT vs no additional treatment							
GOG 99	-0.15	0.25	190	202	15.0%	0.86 [0.53, 1.40]	
PORTEC-1	0.2	0.2	354	360	23.5%	1.22 [0.83, 1.81]	
SUBTOTAL (95% CI)			544	562	38.5%	1.06 [0.76, 1.48]	

Heterogeneity: Tau^2 = 0.01; Chi^2 = 1.20, df = 1 (P = 0.27); I^2 = 16%
Test for overall effect: Z = 0.33 (P = 0.74)

1.1.2 EBRT vs no additional treatment (VBT balanced across groups)							
ASTEC/EN.5 (1)	0.05	0.175	452	453	30.7%	1.05 [0.75, 1.48]	
SORBE 2011 (2)	-0.14	0.23	264	263	17.8%	0.87 [0.55, 1.36]	
Subtotal (95% CI)			716	716	48.4%	0.98 [0.75, 1.29]	

Heterogeneity: Tau^2 = 0.00; Chi^2 = 0.43, df = 1 (P = 0.51); I^2 = 0%
Test for overall effect: Z = 0.14 (P = 0.89)

1.1.3 EBRT vs VBT							
PORTEC-2 (3)	-0.16	0.268	214	213	13.1%	0.85 [0.50, 1.44]	
Subtotal (95% CI)			214	213	13.1%	0.85 [0.50, 1.44]	

Heterogeneity: Not applicable
Test for overall effect: Z = 0.60 (P = 0.55)

Total (95% CI)			1474	1491	100.0%	0.99 [0.82 , 1.20]	

Heterogeneity: Tau^2 = 0.00; Chi^2 = 2.16, df = 4 (P = 0.71); I^2 = 0%
Test for overall effect: Z = 0.06 (P = 0.95)
Test for subgroup differences: Chi^2 = 0.47, df = 2 (P = 0.79); I^2 = 0%
(1) 54% in EBRT group and 52% in the No EBRT group received VBT
(2) All women received VBT. This trial expressed HRs in terms of VBT; we have expressed the HR in terms of EBRT.
(3) This trial expressed HRs in terms of VBT (VBT vs EBRT); we have expressed the HR in terms of EBRT.

Figure 5.2 Forrest plot of comparison: EBRT versus no EBRT. All patients at 5 years—outcome: death from all causes.

Reproduced from Kong, A. *et al.*, Adjuvant Radiotherapy for Stage I Endometrial Cancer: An Updated Cochrane Systematic Review and Meta-analysis, *Journal of the National Cancer Institute*, Volume 104, Issue 21, pp. 1625–1634, Copyright © 2012 by permission of Oxford University Press.

⊕ Clinical tip Toxicity of pelvic radiotherapy

- Acute toxicity:
  - Gastrointestinal (GI): diarrhoea, urgency, rectal bleeding
  - Genitourinary (GU): frequency, urgency, dysuria
  - skin: erythema
  - fatigue.
- Late toxicity:
  - GI: diarrhoea, urgency, rectal bleeding, obstruction, faecal incontinence, fistula
  - GU: frequency, urinary incontinence, fistula
  - vaginal dryness and stenosis
  - femoral head ischaemia
  - secondary cancers
  - poorer QoL scores.

⊘ Evidence base PORTEC 2: vaginal brachytherapy versus pelvic EBRT for patients with endometrial cancer of high-intermediate risk [10]

- Post-operative EBRT versus VBT.
- Open-label, non-inferiority randomized trial, EBRT (46 Gy in 23 fractions) (*n* = 214) versus VBT (21 Gy high dose rate or 30 Gy low dose rate) (*n* = 213).
- Stage I or IIA patients with high-intermediate risk factors (age >60 plus stage 1C, grade 1 or 2 disease; stage 1B, grade 3 disease or stage 2A disease, any age, excluding grade 3 with >50% myometrial invasion).
- Primary endpoint: 5-year vaginal recurrence 1.8% (95% CI 0·6–5·9) VBT versus 1·6% (95% CI 0·5–4·9) EBRT. HR 0·78, 95% CI 0·17–3·49; *p* = 0·74.
- 5-year locoregional recurrence (pelvic or vaginal) HR 2.08; *p* = 0.17.
- No statistically significant difference in rate of distant metastases, OS, DFS.
- Acute grades 1 and 2 GI toxicity less in the VBT group (12.6% versus 53.8%).
- Late grade 3 GI toxicity in 2% EBRT and <1% VBT.
- Significantly more grades 1–3 late vaginal toxicity with VBT versus EBRT.

Source: data from Nout RA, *et al.*, Vaginal brachytherapy versus external beam pelvic radiotherapy for high-intermediate risk endometrial cancer: Results of the randomized PORTEC-2 trial, *Journal of Clinical Oncology*, Volume 26, Number 15S, Copyright © 2008 American Society of Clinical Oncology.

The patient had an uneventful post-operative recovery and was referred to a consultant clinical oncologist for further management. Her risk factors for disease

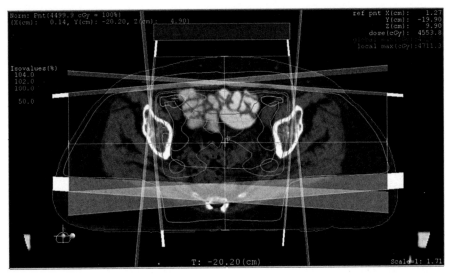

Figure 5.3 Single-slice CT image at the level of the isocentre of conformally planned EBRT using typical 'four-field brick' beam arrangement. Reproduced courtesy of University Hospital Southampton NHS Foundation Trust.

recurrence were deep myometrial invasion, stage III disease, lymphovascular invasion, and age over 60. Following an informed discussion, she elected not to receive adjuvant chemotherapy. She went on to receive pelvic EBRT 45 Gy in 25 fractions over 5 weeks. She did not need brachytherapy. Acutely, she had grade 2 GI toxicity and required oral antibiotics for a urinary tract infection. At 8 weeks' follow-up post-radiotherapy, she had grade 1 GI toxicity only (Figure 5.3).

⊘ **Learning point** Management of locally advanced disease

Surgery

Pelvic lymphadenectomy for stage II disease and above is not controversial. The incidence of involved nodes in a series of 238 women undergoing lymphadenectomy was 22% with cervical involvement and 52% with adnexal involvement. Lymph node involvement is a strong risk factor for recurrence [9]. Patients presenting with extensive pelvic or abdominal disease undergo cytoreductive surgery, if possible. Women with inoperable disease are treated in the same way as metastatic disease.

Patients with stage III disease are at high risk of relapse, so adjuvant treatment is indicated. Adjuvant treatment is also considered in patients with earlier-stage disease with high-risk features.

Adjuvant radiotherapy and chemotherapy

Stage II patients require VBT. For those who have not had pelvic lymphadenectomy, EBRT is offered because of the high risk of occult lymph node involvement.

Given the high recurrence risk in stage III disease, adjuvant EBRT is indicated. Most patients will have had pelvic lymphadenectomy. Additionally, brachytherapy is indicated in patients with cervical invasion. Although widely practised, evidence for the use of adjuvant chemotherapy in advanced disease is lacking. The risk of pelvic recurrence in high-risk disease treated with adjuvant chemotherapy alone was evaluated by Mundt et al [11]. A total of 43 patients with stages I–IV disease (high-risk histology subtype or advanced stages III–IV disease) had surgery, followed by cisplatin and doxorubicin chemotherapy; 67.4% relapsed; of these, 39.5% were in the pelvis. Cervical and adnexal involvement correlated most strongly with pelvic recurrence [11]. Other studies have randomized adjuvant radiotherapy (whole pelvic or whole abdominal) against chemotherapy. Of three RCTs studying this issue, one used doxorubicin and cisplatin

(continued)

Expert comment

To avoid confusion, the term 'high risk' should only be used with stage I disease. The risk to which it alludes is that of pelvic relapse (nodal or otherwise) without adjuvant treatment. Stage III disease carries a much higher risk of relapse than the high-risk stage I patients.

Expert comment

Stage II disease contains a multitude of clinical scenarios, and risk assessment needs to be based on knowledge of these; at one extreme is G1 cancer confined to the inner half, no LVSI, and some cervical stromal involvement, and the other end of the spectrum would be a G3 cancer with deep myometrial involvement and extensive LVSI. For the first patient, VBT may be entirely appropriate, whereas, for the latter case, one would recommend adjuvant chemotherapy followed by EBRT and VBT. There are several variations in between these two extremes, of course.

Expert comment

The EORTC randomized trial of radiotherapy versus CRT in high-risk stage I, i.e. IB, grade 3 (clear cell/serous, etc.), or occult stages II and III has shown an improvement in DFS and a trend towards an improvement in OS.

(AP), and two used doxorubicin, cisplatin, and cyclophosphamide (CAP). Two found no improvement in PFS or OS with chemotherapy over radiotherapy. One found a 12% improvement in 5-year PFS, favouring chemotherapy (50% versus 38%), and OS benefit of 11% (53% versus 42%) [12].

Uncertainties remain over the use of adjuvant chemotherapy and practice varies. The evidence base for the use of adjuvant chemotherapy in serous or clear cell disease is also limited and mixed. The optimal sequencing of radiotherapy and chemotherapy is not clear. Some argue that, as radiotherapy has proven efficacy, it should be given first, and the less proven adjuvant chemotherapy given subsequently. A phase II study has looked at CRT with cisplatin and brachytherapy followed by four cycles of adjuvant cisplatin and paclitaxel [13]. It included 44 patients with stage Ib, grade 2 to stage III. Ninety-eight per cent of patients completed the protocol. The acute grades 3 and 4 toxicities seen were mainly haematological. Late grades 3 and 4 toxicity occurred in 21% of patients (9/44); small bowel toxicity was present in five of these patients. PORTEC 3 has been set up to look at CRT and adjuvant chemotherapy versus RT alone in high-risk patients [12]. It is hoped that PORTEC 3 will provide clear guidance.

Evidence base PORTEC 3: concurrent chemoradiation followed by adjuvant chemotherapy versus adjuvant pelvic radiotherapy alone in high-risk groups after surgery [12]

- Prospective, multicentre phase III study.
- 48.6 Gy in 27 fractions over 5.5 weeks, with brachytherapy boost if cervical involvement, versus same radiotherapy schedule plus cisplatin 50 mg/m^2 on weeks 1 and 4, followed by four cycles of carboplatin (area under the curve, AUC 5) and paclitaxel 175 mg/m^2 every 21 days.
- Completed recruitment in December 2013.

Source: data *from Randomized Phase III Trial Comparing Concurrent Chemoradiation and Adjuvant Chemotherapy with Pelvic Radiation Alone in High Risk and Advanced Stage Endometrial Carcinoma: PORTEC-3, An international Intergroup trial*, CKTO 2006-04, CME P06.031, version 12, Copyright © 2012.

The patient was followed up at 4-monthly intervals for the first year and then 6-monthly thereafter, alternating care with her gynaecologist and oncologist. Eighteen months post-diagnosis, she presented to her GP with lethargy, weight loss, and non-specific abdominal discomfort. Blood tests are shown in Table 5.3.

Her GP arranged an ultrasound of the abdomen that showed multiple liver lesions consistent with liver metastases. She was reviewed urgently in oncology outpatients. Subsequent CT CAP confirmed multiple liver metastases and a small right pleural effusion (Figure 5.4). Her PS was 2.

Assessment of glomerular filtration rate using EDTA predicated a of 70 mL/min. The patient's weight was 71.7 kg and height 163 cm, and body surface area (BSA) 1.81. She was started on carboplatin AUC 5 and paclitaxel which was dose-reduced to 75% of 175 mg/m^2 due to her hepatic impairment. Cycle 1 was well tolerated, with grade 1 nausea and grade 1 peripheral neuropathy. After cycle 2, her LFTs normalized, so

Table 5.3 GP blood test results

Haematology	Renal function	LFTs
Hb 10.8 g/dL	Na 138 mmol/L	Bilirubin 27 μmol/L
WBC 5.6×10^9/L	K 3.6 mmol/L	Alanine aminotransferase (ALT) 60 IU/L
Platelets 365×10^9/L	Urea 7.1 mmol/L	Alkaline phosphatase (ALP) 295 IU/L
Neutrophils 3.1	Creatinine 64 mmol/L	

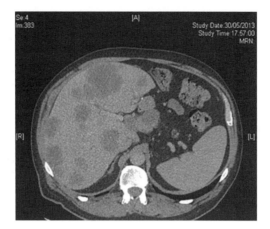

Figure 5.4 CT slice showing multiple liver metastases. Reproduced courtesy of University Hospital Southampton NHS Foundation Trust.

the paclitaxel dose was increased to 100%. Following cycle 3, she reported grade 2 peripheral neuropathy in her fingers, persisting until the next treatment cycle was due. This resolved to grade 1 after 1 week's delay, and so cycle 4 paclitaxel was given with a 25% dose reduction.

Restaging CT scan after three cycles showed a partial response in the liver and resolution of the pleural effusion. She complained of persisting grade 2 peripheral neuropathy, and so the fifth cycle was given as single-agent carboplatin only. She elected to stop chemotherapy after five cycles of treatment. Repeat CT showed a mixed response with stable disease in the liver, but two new lung lesions, measuring 10 mm and 6 mm, suspicious for lung metastases. She opted for medroxyprogesterone, on which she remained for 4 months and lived to attend her daughter's wedding before dying 3 months later.

⭐ **Learning point** Metastatic treatment options

The treatment options for metastatic disease include chemotherapy, hormonal therapy, novel agents, palliative radiotherapy, and best supportive care.

Chemotherapy

A meta-analysis, published in 2012, concluded that combination chemotherapy improves OS and PFS over less intense regimes, but at the expense of additional toxicity. There was insufficient evidence to recommend a specific regime. The triplet regime of doxorubicin, cisplatin, and paclitaxel has been used in fit patients. However, a non-inferiority GOG study, published in abstract form, has show non-inferiority of carboplatin and paclitaxel (TC) over doxorubicin, cisplatin, and paclitaxel in interim analysis [14]. TC has therefore been adopted by many centres as first-line treatment. Single-agent carboplatin is an option for less fit patients. For patients who have had TC adjuvantly, the choice of chemotherapy in the metastatic setting will depend on the disease-free interval. If this is over a year, then patients may be rechallenged with TC, although peripheral neuropathy may limit the number of cycles that can be given. Response rates to second-line chemotherapy tend to be low and short-lived. Cisplatin plus topotecan is one option. Single-agent therapies may be used with various drugs, including weekly docetaxel. Co-morbidities and PS limit the treatment options in a significant proportion of patients.

(continued)

⊕ **Clinical tip** Active chemotherapy agents for endometrial cancer

Active chemotherapy agents in endometrial cancer include doxorubicin, cisplatin, carboplatin, paclitaxel, cyclophosphamide, topotecan, and ifosfamide. Response rates are 30–35% [12].

Hormonal therapy

Progestogens are an alternative to chemotherapy. They are most useful in low-grade disease and ER- or PR-positive disease. Response rates are in the region of 15–25%. Examples are oral medroxyprogesterone acetate. Although the duration of response is usually short, progestogens are well tolerated. Tamoxifen may be helpful in ER-/PR-positive tumours. AIs show minimal activity in endometrial cancer.

Novel agents

There is growing interest in novel agents for endometrial cancer, with most in phase II studies. These include the EGFR inhibitors erlotinib and gefitinib and mammalian target of rapamycin (mTOR) inhibitors temsirolimus and everolimus. The GOG 86P study is a three-arm randomized phase II study, comparing TC plus bevacizumab versus TC plus temsirolimus versus C-plus ixabepilone and bevacizumab. Eligible women have stage III or IVA, stage IVB, or recurrent endometrial cancer and are treated first line. The study is closed to recruitment.

Radiotherapy

Radiotherapy is helpful for pain or vaginal bleeding caused by pelvic recurrence. It also has a role in controlling pain from para-aortic lymphadenopathy. Any previous pelvic radiotherapy needs to be considered when re-treating with radiotherapy.

✪ Learning point Chemotherapy-induced neuropathy

Paclitaxel-induced peripheral neuropathy is common (85% of patients experience some neurotoxicity) and can be dose-limiting. Its grading is shown in Table 5.4.

Chemotherapy agents that cause peripheral neuropathy include:

- platinums—cisplatin, carboplatin, oxaliplatin
- vinca alkaloids—vincristine
- taxanes—paclitaxel, docetaxel
- lenalidomide
- thalidomide
- bortezomib.

Peripheral neuropathy can be sensory, sensory–motor, and/or autonomic, depending on the individual drug, with sensory disturbance the commonest symptom. The risk depends on the drug, infusion time, and cumulative dose. Patients with diabetes or pre-existing neuropathy are at increased risk. It is usually diagnosed clinically, but EMG and blood tests to rule out metabolic or vitamin deficiency causes may be necessary. A typical approach to its management, whilst on chemotherapy, is given in the PORTEC 3 protocol [12]. Whilst many cases resolve, some patients experience permanent sensory loss that can be disabling. There is no effective prophylaxis or treatment. Gabapentin, carbamazepine, and tricyclic antidepressants can be used for painful neuropathic symptoms. Physiotherapy and occupational therapy may be helpful.

Table 5.4 Grading of peripheral sensory neuropathy, according to common terminology criteria for adverse events (CTCAE) version 4.03

	Grade 1	Grade 2	Grade 3	Grade 4	Grade 5
Peripheral sensory neuropathy	Asymptomatic; loss of deep reflexes or paraesthesiae with function	Moderate symptoms; limiting instrumental activities of daily living (ADLs)	Severe symptoms; limiting self-care ADLs	Life-threatening consequences; urgent interventions indicated	Death

Source: data from *Common Terminology Criteria for Adverse Events (CTCAE) Version 4.03*, US Department of Health and Human Service, National Institutes of Health and National Cancer Institute, available from <http://evs.nci.nih.gov/ftp1/CTCAE/CTCAE_4.03_2010-06-14_QuickReference_5x7.pdf>.

Discussion

The majority of women with endometrial cancer present with early disease and have a good prognosis (85% 5-year survival for stage I low-risk disease). Controversy remains over the optimal management of women requiring adjuvant therapy. Current treatment options for metastatic disease are limited.

A final word from the expert

This case highlights some of the issues around decision making in endometrial cancer. The management of early (stage I) disease is particularly contentious, with very little agreement on the use of radiotherapy or chemotherapy in this setting. There is also controversy around what constitutes optimal surgical management; different points of view exist in the UK, compared to the US and the continent of Europe. Advanced and metastatic disease is another area where there is active research ongoing, and hopefully we will see this bear fruit in the next 5 years or so.

References

1. Amant F, Moerman P, Neven P, Timmerman D, Van Limbergen E, Vergote I, Endometrial cancer. *The Lancet* 2005; **366**(9484): 491–505.
2. Dijkhuizen FP, Mol BW, Brölmann HA, Heintz AP. The accuracy of endometrial sampling in the diagnosis of patients with endometrial carcinoma and hyperplasia: a meta analysis. *Cancer* 2000; **89**(8): 1765–72.
3. Pecotelli S. Revised FIGO staging for carcinoma of the vulva, cervix and endometrium. *International Journal of Gynecology and Obstetrics* 2009; **105**(2): 103–4.
4. ASTEC Study Group, Blake P, Swart AM *et al*. Efficacy of systematic pelvic lymphadenectomy in endometrial cancer (MRC ASTEC trial): a randomized study. *The Lancet* 2009; **373**(9658): 125–36.
5. Creasman WT, Morrow CP, Bundy BN, Homesley HD, Graham JE, Heller PB, Surgical pathologic spread patterns of endometrial cancer. A Gynecologic Oncology Group Study. *Cancer* 1987; **60**(8 Suppl): 2035–41.
6. Kong A, Johnson N, Kitchener HC, Lawrie TA, Adjuvant radiotherapy for stage I endometrial cancer. *Cochrane Database of Systematic Reviews* 2012; 4 CD003916
7. Creutzberg CL, van Putten WL, Koper PC *et al*. Surgery and postoperative radiotherapy versus surgery alone for patients with stage-1 endometrial carcinoma: multicentre randomised trial. PORTEC Study Group. Post Operative Radiation Therapy in Endometrial Carcinoma. *The Lancet* 2000; **355**(9213): 1404–11.
8. Keys HM, Roberts JA, Brunetto VL *et al*. A phase III trial of surgery with or without adjunctive external pelvic radiation therapy in intermediate risk endometrial adenocarcinoma: a Gynecologic Oncology Group study. *Gynecologic Oncology* 2004; **92**(3): 744–51.
9. COSA-NZ-UK Endometrial Cancer Study Groups. Pelvic lymphadenectomy in high risk endometrial cancer. *International Journal of Gynecological Cancer* 1996; **6**(2): 102–7.
10. Nout RA, Putter H, Jürgenliemk-Schulz IM *et al*. Vaginal brachytherapy versus external beam pelvic radiotherapy for high-intermediate risk endometrial cancer: Results of the randomized PORTEC-2 trial. *Journal of Clinical Oncology* 2008; **26**(15 Suppl): LBA5503
11. Mundt AJ, McBride R, Rotmensch J, Waggoner SE, Yamada SD, Connell PP. Significant pelvic recurrence in high-risk pathologic stage I–IV endometrial carcinoma patients after adjuvant chemotherapy alone: implications for adjuvant radiation therapy. *International Journal of Radiation Oncology*Biology*Physics* 2001; **50**(5): 1145–53.

12. *Randomized phase III trial comparing concurrent chemoradiation and adjuvant chemotherapy with pelvic radiation alone in high risk and advanced stage endometrial carcinoma: PORTEC-3. An international Intergroup trial.* CKTO 2006-04, CME P06.031, version 12 April 2012. Available at: <https://www.clinicalresearch.nl/portec3/protocol_portec3_final_amendments_fin_120412.pdf>.

13. Greven K, Winter K, Underhill K, Fontenesci J.Cooper J, Burke T. Final analysis of RTOG 9708: Adjuvant postoperative irradiation combined with cisplatin/paclitaxel chemotherapy following surgery for patients with high-risk endometrial cancer. *Gynecologic Oncology* **103**(1): 2006 155–9.

14. Miller D, Filiaci V, Fleming G *et al* Randomized phase III noninferiority trial of first line chemotherapy for metastatic or recurrent endometrial carcinoma: A Gynecologic Oncology Group study. *Gynecologic Oncology* 2012; **125**(3): 771

6 Ovarian cancer and malignant bowel obstruction

Caroline Chau

⏱ **Expert commentary** Iain McNeish

Case history

A 60-year-old lady presented to her GP with a 3-month history of malaise, abdominal swelling, and pain. She was previously fit and well, with no significant past medical history. She became aware of her symptoms when they started to interfere with her work as a cleaner, becoming increasingly tired and needing to reduce her hours. She felt bloated and nauseated, with a loss of appetite. In the 4 weeks prior to presentation, she noticed a change in her bowel habit and a new pain in the right iliac fossa. The pain was sharp, stabbing, and severe, increasing in frequency and intensity, to the point that she had to stop work. She was on no regular medication and had no family history of cancer. She had never smoked and consumed alcohol within the recommended limit.

Clinical examination revealed ascites. Bowel sounds were present, and there was no hepatosplenomegaly. Cardiac and respiratory examination was unremarkable, and no stigmata of liver disease were found.

She was referred for an urgent abdominal ultrasound and blood test.

✪ Learning point How to diagnose ovarian cancer

Suspicious symptoms and signs (especially in women aged 50 or over) that warrant further investigation:

- Persistent or frequent (>12 times per month) abdominal distension/bloating.
- Early satiety, loss of appetite, weight loss, fatigue.
- Pelvic or abdominal pain.
- Increased urinary frequency and/or urgency.
- New symptoms suggestive of irritable bowel syndrome (IBS) in any woman over 50, as IBS rarely presents for the first time in women of this age group.

Investigations

- Measure serum CA125. If >35 IU/mL, organize an ultrasound scan (USS) of the abdomen and pelvis.
- In women under 40 with suspected ovarian cancer, in addition to serum CA125, measure levels of beta-HCG and AFP to exclude germ cell ovarian cancer.
- Calculate a risk of malignancy index (RMI) score, and refer if the RMI score is >200 to a specialist MDT.
- Tissue diagnosis by either percutaneous image-guided or laparoscopic biopsy. Cytological diagnosis is not considered adequate, unless biopsy is contraindicated.
- CT of the abdomen and pelvis with contrast is the imaging of choice for staging ovarian cancer, both pretreatment and for post-treatment surveillance.
- MRI may be useful for the characterization of adnexal masses, following equivocal CT, but is usually not the best initial procedure for ovarian cancer staging.

> **⊕ Clinical tip** RMI [1]
>
> A useful tool for predicting whether or not an ovarian mass is likely to be malignant.
>
> **RMI = U (ultrasound score) × M (menopausal status) × CA125**
>
> *Ultrasound score:*
>
> - abnormality defined as multilocular cysts, solid areas, bilateral lesions, ascites, or metastases
> - U = 0, for no abnormality
> - U = 1, for one abnormality
> - U = 3, for two or more abnormalities.
>
> *Menopausal status:*
>
> - M = 1, pre-menopausal
> - M = 3, post-menopausal (defined as a women who has had no period for >1 year or a women over 50 who has had a hysterectomy).
>
> *Serum CA125 measured in IU/mL.*
>
> *If RMI ≥200, the patient must be referred to a specialist MDT.*
>
> *Source*: data from Jacobs I *et al.*, A risk of malignancy index incorporating CA125, ultrasound and menopausal status for the accurate preoperative diagnosis of ovarian cancer, *BJOG: An International Journal of Obstetrics and Gynaecology,* Volume 97, Issue 10, pp. 922–929, Copyright © 1990 John Wiley & Sons, Inc.

CA125 was raised at 1604 IU/mL (normal range <35), and the USS confirmed a large volume of ascites and a pelvic mass. Her other blood tests were unremarkable. Her calculated RMI score was 14 436. She was therefore urgently referred to the 2-week wait combined gynaecology/oncology clinic.

A staging CT scan revealed omental thickening, ascites, diffuse serosal disease surrounding the sigmoid colon, multiple peritoneal and subcapsular liver deposits, and a mass measuring $58 \times 48 \times 50$ mm. Omental biopsy confirmed high-grade serous carcinoma of likely ovarian origin—CK7-, WT1-, and PAX8-positive; CK20-negative.

In light of these test results, the patient was diagnosed with probable stage IIIc ovarian cancer.

> **✪ Learning point** FIGO staging of ovarian cancer [2]
>
> | Stage | Description |
> |---|---|
> | I | Tumour confined to ovaries |
> | | Ia—one ovary |
> | | Ib—both ovaries |
> | | Ic—either or both with capsule breached/ascites |
> | II | Tumour involves one or both ovaries, with extension into the uterus or other pelvic organs |
> | | IIa—uterus |
> | | IIb—other pelvic tissues |
> | | IIc—IIa or IIb plus ascites |
> | III | A—tumour involves one or both ovaries, with microscopically confirmed peritoneal metastasis outside the pelvis |
> | | B—tumour involves one or both ovaries, with implants on peritoneal surfaces <2 cm |
> | | C—tumour involves one or both ovaries, with peritoneal deposits >2 cm or positive lymph nodes |
> | IV | Distant metastasis beyond the peritoneal cavity |
>
> Reprinted from *International Journal of Gynecology and Obstetrics*, Volume 70, Number 2, Benedet JL *et al.*, FIGO staging classifications and clinical practice guidelines in the management of gynecologic cancers, FIGO Committee Tsciencedirect.com/science/journal/00207292>.

⊗ **Learning point** Histological classification of ovarian cancer [3]

Epithelial (90%)	High-grade serous (50–70%)
	Low-grade serous (10–15%)
	Endometrioid (10–20%)
	Mucinous (1–2%)
	Clear cell (10–12%)
	Carcinosarcomas (2–3%)
	Transitional cell (Brenner tumours)
	Squamous cell
	Mixed epithelial—these are probably variants of high-grade serous
	Undifferentiated
Germ cell/stromal (10%)	

Source: data from Kaku T *et al.*, Histological classification of ovarian cancer, *Medical Electron Microscopy*, Volume 36, Issue 1, pp. 9–17, Copyright © The Clinical Electron Microscopy Society of Japan 2003.

ℹ **Expert comment**

There has been a great change in our understanding of ovarian cancer biology in recent years. The commonest histological subtype high-grade serous seems to arise in the distal fimbria of the Fallopian tube, rather than the ovarian surface epithelium itself. Historically, the frequency of mucinous ovarian cancers was reported to be as high as 10%. However, advances in pathology, especially IHC, have revealed that the true frequency is much lower; many mucinous tumours are metastases from GI malignancies, especially colorectal and stomach primaries. Ovarian primaries are usually positive for cytokeratin 7 and negative for CK20.

⊗ **Learning point** Histological subtypes of ovarian carcinoma are actually different diseases

The rare histological subtypes, such as low-grade serous and clear cell tumours, are recognized to be more chemoresistant, leading to poorer prognosis. In particular, clear cell carcinoma (CCC) of the ovary is a distinctive tumour, frequently arising from endometriosis or clear cell adenofibroma, and the response rate to platinum-based therapy is extremely low. GCIG/JCOG (Gynecologic Cancer Intergroup/Japanese Gynecologic Oncology Group) 3017 [4] is an ongoing international prospective clinical study, comparing irinotecan plus cisplatin and carboplatin plus paclitaxel as the first-line chemotherapy for CCC. In addition, molecular-targeting agents are also being evaluated for advanced or recurrent CCC in clinical trials.

	High-grade serous	Low-grade serous	Low-grade endometrioid	Clear cell
Prevalence	Commonest	Uncommon	Uncommon	Uncommon
FIGO stage at presentation	Advanced (mostly stages III/IV)	Early (mostly stage I)	Early (mostly stages I and II)	Early (mostly stages I and II)
Clinical course	Aggressive	Indolent	Indolent	Aggressive
Cytogenetic profile	Universal *TP53* mutation (97%), 20% mutations in *BRCA1/2*, 30% mutations in other genes associated with homologous recombination, Rb pathway abnormalities in about 70%	Frequent *K-ras*, *BRAF* and erb-B2 (HER2) mutations	ER/PR and nuclear beta-catenin expression, lack of WT-1 and p53 expression, *CTNNB-1* (beta-catenin), PTEN mutation and *PIK3CA* mutation, microsatellite instability-high (MSI-H)	*ARID1A* and *PIK3CA* mutations, HNF-1 beta upregulation, absence of WT-1 and ER expression

(continued)

Prognosis	Poor	Better (but very poor if advanced stage or relapsed)	Better (most favourable among all subtypes)	Variable—excellent in stage I, poor in stages II–IV
Platinum response	Sensitive initially, relapse frequent with acquired platinum resistance	Less sensitive (recurrent tumours are often resistant to platinum therapy)	Variable	Resistant

Source: data from McCluggage WG, Morphological subtypes of ovarian carcinoma: a review with emphasis on new developments and pathogenesis, *Pathology*, Volume 43, Issue 5, pp. 420–432, Copyright © 2011 Royal College of Pathologists of Australasia.

The patient has a PS of 1, and, in view of the extent of her disease, the treatment proposed was three cycles of neoadjuvant carboplatin and paclitaxel, followed by interval debulking surgery and three further cycles of carboplatin and paclitaxel.

⭐ Learning point Primary debulking surgery versus neoadjuvant chemotherapy in advanced ovarian cancer

EORTC-55971 [5] was a randomized, multicentre phase III study of 670 women with stage IIIc or IV ovarian cancer, which demonstrated non-inferiority of neoadjuvant platinum-based chemotherapy followed by interval debulking surgery, when compared with primary surgery followed by platinum-based chemotherapy. However, post-operative mortality and morbidity (severe haemorrhage, infection, venous complications), and length of stay tended to be higher in the primary debulking group than the interval debulking group.

	Primary debulking surgery followed by chemotherapy	Neoadjuvant chemotherapy followed by interval debulking surgery
Patient number (*n*)	336	334
Median age (range)	62 (25–86)	63 (33–81)
Stage IIIc	257 (76.5%)	253 (75.7%)
Stage IV	77 (22.9%)	81 (24.3%)
Other	2 (0.6%)	0 (0%)
Median OS (months)	29	30
Median PFS (months)	12	12
Post-operative mortality (%)	2.5	0.7
Grade 3–4 haemorrhage (%)	7.4	4.1

Source: data from Vergote I *et al.*, Neoadjuvant chemotherapy or primary surgery in stage IIIC or IV ovarian cancer, *New England Journal of Medicine*, Volume 363, Number 10, pp. 943–53, Copyright © 2010 Massachusetts Medical Society. All rights reserved.

Importantly, this study, amongst many others, confirmed that the extent of residual disease following cytoreductive surgery is a determinant of outcome [6].

	Microscopic residual disease	Gross-optimal ≤1 cm	Suboptimal >1 cm
Median PFS (months)	29	16	13
Median OS (months)	68	40	33

Source: data from Bookman MA *et al.*, Evaluation of new platinum-based treatment regimens in advanced-stage ovarian cancer: a Phase III Trial of the Gynecologic Cancer Intergroup, *Journal of Clinical Oncology*, Volume 27, Number 9, pp. 1419–25, Copyright © 2009 by American Society of Clinical Oncology.

She had a good response to her neoadjuvant chemotherapy, both radiologically (confirmed on interim CT scan) and biochemically (a marked fall in CA125). Her disease was optimally debulked at interval surgery, with no visible residual tumour. She received three further cycles of chemotherapy, with no significant adverse events, and her CA125 returned to normal at treatment completion (21 IU/mL).

> **✆ Expert comment**
>
> The role of primary chemotherapy with delayed debulking surgery remains controversial. A second study CHORUS has reiterated the findings of EORTC-55971. However, critics of these two studies point out that the survival for all participants in the study was poor (median PFS of 12 months in both arms), suggesting that these were trials in women with very poor-prognosis disease. Proponents of primary chemotherapy argue that these studies indicate that delayed surgery is not detrimental to patient outcome and is associated with reduced surgical morbidity.

⊘ Evidence base Trials which have assessed the benefit of additional bevacizumab in a front-line setting

ICON7 trial [7]

- International, multicentre, randomized phase III study of 1528 women with FIGO high-risk stages I–IV epithelial ovarian cancer.
- Carboplatin AUC 5/6 plus paclitaxel (CP) 175 mg/m^2 every 3 weeks for six cycles versus CP with concurrent bevacizumab (BV) (7.5 mg/kg) every 3 weeks for six cycles and 12 further cycles of maintenance BV every 3 weeks or until disease progression.
- Improvement in median PFS (19 months versus 17.3 months; $p = 0.004$) in favour of the BV group.
- Positive BV treatment effect was also greater in advanced-stage patients.
- More cases of hypertension, GI perforation, and proteinuria reported in the BV group, but overall it was well tolerated.

Gynecologic Oncology Group (GOG) 218 trial [8]

- International, multicentre, double-blind, placebo-controlled, three-arm phase III study of 1873 women with previously untreated, incompletely resected stage III or stage IV ovarian cancer.
- Six cycles of carboplatin AUC 6 plus paclitaxel (175 mg/m^2) plus placebo every 3 weeks followed by placebo maintenance every 3 weeks versus six cycles of CP plus BV (15 mg/kg) every 3 weeks followed by placebo maintenance every 3 weeks versus six cycles of CP plus BV followed by BV maintenance (15 mg/kg) every 3 weeks.
- Improvement in median PFS (14.1 months versus 10.3 months, control arm; $p < 0.001$), in favour of the BV-throughout group. The BV-initiation group had a median survival of 11.2 months ($p = 0.16$).
- No significant improvement in median OS (39.3, 38.7, 39.7 months for the control group, BV-initiation group, and BV-throughout group, respectively).
- There was a 28% reduction in risk of progression in the BV-throughout group, as compared with the placebo group.
- BV-related toxic effects after chemotherapy were not associated with a reduction in QoL.

Source: data from Perren TJ *et al.*, A phase 3 trial of bevacizumab in ovarian cancer, *New England Medical Journal*, Volume 365, Number 26, pp. 2484–96, Copyright © 2011 Massachusetts Medical Society. All rights reserved.
Source: data from Burger RA *et al.*, Incorporation of bevacizumab in the primary treatment of ovarian cancer, *New England Medical Journal*, Volume 365, Number 26, pp. 2373–83, Copyright © 2011 Massachusetts Medical Society. All rights reserved.

> **✪ Learning point**
> Bevacizumab in ovarian cancer
>
> Bevacizumab is a humanized mAb, selective for vascular endothelial growth factor A (VEGF-A), that has demonstrated activity in phase III studies in ovarian cancer.

She returned to full-time work and remained asymptomatic. She was reviewed at the oncology follow-up clinic at 8 months when her CA125 was found to be raised at 141 IU/mL. However, as the patient was symptom-free, with a PS of 0, the decision was made for her to be closely monitored and to commence treatment only when she developed symptoms.

Two months later, she re-presented to the clinic with a 2-week history of increasing fatigue, bloating, and abdominal discomfort. Clinical examination revealed ascites and generalized abdominal tenderness. CA125 had further increased to 398 IU/mL. A restaging CT scan confirmed disease relapse, with the recurrence of ascites and multiple peritoneal deposits.

⭐ **Learning point**   Patient follow-up and the role of CA125 monitoring

A falling CA125 is an established surrogate marker for response to chemotherapy treatment in the majority of patients with epithelial ovarian cancer.

A confirmed rise in CA125 to more than twice the upper limit of normal (ULN) can also predict relapse with a sensitivity of 86% and a positive predictive value of 95% [9]. Interestingly, the rise in CA125 is usually several months prior to the presentation of symptoms or radiological signs of recurrence. The rate of increase may also be important; a CA125 doubling time of <3 weeks has a median survival of 9.5 months, compared to a doubling time of over 11 weeks, which has a median survival of 34.5 months [10].

✔ **Evidence base**   MRC OV05/EORTC 55955 trial [11]

Multicentre randomized study comparing early versus delayed treatment of relapsed ovarian cancer:

- a total of 1442 women with ovarian cancer in complete remission after first-line platinum-based chemotherapy and a normal CA125 concentration were enrolled
- a total of 529 women were randomized to either early treatment (chemotherapy started as soon as possible within 28 days of CA125 rise) or delayed treatment (chemotherapy started at symptomatic or clinical relapse)
- the study demonstrated no evidence of survival benefit with early treatment of relapse on the basis of a raised CA125 alone (HR 0.98, 95% CI 0.80–1.20; $p = 0.85$). The median survival from randomization was 27.1 months for patients on delayed treatment and 25.7 months for those on early treatment.

The authors did not recommend routine CA125 monitoring in the follow-up of patients with ovarian cancer in complete remission and concluded that there is no benefit in early intervention with chemotherapy for disease relapse based on a rising CA125 alone.

Source: data from *The Lancet*, Volume 376, Issue 9747, Rustin GJ *et al.*, Early versus delayed treatment of relapsed ovarian cancer (MRC OV05/EORTC 55955): a randomised trial, pp. 1155–63, Copyright © 2010 Elsevier Ltd. All rights reserved.

⭐ **Learning point**   Patients with relapsed ovarian cancer can be categorized according to their response to platinum-based therapy and subsequent platinum-free interval [12]

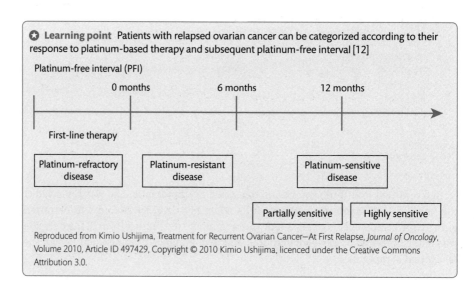

Reproduced from Kimio Ushijima, Treatment for Recurrent Ovarian Cancer—At First Relapse, *Journal of Oncology*, Volume 2010, Article ID 497429, Copyright © 2010 Kimio Ushijima, licenced under the Creative Commons Attribution 3.0.

This patient had a symptomatic relapse, 10 months after responding to her primary platinum-based therapy; she therefore had platinum-sensitive disease. As she tolerated first-line chemotherapy well, with no significant side effects, and her current PS is 1, her re-treatment options include platinum-based combinations of chemotherapy.

⊘ **Evidence base** Combination chemotherapy options in recurrent platinum-sensitive ovarian cancer

ICON4/AGO-OVAR-2.2 trial: carboplatin plus paclitaxel [13]

- International, multicentre, randomized phase III study of 802 women with platinum-sensitive recurrent ovarian cancer.
- Platinum (carboplatin or cisplatin) plus paclitaxel versus platinum alone.
- Improvement in median OS (29 months versus 24 months; $p = 0.02$) and median PFS (13 months versus 10 months; $p = 0.0004$), in favour of the combination group.

AGO-OVAR, the NCIC CTG, the EORTC GCG intergroup trial: carboplatin plus gemcitabine [14]

- International, open-label, randomized phase III study of 356 women with platinum-sensitive recurrent ovarian cancer.
- Carboplatin AUC 4 day 1 plus gemcitabine 1000 mg/m^2 days 1 and 8 (GC) versus carboplatin AUC 5 alone.
- Improvement in response rate (47.2% versus 30.9%; $p = 0.0016$) and median PFS (8.6 months versus 5.8 months; $p = 0.0031$), in favour of the GC group.
- More reported cases of grades 3–4 haematological toxicities in the GC group.
- No statistically significant difference in QoL scores between groups detected.

Gynecologic Cancer Intergroup (GCIG) CALYPSO trial: carboplatin plus pegylated liposomal doxorubicin (PLD) [15]

- Multicentre, randomized, non-inferiority phase III study of 976 women with platinum-sensitive recurrent ovarian cancer.
- Carboplatin AUC 5 plus PLD 30 mg/m^2 (CD) versus carboplatin AUC 5 plus paclitaxel 175 mg/m^2 (CP).
- CD definitely not inferior to CP ($p \leq 0.001$). In a superiority analysis, CD improved PFS (median 11.3 months versus 9.4 months; $p = 0.005$).
- The CP group experienced more grades 3–4 neutropenia, grade 2 alopecia, neuropathy, and hypersensitivity reactions. Palmar–plantar erythema was commoner in the CD group.

OCEANS trial: addition of bevacizumab in platinum-sensitive relapse [16]

- Multicentre, randomized phase III study of 484 women with platinum-sensitive relapsed ovarian cancer.
- BV plus gemcitabine and carboplatin (GC) versus GC plus placebo.
- Improvement in median PFS (12.4 months versus 8.4 months; $p < 0.0001$) and response rate (78.5% versus 57.4%; $p < 0.0001$), in favour of the BV group.
- No improvement in OS in two interim analyses, but final data still awaited.
- More reported cases of grades 3–4 hypertension (17.4% versus <1%) and proteinuria (8.5% versus <1%) in the BV group, and two patients had GI perforation after study treatment was discontinued.
- No new safety concerns found in the BV group, and the rates of febrile neutropenia and neutropenia were similar between the groups.

❝ Expert comment

The AGO group in Germany conducted the DESKTOP I and II trials. In DESKTOP I, the criteria for achieving complete debulking (no ascites, good PS, and no macroscopic residual disease at primary surgery) were defined and tested prospectively in DESKTOP II; women who met these three criteria had a 75% chance of complete macroscopic resection. DESKTOP 3 will randomize women who meet these three criteria to have attempted debulking surgery followed by chemotherapy versus chemotherapy alone.

✪ Learning point The role of secondary surgery in disease relapse

The role of secondary cytoreductive surgery remains controversial. At present, a Cochrane review has found no evidence of survival benefit from randomized clinical trials to support secondary surgical cytoreduction and chemotherapy, compared to chemotherapy alone, for women with recurrent epithelial ovarian cancer. The DESKTOP III trial by the AGO group is a randomized phase III study which has been set up to answer this question. However, secondary cytoreductive surgery may be beneficial in patients with no ascites, good PS, and no macroscopic residual disease at primary surgery.

The decision was made for the patient to be treated with six cycles of carboplatin plus PLD. Her symptoms resolved after two cycles of chemotherapy, and her CA125 returned to normal (17 IU/mL).

Four months after the completion of her second-line chemotherapy, she presented to the ED with a 10-day history of intermittent nausea and vomiting, abdominal distension, and pain. She had last opened her bowels 7 days previously but was still passing flatus.

On examination, she appeared distressed; she was haemodynamically stable; her abdomen was soft, but distended, with generalized tenderness. There were no guarding or other signs of peritonism. Bowel sounds were present. A plain abdominal X-ray showed dilated loops of bowels. An erect CXR did not show air under the diaphragm. Her CA125 had risen to 1764 IU/mL.

The patient was diagnosed with subacute bowel obstruction, secondary to probable underlying disease relapse. She was admitted to the oncology ward and kept nil by mouth. She received regular IV fluids, cyclizine, and dexamethasone and was commenced on senna and magnesium hydroxide. A CT scan confirmed disease progression and loops of dilated small bowel, with multiple sites of serosal disease and no obvious single transition point. Her symptoms partially improved with conservative management.

✪ Learning point (Acute Oncology) Conservative management of bowel obstruction

Retrospective and autopsy studies have shown the overall incidence of malignant bowel obstruction in relapsed advanced ovarian cancer to be as high as 51% [17]. Published surgical series, albeit over 15 years ago, showed surgery to be detrimental to survival and QoL, with a perioperative mortality of 5–32% [18]. Conservative management is therefore the mainstay of treatment, with the aim of relieving symptoms of nausea, vomiting, and pain.

Corticosteroids

A Cochrane review [19] concluded that there is a statistical trend towards a more rapid resolution of symptoms and bowel obstruction with the usage of IV dexamethasone (6–16 mg). This is well tolerated, with few side effects. However, there is no positive effect on OS.

Anti-emetics

Commonly used anti-emetics include cyclizine, haloperidol, levomepromazine, phenothiazines, metoclopramide (has promotility action and is not suitable for complete obstruction).

Anti-secretory agents

Octreotide and hyoscine butylbromide have both been shown to be effective. Studies have shown octreotide to be superior to hyoscine butylbromide in reducing GI secretions, nausea, and vomiting [20].

Analgesia

Colic usually responds best to hyoscine butylbromide, whereas strong opioid and anti-neuropathic agents (gabapentin) are more effective with visceral pain.

> **❻ Expert comment**
>
> Management of bowel obstruction is extremely difficult. The use of surgery remains controversial—most centres will only offer surgery in very selected cases, usually those with a single site of disease in the distal small bowel. It is also important to differentiate between complete mechanical obstruction and diffuse serosal disease causing functional obstruction. Promotility agents can be helpful in the latter but will exacerbate pain and discomfort in the former. Early liaison with both surgical and palliative care teams is essential in the management of small bowel obstruction. Finally, the use of total parenteral nutrition in patients with small bowel obstruction is also a difficult subject and raises many ethical issues.

This patient now had platinum-resistant relapse, and the decision was for her to be treated with weekly paclitaxel chemotherapy.

> **✪ Learning point** Chemotherapy for platinum-resistant disease
>
> Phase II studies showed single-agent response rate to be between 5% and 25% [12].
>
> | | Paclitaxel [21] | PLD [22] | Topotecan [23] | PLD versus topotecan [24] | PLD versus gemcitabine [25] |
> |---|---|---|---|---|---|
> | Number of patients | 53 | 82 | 112 | 130 versus 124 | 96 versus 99 |
> | Dose | 80 mg/m^2/1 week | 50 mg/m^2/4 weeks | 1.5 mg/m^2 days 1–5/3 weeks | 50 mg/m^2/4 weeks 1.5 mg/m^2 for 5 days/3 weeks | 50 mg/m^2/ 4 weeks 1 g/m^2/3 weeks |
> | RR (CR + PR) (%) | 25 | 18.3 | 12.4 | 12.3 versus 6.5 | 8.3 versus 6.1 |
> | PFS (weeks) | 24 | 17 | 12.1 | 9.1 versus 13.6 | 12.4 versus 14.4 |
> | OS (weeks) | 58 | N/A | 47 | 35.6 versus 41.3 | 50.8 versus 54 |
> | Most frequent side effects | Peripheral neuropathy, myelo-suppression | Palmar–plantar erythema, mucositis | Neutropenia | PPE/neutropenia | Fatigue/fatigue |
>
> Adapted from Kimio Ushijima, Treatment for Recurrent Ovarian Cancer—At First Relapse, *Journal of Oncology*, Volume 2010, Article ID 497429, Copyright © 2010 Kimio Ushijima, licenced under the Creative Commons Attribution 3.0.

> **✔ Evidence base** AURELIA Trial: addition of bevacizumab in platinum-resistant relapse [26]
>
> - Multicentre, randomized phase III study of 361 women with ovarian cancer that progressed within 6 months of completing at least four cycles of platinum-based therapy and no history of bowel complications.
> - BV plus single-agent chemotherapy of investigators' choice (weekly paclitaxel, topotecan, or PLD) versus chemotherapy alone.
> - Improvement in median PFS (6.7 months versus 3.4 months; $p < 0.001$), in favour of the BV group.
> - Subgroup analysis indicated that PFS benefit is independent of age, relapse-free interval, type of chemotherapy administered, extent of disease, or presence of ascites.
> - Median PFS benefit is greatest when BV was added to weekly paclitaxel (10.4 months versus 3.9 months), followed by topotecan (5.8 months versus 2.1 months), then PLD (5.4 months versus 3.5 months).
> - Overall response rate was superior when BV was added to chemotherapy, with the greatest improvement with weekly paclitaxel (51.7% versus 28.8%), followed by topotecan (22.8% versus 3.3%) and PLD (18.3% versus 7.9%).
>
> *Source*: data from Pujade-Lauraine *et al.*, Bevacizumab combined with chemotherapy for platinum-resistant recurrent ovarian cancer: The AURELIA open-label randomized phase III trial, *Journal of Clinical Oncology*, Volume 32, Number 13, pp. 1302–8, Copyright © 2014 by American Society of Clinical Oncology.

> ⭐ **Learning point** Future directions
>
> **Defective homologous recombination repair**
>
> Approximately 20% of high-grade serous ovarian carcinomas (HGSCs) have *BRCA1/2* mutations, resulting in defects or deficiency in homologous recombination repair [27]. A further 30% of HGCS may also have defective HR due to other mechanisms, including BRCA1 methylation and mutation in other HR genes, such as *RAD51C*. Selective tumour cell cytotoxicity, can be achieved using PARP (poly (adenosine diphosphate-ribose) polymerase) inhibitors.
>
> Olaparib is a potent oral PARP inhibitor, with selective anti-tumour activity in *BRCA1/2* mutation carriers. A phase II study of olaparib monotherapy has demonstrated an objective response rate of 41% for HGSC patients with *BRCA1/2* mutations, and 24% for those without [28].
>
> Ledermann *et al.* conducted a randomized, double-blind, placebo-controlled phase II study, evaluating olaparib maintenance therapy in 265 women with platinum-sensitive relapsed HGSC [27]. Patients who had responded to at least four cycles of second- or third-line platinum-based chemotherapy were randomized to either olaparib (400 mg PO bd) or placebo, given until disease progression. Median PFS was improved in the olaparib group (8.4 months versus 4.8 months; p <0.001). Subgroup analyses showed the PFS benefit to be across all subgroups. Mature data on OS are not yet available. Adverse events are commoner in the olaparib group, namely fatigue, nausea, vomiting, and anaemia.
>
> Selection for germline *BRCA1/2* testing in ovarian cancer patients has primarily been for patients with a positive family history. However, the Australian Ovarian Cancer Study [29] (a population-based case control study of 1001 women with non-mucinous ovarian cancer) and the Cancer Genome Atlas consortium study [30] of 489 women with high-grade serous ovarian cancer demonstrated that rates of germline mutation in *BRCA1* and *BRCA2* in patients with high-grade serous disease were approximately 15–20%. Moreover, long-term cohort studies have suggested a highly significant improvement in OS for patients carrying germline *BRCA1/2* mutations, especially *BRCA2* [31]. Many centres are now recommending that all patients with high-grade serous ovarian cancer be offered *BRCA1/2* germline mutation testing.

> 🕪 **Expert comment**
>
> There is huge interest in the use of PARP inhibitors in high-grade ovarian cancer. The data from the olaparib phase II trial suggest that the benefit is particularly striking in women with germline mutations in *BRCA1* and *2* (HR for PFS 0.11). Olaparib is now being evaluated in phase III trials in women with germline *BRCA1* and *2* mutations both in first-line and platinum-sensitive relapse.
>
> In sporadic high-grade serous disease, there is also great interest. Functional and genomic data suggest that up to 50% of high-grade serous ovarian cancers may have defective homologous recombination (HRD), with only 10–15% due to germline mutations. Because HRD is a complex phenotype and there are no adequate functional assays, many investigators are keen to identify mutation signatures that can be applied prospectively in ongoing phases II and III trials of other PARP inhibitors.

Discussion

Ovarian cancer is the fifth commonest cancer in women in the UK, with a lifetime risk of approximately 2%. It is the leading cause of death in gynaecological cancers, because most women present late with advanced disease and little prospect for cure. Despite some improvements in survival over the last 20 years, due to the routine use of platinum–taxane chemotherapy and more aggressive surgical techniques, OS at 5 years remains <35% for patients with FIGO stages III/IV disease.

Targeted therapy, including anti-angiogenic agents and PARP inhibitors, has shown encouraging results as a treatment adjunct. Together with a clearer understanding of the molecular changes driving this disease, and better patient stratification using selective germline *BRCA1/2* testing and accurate histological diagnosis, the future of ovarian cancer remains hopeful.

A final word from the expert

There has been a huge increase in our understanding of the basic biology of ovarian cancer in the past 5 years. It has been recognized for many years that the different subtypes of ovarian cancer behave differently—the large-scale sequencing efforts have been able to confirm this at a mutation level, as well as identify potential targets for new therapies. The key breakthrough has been the realization that high-grade serous disease appears to arise not in the ovary, but in the fimbria of the distal Fallopian tube.

The key challenge in the next 5 years is to turn this new knowledge into treatments. Most pressing is the need to run clinical trials in specific subtypes; such studies are in set-up in both low-grade serous and clear cell carcinomas. In addition, given the cost and complexity of novel therapies, it is utterly vital that companion diagnostics and biomarkers are developed alongside these novel therapies, rather than retrospectively; bevacizumab is a good case in point—the benefit in unselected first-line populations is relatively modest. However, there was greater benefit in ICON7 in patients with clinically poor prognosis features (especially suboptimal debulking)—the challenge remains to identify robust molecular markers that can be easily assessed in routine diagnostic laboratories using tumour material or serum.

References

1. Jacobs I, Oram D, Fairbanks J, Turner J, Frost C, Grudzinskas JG. A risk of malignancy index incorporating CA125, ultrasound and menopausal status for the accurate preoperative diagnosis of ovarian cancer. *British Journal of Obstetrics and Gynaecology* 1990; **97**(10): 922–9.
2. Benedet JL, Bender H, Jones H, 3rd, Ngan HY, Pecorelli S. FIGO staging classifications and clinical practice guidelines in the management of gynecologic cancers. FIGO Committee on Gynecologic Oncology. *International Journal of Gynaecology and Obstetrics* 2000; **70**(2): 209–62.
3. Kaku T, Ogawa S, Kawano Y *et al.* Histological classification of ovarian cancer. *Medical Electron Microscopy* 2003; **36**(1): 9–17.
4. Takano M, Tsuda H, Sugiyama T. Clear cell carcinoma of the ovary: is there a role of histology-specific treatment? *Journal of Experimental and Clinical Cancer Research* 2012; **31**: 53.
5. Vergote I, Trope CG, Amant F *et al.* Neoadjuvant chemotherapy or primary surgery in stage IIIC or IV ovarian cancer. *The New England Journal of Medicine* 2010; **363**(10): 943–53.
6. Bookman MA, Brady MF, McGuire WP *et al.* Evaluation of new platinum-based treatment regimens in advanced-stage ovarian cancer: a Phase III Trial of the Gynecologic Cancer Intergroup. *Journal of Clinical Oncology* 2009; **27**(9): 1419–25.
7. Perren TJ, Swart AM, Pfisterer J *et al.* A phase 3 trial of bevacizumab in ovarian cancer. *The New England Journal of Medicine* 2011; **365**(26): 2484–96.
8. Burger RA, Brady MF, Bookman MA *et al.* Incorporation of bevacizumab in the primary treatment of ovarian cancer. *The New England Journal of Medicine* 2011; **365**(26): 2473–83.
9. Rustin GJ, Nelstrop AE, Tuxen MK, Lambert HE. Defining progression of ovarian carcinoma during follow-up according to CA 125: a North Thames Ovary Group Study. *Annals of Oncology* 1996; **7**(4): 361–4.

➕ **Clinical tip** Management of dysphagia

- The management of dysphagia requires a multimodality approach that is dependent on whether the paradigm of care is curative or palliative. Treatments include dietary modification and supplementation, oesophageal dilatation, laser therapy, photodynamic therapy, endoscopic stenting, feeding tubes, chemotherapy, radiotherapy, and brachytherapy.
- Expandable metal stents provide palliation for dysphagia secondary to mechanical compression from intrinsic tumours [20]. They are less effective in resolving dysphagic symptoms due to extrinsic compression and are more effective in proximal and mid-oesophageal lesions than distally obstructing tumours.
- Expandable stents are metallic, plastic, or biodegradable (Figure 7.2). Self-expanding metallic stents are the most widely used and are either uncovered, partially covered, or fully covered [21]. Covered stents can be used over oesophageal fistulae and have the advantage of preventing tumour overgrowth and being removable; however, they are more prone to migration, compared to uncovered stents.
- After stent placement, a soft or liquid diet is recommended, whilst avoiding fibrous or dense foods, such as broccoli or meat, to prevent food impaction. Distal stents involving the GOJ can induce reflux symptoms or aspiration, which can be combatted using an anti-reflux valve within the stent or with high-dose proton pump inhibitors.
- Specialist dietician input is critical to maintaining weight and ensuring the delivery of food products that provide specific nutritional values required for the basal metabolic rate and physical activity. Nutritional support prevents and treats malnutrition, improves subjective QoL, enhances anti-tumour treatment effects, and reduces adverse effects of anti-cancer therapy [22].
- Dieticians assess the degree of dysphagia, food portion size, consistency, volume, hydration, diabetic considerations, patient preferences, and treatment-induced cachexia, anorexia, or nausea. Dietetic input may involve food fortification, consistency modification, or nutritional supplementation to increase calorie, protein, mineral, or vitamin intake. There are a wide variety of supplements with variable contents of nutritional additives and in various forms and volumes (e.g. milkshake-based drinks, high-calorie shots, fruit-based drinks, puddings, soups, etc.).
- Dysphagic patients who are unable to maintain adequate oral intake may benefit from enteral feeding. This can be delivered using multiple devices: NG tubes, gastrostomy tubes (e.g. percutaneous endoscopic gastrotomy (PEG), radiologically inserted gastrostomy (RIG)), nasojejunostomy tubes, etc. The risk of refeeding syndrome needs to be assessed, and appropriate vitamin replacement given.

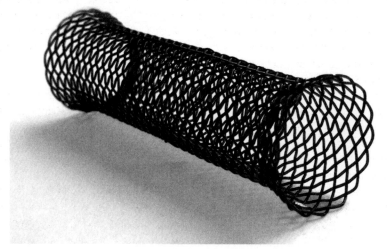

Figure 7.2 Endoscopic biodegradable oesophageal stent. An example of a biodegradable stent inserted for dysphagia, suitable for patients receiving CRT for locally advanced oesophageal cancer.

van Boeckel PG, Vleggaar FP, Siersema PD, Biodegradable stent placement in the esophagus, *Expert Review of Medical Devices*, 2013, **10**(1), 37–43. doi: 10.1586/erd.12.45.

Discussion

In the UK, oesophageal cancer is the fourth commonest cause of cancer death in men, and the sixth commonest in women. Since the 1960s, there has been a dramatic rise in the incidence of upper GI adenocarcinoma, compared to SCC, in Western countries. Adenocarcinoma typically arises from an area of Barrett's metaplasia on a background of gastro-oesophageal reflux. However, the majority of patients who develop adenocarcinoma have no history of symptomatic reflux disease.

An endoscopic surveillance approach is commonly adopted in patients with Barrett's oesophagus, since acid suppression or anti-reflux surgery has not been proven to prevent the progression to cancer. Patients with high-grade dysplasia are managed with active surveillance, endoscopic procedures, or surgical resection.

Advanced oesophageal cancer is associated with a poor prognosis. Despite an initial good partial response, disease progression on first-line palliative chemotherapy is not uncommon. The degree of tumour response and its duration, both on and off treatment, can help to inform about the tumour biology, with long treatment-free intervals being favourable whilst progression on treatment being a poor prognostic sign.

The 1-year median survival remains under 50% for metastatic disease treated with palliative chemotherapy. Molecularly targeted therapies have been investigated in the treatment of oesophageal cancers; however, to date, there is only one approved novel agent trastuzumab. There is a survival advantage of several months with trastuzumab combined with platinum-based chemotherapy in upper GI adenocarcinomas overexpressing HER2 (see ToGa trial [23]) (see Chapter 8 for more details (page 94)). Trials are currently investigating the role for trastuzumab alongside neo-adjuvant chemotherapy or chemoradiation in locally advanced adenocarcinomas overexpressing HER2.

The anti-angiogenesis VEGF inhibitor bevacizumab has been shown to increase treatment response rates when combined with chemotherapy. To date, however, it has failed to demonstrate a statistically significant survival (AVAGAST [24]). The addition of the mAb against EGFR panitumumab resulted in a statistically inferior outcome than with chemotherapy alone (see REAL-3 trial [25]). There are several large phases II–III clinical trials in progress, assessing how best to optimize perioperative treatment for adenocarcinomas (e.g. OE05 and ST03 trials). Concern over leak rates in ST03 led to early closing of the trial [26].

New molecular targets involved in alternative cell signalling pathways are currently under review and include mesenchymal–epithelial transition factor (MET) inhibitors, hepatocyte growth factor (HGF) inhibitors, and heat shock protein 90 (Hsp90) inhibitors. The relative lack of progress with targeted agents, compared to other tumour types, may be due to the infrequent occurrence of driver mutations found in genomic sequencing of oesophageal cancers.

Much of the relevant published clinical trials combine patients with lower oesophageal tumours, GOJ tumours, and primary gastric tumours in their studies. It is unclear whether these anatomical differences are relevant to therapeutic approaches, since subgroup analyses have frequently been underpowered.

The most effective treatment strategy remains early detection to enable a curative approach. There remains a lack of clinical consensus as to which combination of multimodality therapies achieves optimal downstaging, enabling curative surgery that delivers clear resection margins and a long-term disease-free state. Treatment planning needs to take account of the histology and staging information alongside patient factors such as nutritional status, co-morbidities, and patient preference.

Current curative treatment recommendations for oesophageal squamous carcinomas are definitive chemoradiation for proximal oesophageal tumours and chemoradiation, either alone or combined with surgery, for tumours of the mid or lower oesophagus. For oesophageal adenocarcinomas and GOJ tumours, preoperative chemotherapy or preoperative chemoradiation improves long-term survival, compared to surgery alone. Perioperative chemotherapy increases survival in Siewert II and III tumours of the GOJ.

A final word from the expert

The management of oesophageal cancer is highly reliant on effective and appropriately skilled multidisciplinary teamwork. Accurate staging, using multiple modalities and skills, is essential. The curative managements of oesophageal adenocarcinoma and squamous carcinoma differ. The management of adenocarcinoma is similar to that of stomach cancer. For squamous oesophageal cancers, the use of CRT alone or with surgery requires careful assessment. Successful palliation also requires close teamwork.

References

1. Hurt CN, Nixon LS, Griffiths GO et al. SCOPE1: a randomised phase II/III multicentre clinical trial of definitive chemoradiation, with or without cetuximab, in carcinoma of the oesophagus. *BMC Cancer* 2011; **11** 466
2. Schwartz LH, Bogaerts J, Ford R et al. Evaluation of lymph nodes with RECIST 1.1. *European Journal of Cancer* 2009; **45**(2): 261–7.
3. Siewert JR, Feith M, Stein HJ. Biologic and clinical variations of adenocarcinoma at the esophago-gastric junction: relevance of a topographic-anatomic subclassification *Journal of Surgical Oncology* 2005; **90**(3): 139–46; discussion 146.
4. Lordick F, Ott K, Krause BJ et al. PET to assess early metabolic response and to guide treatment of adenocarcinoma of the oesophagogastric junction: the MUNICON phase II trial *The Lancet Oncology* 2007; **8**(9): 797–805.
5. Mandard AM, Dalibard F, Mandard JC et al. Pathologic assessment of tumor regression after preoperative chemoradiotherapy of esophageal carcinoma Clinicopathologic correlations. *Cancer* 1994; **73**(11): 2680–6.
6. Cunningham D, Starling N, Rao S et al. Upper Gastrointestinal Clinical Studies Group of the National Cancer Research Institute of the United Kingdom Capecitabine and oxaliplatin for advanced esophagogastric cancer. *The New England Journal of Medicine* 2008; **358**(1): 36–46.
7. Hofstetter W, Correa AM, Bekele N et al. Proposed modification of nodal status in AJCC esophageal cancer staging system. *The Annals of Thoracic Surgery* 2007; **84**(2): 365–73; discussion 374–5.
8. Stein HJ, Feith M, Bruecher BL, Naehrig J, Sarbia M, Siewert JR. Early esophageal cancer: pattern of lymphatic spread and prognostic factors for long-term survival after surgical resection. *Annals of Surgery* 2005; **242**(4): 566–73; discussion 573–5.
9. Cooper JS, Guo MD, Herskovic A et al. Chemoradiotherapy of locally advanced esophageal cancer: long-term follow-up of a prospective randomized trial (RTOG 85-01) Radiation Therapy Oncology Group. *JAMA* 1999; **281**(17): 1623–7.

10. Herskovic A, Martz K, al-Sarraf M *et al*. Combined chemotherapy and radiotherapy compared with radiotherapy alone in patients with cancer of the esophagus. *The New England Journal of Medicine* 1992; **326**(24): 1593–8.

11. Cunningham D, Allum WH, Stenning SP *et al*. Perioperative chemotherapy versus surgery alone for resectable gastroesophageal cancer *The New England Journal of Medicine* 2006; **355**(1): 11–20.

12. van Hagen P, Hulshof MC, van Lanschot JJ *et al*. Preoperative chemoradiotherapy for esophageal or junctional cancer. *The New England Journal of Medicine* 2012; **366**(22): 2074–84.

13. Macdonald JS, Smalley SR, Benedetti J *et al*. Chemoradiotherapy after surgery compared with surgery alone for adenocarcinoma of the stomach or gastroesophageal junction *The New England Journal of Medicine* 2001; **345**(10): 725–30.

14. Medical Research Council Oesophageal Cancer Working Group. Surgical resection with or without preoperative chemotherapy in oesophageal cancer: a randomised controlled trial. *The Lancet* 2002; **359**(9319): 1727–33.

15. Ando N, Iizuka T, Ide H *et al*. Surgery plus chemotherapy compared with surgery alone for localized squamous cell carcinoma of the thoracic esophagus: a Japan Clinical Oncology Group Study—JCOG9204 *Journal of Clinical Oncology* 2003; **21**(24): 4592–6.

16. Tepper J, Krasna MJ, Niedzwiecki D *et al*. Phase III trial of trimodality therapy with cisplatin, fluorouracil, radiotherapy, and surgery compared with surgery alone for esophageal cancer: CALGB 9781 *Journal of Clinical Oncology* 2008; **26**(7): 1086–92.

17. Sjoquist KM, Burmeister BH, Smithers BM *et al*.; Australasian Gastro-Intestinal Trials Group. Survival after neoadjuvant chemotherapy or chemoradiotherapy for resectable oesophageal carcinoma: an updated meta-analysis. *The Lancet Oncology* 2011; **12**(7): 681–92.

18. Bedenne L, Michel P, Bouché O *et al*. Chemoradiation followed by surgery compared with chemoradiation alone in squamous cancer of the esophagus: FFCD 9102 *Journal of Clinical Oncology* 2007; **25**(10): 1160–8.

19. Stahl M, Stuschke M, Lehmann N *et al*. Chemoradiation with and without surgery in patients with locally advanced squamous cell carcinoma of the esophagus. *Journal of Clinical Oncology* 2005; **23**(10): 2310–17.

20. Boyce HW.Jr. Stents for palliation of dysphagia due to esophageal cancer. *The New England Journal of Medicine* 1993; **329**(18): 1345–6.

21. Conio M, Repici A, Battaglia G *et al*. A randomized prospective comparison of self-expandable plastic stents and partially covered self-expandable metal stents in the palliation of malignant esophageal dysphagia *American Journal of Gastroenterology* 2007; **102**(12): 2667–77.

22. Arends J, Bodoky G, Bozzetti F *et al*. DGEM (German Society for Nutritional Medicine) ESPEN (European Society for Parenteral and Enteral Nutrition). ESPEN Guidelines on Enteral Nutrition: Non-surgical oncology. *Clinical Nutrition* 25(2): 2006, 245–59.

23. Bang YJ, Van Cutsem E, Feyereislova A *et al*. ToGA Trial Investigators. Trastuzumab in combination with chemotherapy versus chemotherapy alone for treatment of HER2-positive advanced gastric or gastro-oesophageal junction cancer (ToGA): a phase 3, open-label, randomised controlled trial *The Lancet* 2010; **376**(9742): 687–97.

24. Ohtsu A, Shah MA, Van Cutsem E *et al*. Bevacizumab in combination with chemotherapy as first-line therapy in advanced gastric cancer: a randomized, double-blind, placebo-controlled phase III study. *Journal of Clinical Oncology* 2011; **29**(30): 3968–76.

25. Waddell T, Chau I, Cunningham D *et al*. Epirubicin, oxaliplatin, and capecitabine with or without panitumumab for patients with previously untreated advanced oesophagogastric cancer (REAL3): a randomised, open-label phase 3 trial. *The Lancet Oncology* 2013; **14**(6): 481–9.

26. Okines AF, Langley RE, Thompson LC *et al*. Bevacizumab with peri-operative epirubicin, cisplatin and capecitabine (ECX) in localised gastro-oesophageal adenocarcinoma: a safety report. *Annals of Oncology* 2013; **24**(3): 702–9.

Gastric cancer and complications of relapsed disease

Imran Petkar

 Expert commentary John Bridgewater

Case history

A 67-year-old man presented to his GP with a 6-week history of dyspepsia and 2 kg weight loss. He did not report any abdominal pain, dysphagia, vomiting, or melaena. Co-morbidities included hypertension and hypercholesterolaemia, which were well controlled with lisinopril and simvastatin, respectively. There was no family history of cancer. He was a retired IT engineer with a 30-pack year smoking history and occasional alcohol consumption. Systemic examination was unremarkable.

The patient was referred to the gastroenterology team under the urgent 2-week rule for suspected cancer. The only abnormality on baseline blood tests was a normocytic anaemia. An OGD showed a malignant-appearing lesion in the gastric antrum, which was biopsied and confirmed to be a HER2-negative, moderately differentiated adenocarcinoma diffuse subtype. A CT CAP scan staged the tumour as T3N2M0. A PET scan confirmed no distant metastasis, and a staging laparoscopy showed a localized gastric tumour, with no evidence of obvious peritoneal spread or hepatic metastasis. The patient's disease was considered suitable for radical treatment, following MDT review, and a decision was made to recommend neoadjuvant chemotherapy, followed by definitive surgery and adjuvant chemotherapy.

The patient was seen in the oncology outpatient clinic where the benefits and toxicities of chemotherapy were discussed. He was also reviewed by the dietician and commenced on nutritional supplements. Baseline echocardiogram, EDTA, and electrocardiogram (ECG) were all within normal limits. The patient was offered systemic chemotherapy within the context of a clinical trial, which he declined, and so proceeded with three cycles of neoadjuvant epirubicin, cisplatin, and capecitabine (ECX) chemotherapy. He required an overnight inpatient admission immediately following his first cycle of chemotherapy due to severe vomiting. Subsequent cycles were administered with aprepitant support and were better tolerated. A dose reduction of capecitabine was required, however, due to the development of grade 2 palmar–plantar erythrodysaesthesia (PPE) of the hands and feet.

Following his third cycle of chemotherapy, a CT scan showed stable appearances, and the patient therefore went on to have a subtotal distal gastrectomy with D2 LND. Histology was reported as ypT2N1 moderately differentiated adenocarcinoma diffuse subtype with clear resection margins. Post-operative recovery was, however, complicated by anastomotic leakage, leading to sepsis requiring IV antibiotics and prolonged hospitalization.

Expert comment

Gastric cancer levels are very high in Japan. A diet high in salty food is thought to be one explanation for this. the overall survival in Japan for gastric cancer is significantly higher than in the UK. This may relate to the use of screening, resection of mostly early-stage disease, surgery involving extensive nodal resection, and the extensive use of adjuvant chemotherapy. This contrasts with more advanced disease presentation, neoadjuvant chemotherapy, limited surgery, and limited adjuvant chemotherapy in the UK.

Expert comment

In families with germline *CDH1* mutations, prophylactic gastrectomy is indicated. Even in the absence of any macroscopic lesion, intramucosal cancers are found.

✛ Clinical tip Symptoms and risk factors in suspected gastric cancer

- Anyone over the age of 55 years with a history of recent-onset unexplained dyspepsia should be referred for an urgent endoscopy.
- Red flag symptoms include unintentional weight loss, early satiety, melaena, epigastric bloating or discomfort, dysphagia, and persistent vomiting.
- Always remember familial cancer syndromes such as Lynch syndrome, Li–Fraumeni syndrome, and Peutz–Jeghers syndrome
- Hereditary diffuse gastric cancer (HDGC) is an inherited condition due to germline mutation in the tumour suppression gene CDH1 which encodes the cell adhesion molecule E-cadherin; HDGC usually presents late and carries a poor prognosis.
- Environmental risk factors include low socio-economic status, high salt intake, previous *Helicobacter pylori* infection, obesity, chronic gastritis, pernicious anaemia, smoking, and reflux disease.

✪ Learning point Pathology of gastric adenocarcinoma

Intestinal and diffuse types are the two subtypes of gastric adenocarcinoma with different pathogenesis patterns. The intestinal subtype, which carries a better prognosis, is felt to develop as a result of chronic inflammation of any cause that subsequently leads to intestinal dysplasia and eventually adenocarcinoma. On the other hand, germline or somatic mutations in the *CDH1* gene appear to play a role in the carcinogenesis of the diffuse subtype. On IHC, gastric tumours are usually CK7- and CK20-positive. Between 7 and 34% of OGJ and gastric tumours overexpress HER2, with intestinal-subtype tumours more likely to be HER2-positive, compared to the diffuse subtype [1]. The association between HER2 status and the prognosis of gastric tumours is, however, still unclear at present.

✛ Clinical tip Nutrition in gastric cancer

The majority of patients with gastric cancer have poor nutritional status at presentation, with consequently poor PS. Toxicities from chemotherapy, such as vomiting and diarrhoea, can have a further impact on their oral intake. Early dietary assessment by a dietician, with the use of oral supplements, if required, is vital to maintain an adequate nutritional status, which, in turn, can lead to an improvement in general fitness and PS prior to major surgery. It is important to make sure there are regular follow-up assessments with the dietician during the course of their systemic treatment.

✪ Learning point Neoadjuvant chemotherapy for gastric cancer

The concept of neoadjuvant treatment in gastric cancer mainly arose as a result of difficulties in delivering adjuvant chemotherapy following primary surgical resection. The causes for this were multifactorial, including poor nutritional status and poor post-operative PS, leading to delayed initiation of systemic chemotherapy due to prolonged hospitalization. Failure of administration of adequate therapeutic systemic treatment is associated with an increased risk of locoregional and distant relapse. Neoadjuvant chemotherapy, in contrast, is better tolerated and can potentially downsize tumours, increasing the rates of R0 resection and improving survival, potentially because of the elimination of distant micrometastasis (Figure 8.1). Potential pitfalls include a delay in surgery secondary to chemotherapy toxicity or progression of the disease.

Following recovery from this surgery, the patient commenced adjuvant ECX, with a 25% reduction in the capecitabine dose due to previous toxicities. Towards the end of the second week of the treatment, he was admitted to hospital with dehydration due to grade 3 diarrhoea, and capecitabine was stopped. The patient improved with IV rehydration and was discharged 7 days later. Due to the severity of his symptoms and subsequent profound lethargy, it was decided to discontinue his adjuvant chemotherapy.

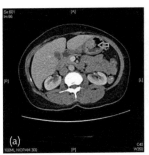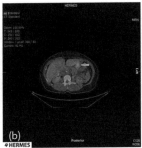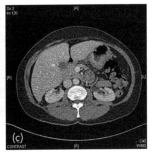

Figure 8.1 A polypoidal gastric tumour at diagnosis on (A) CT and (B) PET scan (arrowhead), and (C) a radiological complete response of the tumour following neoadjuvant chemotherapy.

> ⭐ **Learning point** Surgery and LND in gastric cancer
>
> Total gastrectomy is recommended for tumours of the cardia, fundus, or body, whilst antral tumours can be managed with distal subtotal gastrectomy alone. Whilst there is general consensus regarding the extent of surgery for the primary tumour, the extent of lymphadenectomy is a topic of debate. A D1 LND involves the removal of perigastric nodes only; in a D2 dissection, additionally, nodes along the left gastric, hepatic, and splenic artery are removed. A D3 dissection is an extended D2 lymphadenectomy, with the removal of para-aortic lymph nodes. Accurate staging of the tumour requires at least 15 lymph nodes to be removed.
>
> Based on initial results from a large Dutch trial and a British trial that showed increased morbidity and mortality, with no survival advantage for D2 dissection over D1 dissection, D2 LND was not routinely practised in the Western world [2]. However, a recent update of the Dutch trial showed that gastric cancer-related deaths were significantly higher in the D1 group after a median follow-up of 15 years, and, as such, D2 dissection is now recommended [3]. In Japan, where D2 dissection has always been considered as the standard of care, an RCT showed no significant improvement for D3 dissection over D2 dissection [4].

> ⭐ **Learning point** Perioperative chemotherapy for gastric cancer
>
> Perioperative chemotherapy for operable gastric, OGJ, and lower oesophageal tumours was successfully investigated in the MAGIC trial which randomized over 500 patients to surgery alone or perioperative epirubicin, cisplatin, and 5-FU (ECF) chemotherapy [5]. A significant 13% absolute survival improvement in the 5-year survival made perioperative chemotherapy the treatment of choice for the management of gastric and OGJ tumours in the UK and Europe. Adjuvant chemotherapy was given in 54.8% of patients, and 41.6% completed all six cycles of chemotherapy, reflecting the difficulty in administering adjuvant treatment following surgery. It is important to note that the trial was not designed to assess the relative benefits of neoadjuvant and adjuvant chemotherapy.
>
> Further evidence for the use of perioperative chemotherapy came from the FNCLCC ACCORD07-FFCD study which showed improved 5-year OS rates, PFS, and R0 resections, compared to surgery alone [6].

The patient was reviewed in the oncology clinic 3 months later. He was generally well, with no worrying symptoms to report. A surveillance CT scan did not show any evidence of disease recurrence. Three months later, he presented with ascites, malaise, and loss of appetite. He underwent a therapeutic and diagnostic paracentesis, with cytology confirming relapse of his disease. Restaging CT scan showed peritoneal deposits and two liver metastases. He was started on second-line irinotecan. Following two cycles of irinotecan, the ascites re-accumulated, and a CT scan confirmed progressive disease. Following further therapeutic paracentesis, his PS was 1. His tumour showed fibroblast growth factor receptor (FGFR) amplification, and he was referred to the phases I/II unit for consideration of the AZD4547 trial.

> 💬 **Expert comment**
>
> In continental Europe and the US, epirubicin is uncommonly used as an adjunct to platinum and fluoropyrimidine. In Japan, S-1 has been demonstrated to have a survival benefit in gastric cancers and is the adjuvant systemic treatment of choice.

> ✅ **Evidence base** MAGIC: perioperative chemotherapy for operable gastric cancers [5]
>
> A total of 503 patients with stages II–IV lower oesophageal, OGJ, or gastric adenocarcinomas randomized to surgery alone (*n* = 253) or perioperative chemotherapy (*n* = 250) consisting of three preoperative and three post-operative cycles of ECF (epirubicin 50 mg/m^2 IV, cisplatin 60 mg/m^2 IV, and 5-FU 200 mg/m^2/day continuous infusion administered 3-weekly).
>
> - 92% of patients in the perioperative arm proceeded to surgery, with 86% having completed all three cycles of preoperative chemotherapy.
> - No difference in post-operative morbidity or mortality between the two arms.
> - The 5-year OS significantly improved in the perioperative arm 36% versus 23% in the surgery-alone arm (HR 0.75, 95% CI 0.60–0.93; *p* = 0.009).
> - Significant improvement in PFS (HR 0.66, 95% CI 0.53–0.81; *p* <0.001).
> - No evidence of heterogeneity of treatment effect between the three primary tumour sites in the study.
>
> *Source*: data from Cunningham D *et al.*, Perioperative chemotherapy versus surgery alone for resectable gastroesophageal cancer, *New England Journal of Medicine*, Volume 355, Number 1, pp. 11–20, Copyright © 2006 Massachusetts Medical Society. All rights reserved.

> ⭐ **Learning point** Adjuvant CRT
>
> - Adjuvant CRT, following surgical resection of the primary tumour, is widely practised in the US and largely based on the US Intergroup 0116 trial. This trial randomized 556 patients with adenocarcinoma of the stomach or OGJ to either 5-FU/leucovorin-based CRT to the tumour bed and regional nodes (45 Gy/25 fractions) or observation alone following R0 surgical resection. Both median OS (36 months versus 27 months) and PFS (30 months versus 19 months) were significantly improved in the CRT arm [7]. However, as 54% of patients underwent <D1 resection, it can be argued that chemoradiation may be compensating for suboptimal surgery. In addition, only 64% completed the adjuvant treatment, with 17% stopping treatment early due to significant toxicities. As a result, adjuvant CRT as a treatment modality is not used routinely in the UK for gastric and OGJ tumours.
> - Comparisons between the MAGIC trial and the Intergroup 0116 trial cannot be made, as the US study only included patients with R0 resected gastric and OGJ tumours, compared to the MAGIC study in which not all patients ultimately underwent curative surgery, despite being deemed operable at the point of trial entry. The CRITICS trial is an ongoing phase III RCT, in which patients with resectable gastric cancers are randomized to either perioperative ECX chemotherapy or neoadjuvant ECX followed by adjuvant concomitant chemoradiation (45 Gy/25 fractions with cisplatin and capecitabine), and may help answer the question of whether either strategy is superior [8].

Table 8.1 Key phase III trials for first-line management of advanced gastric/OGJ tumours

Study	Treatment	ORR (%)	Median PFS (months)	Median OS (months)	HR
REAL-2 [15]	ECF,ECX, EOF, EOX	41–48		9.9–11.2	
V325 [13]	Cisplatin/5-FU (CF)	25	3.7	8.6	1.29
	Docetaxel + CF	37	5.6	9.2	*p* = 0.02
REAL-3 [16]	EOX	42	7.4	11.3	1.37
	EOX + panitumumab	46	6	8.8	*p* = 0.01
EXPAND [17]	Cisplatin/capecitabine (CX)	29	5.6	10.7	1.00
	CX + cetuximab	30	4.4	9.4	*p* = 0.95
TRIO-013/LOGIC [19]	CapeOx + placebo	40	5.4	10.5	0.91
	CapeOx + lapatinib	53	6.0	12.2	*p* = 0.35
AVAGAST [18]	CX + placebo	37.4	5.3	10.1	0.87
	CX + bevacizumab	46.0	6.7	12.1	*p* = 0.1
ToGA [14]	CX/CF	35	5.5	11.1	0.74
	CX/CF + trastuzumab	47	6.7	13.8	*p* = 0.004

ORR, overall response rate.
Source: data from Van Cutsem E *et al.*, 2006; Bang YJ *et al.*, 2010; Cunningham D *et al.*, 2008; Waddell T *et al.*, 2013; Lordick F *et al.*, 2013; Ohtsu A *et al.*, 2011; and Hecht JR *et al.*, 2013.

> ➕ **Clinical tip** Management of malignant ascites
>
> - Malignant ascites should be drained as much as possible, within the context of clinical stability of the patient. There is no clinical requirement to remove a drain on the same day, as in non-malignant ascites.
> - Human albumin replacement is not normally necessary as an adjunct to the procedure.
> - An indwelling catheter can be considered in the palliative setting for refractory ascites to allow paracentesis to be performed at home.

Table 8.2 Key phase III trials for second-line management of advanced gastric/OGJ tumours

Study	Treatment	Median PFS (months)	Median OS (months)	HR
Kang et al. [20]	BSC	–	3.8	0.657
	BSC + docetaxel or irinotecan	–	5.3	p = 0.007
COUGAR-02 [21]	ASC	–	3.6	0.67
	ASC + docetaxel	–	5.2	p = 0.01
REGARD [22]	BSC	1.3	3.8	0.776
	BSC + ramucirumab	2.1	5.2	p = 0.04
GRANITE-1 [23]	BSC + P	1.4	4.3	0.90
	BSC + everolimus	1.7	5.4	p = 0.124
TyTAN [24]	Paclitaxel	4.4	8.9	0.85
	Paclitaxel+ lapatinib	5.4	11	

Source: data from Kang JH et al., 2012; Ford H et al., 2013; Fuchs CS et al., 2013; Van Cutsem E et al., 2013; and Bang YJ et al., 2012.

✪ Learning point Management of advanced gastric cancer

The median survival for a patient presenting with metastatic disease is approximately 3 months with best supportive care [9,10]. Palliative combination chemotherapy has been shown to improve survival, as well as QoL, when compared to best supportive care or monotherapy [11]. Platinum–fluoropyrimidine doublet forms the backbone of any first-line regimen for advanced gastric cancer, with a response rate of 32–40% and a median OS of 8–9 months [12]. Although the addition of docetaxel to platinum–fluoropyrimidine is associated with an improvement in survival, it has not been adopted by UK oncologists into routine clinical practice due to increased toxicities associated with this regimen [13].

A number of trials have been conducted, investigating the efficacy of biological agents to improve survival, with mixed results. The ToGA trial showed that the addition of trastuzumab to a platinum–fluoropyrimidine combination in the first-line setting resulted in a 26% reduction in the death rate [14]. The combination treatment also resulted in significantly improved response rates, time to progression, and duration of response, with no worsening of toxicities, including cardiac adverse events.

This study led to a change in the treatment paradigm for advanced gastric and OGJ tumours. Patients with HER2-positive advanced gastric tumours are now offered trastuzumab with platinum–fluoropyrimidine, as per the ToGA trial, whereas patients with HER2-negative tumours are commenced on epirubicin, oxaliplatin, and capecitabine (EOX) in the UK, as per the REAL2 data.

With the exception of the ToGA study, results of other trials evaluating targeted agents in advanced gastric cancers in the first-line setting have been largely disappointing, with no survival benefits demonstrated (Table 8.1) [13–19].

There have been few studies looking at second-line options for gastric cancer (Table 8.2) [20–24]. Second-line irinotecan (150 mg/m^2 every 2 weeks) or docetaxel (60–75 mg/m^2 every 3 weeks) for pretreated gastric/OGJ cancers is associated with a modest, but significant, improvement in median OS [20,21]. Less than 25% completed all six cycles of chemotherapy in the COUGAR-02 study, however, either due to toxicities or progressive disease. Of the targeted agents, the use of the mAb against VEGF receptor 2 (VEGFR2) ramucirumab resulted in a 23% reduction in the risk of death in the second-line setting.

3. Songun I, Putter H, Kranenbarg EM, Sasako M, van de Velde CJ. Surgical treatment of gastric cancer: 15-year follow-up results of the randomised nationwide Dutch D1D2 trial. *The Lancet Oncology* 2010; **11**(5): 439–49.

4. Sasako M, Sano T, Yamamoto S *et al.*; Japan Clinical Oncology Group. D2 lymphadenectomy alone or with para-aortic nodal dissection for gastric cancer. *The New England Journal of Medicine* 2008; **359**(5): 453–62.

5. Cunningham D, Allum WH, Stenning SP *et al.* Perioperative chemotherapy versus surgery alone for resectable gastroesophageal cancer. *The New England Journal of Medicine* 2006; **355**(1): 11–20.

6. Ychou M, Boige V, Pignon JP *et al.* Perioperative chemotherapy compared with surgery alone for resectable gastroesophageal adenocarcinoma: an FNCLCC and FFCD multicenter phase III trial. *Journal of Clinical Oncology* 2011; **29**(13):1715–21.

7. Macdonald JS, Smalley SR, Benedetti J *et al.* Chemoradiotherapy after surgery compared with surgery alone for adenocarcinoma of the stomach or gastroesophageal junction. *The New England Journal of Medicine* 2001; **345**(10): 725–30.

8. Dikken JL, van Sandick JW, Maurits Swellengrebel HA *et al.* Neo-adjuvant chemotherapy followed by surgery and chemotherapy or by surgery and chemoradiotherapy for patients with resectable gastric cancer (CRITICS). *BMC Cancer* 2011; **11**: 329.

9. Murad AM, Santiago FF, Petroianu A, Rocha PR, Rodrigues MA, Rausch M. Modified therapy with 5-fluorouracil, doxorubicin, and methotrexate in advanced gastric cancer. *Cancer* 1993; **72**(1): 37–41.

10. Pyrhönen S., Kuitunen T., Nyandoto P, Kouri M. Randomised comparison of fluorouracil, epidoxorubicin and methotrexate (FEMTX) plus supportive care with supportive care alone in patients with non-resectable gastric cancer. *British Journal of Cancer* 1995; **71**(3): 587–91.

11. Wagner AD, Unverzagt S, Grothe W *et al.* Chemotherapy for advanced gastric cancer. *Cochrane Database of Systematic Reviews* 2010; **3**: CD004064.

12. Kang YK, Kang WK, Shin DB *et al.* Capecitabine/cisplatin versus 5-fluorouracil/cisplatin as first-line therapy in patients with advanced gastric cancer: a randomised phase III noninferiority trial. *Annals of Oncology* 2009; **20**(4): 666–73.

13. Van Cutsem E, Moiseyenko VM, Tjulandin S *et al.*; V325 Study Group. Phase III study of docetaxel and cisplatin plus fluorouracil compared with cisplatin and fluorouracil as first-line therapy for advanced gastric cancer: a report of the V325 Study Group. *Journal of Clinical Oncology* 2006; **24**(31): 4991–7.

14. Bang YJ, Van Cutsem E, Feyereislova A *et al.*; ToGA Trial Investigators. Trastuzumab in combination with chemotherapy versus chemotherapy alone for treatment of HER2-positive advanced gastric or gastro-oesophageal junction cancer (ToGA): a phase 3, open-label, randomised controlled trial. *The Lancet* 2010; **376**(9742): 687–97.

15. Cunningham D, Starling N, Rao S *et al.*; Upper Gastrointestinal Clinical Studies Group of the National Cancer Research Institute of the United Kingdom. Capecitabine and oxaliplatin for advanced esophagogastric cancer. *The New England Journal of Medicine* 2008; **358**(1): 36–46.

16. Waddell T, Chau I, Cunningham D *et al.* Epirubicin, oxaliplatin, and capecitabine with or without panitumumab for patients with previously untreated advanced oesophagogastric cancer (REAL3): a randomised, open-label phase 3 trial. *The Lancet Oncology* 2013; **14**(6): 481–9.

17. Lordick F, Kang YK, Chung HC *et al.*; Arbeitsgemeinschaft Internistische Onkologie and EXPAND Investigators. Capecitabine and cisplatin with or without cetuximab for patients with previously untreated advanced gastric cancer (EXPAND): a randomised, open-label phase 3 trial. *The Lancet Oncology* 2013; **14**(6): 490–9.

18. Ohtsu A, Shah MA, Van Cutsem E *et al.* Bevacizumab in combination with chemotherapy as first-line therapy in advanced gastric cancer: a randomized, double-blind, placebo-controlled phase III study. *Journal of Clinical Oncology* 2011; **29**(30): 3968–76.

19. Hecht JR, Bang YJ, Qin S *et al.* Lapatinib in combination with capecitabine plus oxaliplatin (CapeOX) in HER2-positive advanced or metastatic gastric, esophageal, or gastroesophageal adenocarcinoma (AC): The TRIO-013/LOGiC Trial. *Journal of Clinical Oncology* 2013; **31**(Suppl): LBA4001.

20. Kang JH, Lee SI, Lim do H *et al.* Salvage chemotherapy for pretreated gastric cancer: a randomized phase III trial comparing chemotherapy plus best supportive care with best supportive care alone. *Journal of Clinical Oncology* 2012; **30**(13): 1513–18.

21. Ford H, Marshall A, Wadsley J *et al.* COUGAR-02: A randomized phase III study of docetaxel versus active symptom control in patients with relapsed esophagogastric adenocarcinoma. *Journal of Clinical Oncology* 2013; **31**(Suppl 4): LBA4.

22. Fuchs CS, Tomasek J, Cho JY *et al.* REGARD: A phase III, randomized, double-blinded trial of ramucirumab and best supportive care (BSC) versus placebo and BSC in the treatment of metastatic gastric or gastroesophageal junction (GEJ) adenocarcinoma following disease progression on first-line platinum- and/or fluoropyrimidine-containing combination therapy. *Journal of Clinical Oncology* 2013; **31**(Suppl 4): LBA5.

23. Van Cutsem E, Yeh KH, Bang YJ *et al.* Phase III trial of everolimus (EVE) in previously treated patients with advanced gastric cancer (AGC): GRANITE-1. *Journal of Clinical Oncology* 2012; **30**(Suppl 4): LBA3.

24. Bang YJ. A randomized, open-label, phase III study of lapatinib in combination with weekly paclitaxel versus weekly paclitaxel alone in the second-line treatment of HER2 amplified advanced gastric cancer (AGC) in Asian population: Tytan study. *Journal of Clinical Oncology* 2013; **31**(Suppl 4): abstr 11.

25. Ferlay J, Shin HR, Bray F, Forman D, Mathers C, Parkin DM. Estimates of worldwide burden of cancer in 2008: GLOBOCAN 2008. *International Journal of Cancer* 2010; **127**(12): 2893–917.

26. Sakuramoto S, Sasako M, Yamaguchi T *et al.*; ACTS-GC Group. Adjuvant chemotherapy for gastric cancer with S-1, an oral fluoropyrimidine. *The New England Journal of Medicine* 2007; **357**(18): 1810–20.

27. Bang YJ, Kim YW, Yang HK *et al.*; CLASSIC trial investigators. Adjuvant capecitabine and oxaliplatin for gastric cancer after D2 gastrectomy (CLASSIC): a phase 3 open-label, randomised controlled trial. *The Lancet* 2012; **379**(9813): 315–21.

28. Lee J, Lim do H, Kim S *et al.* Phase III trial comparing capecitabine plus cisplatin versus capecitabine plus cisplatin with concurrent capecitabine radiotherapy in completely resected gastric cancer with D2 lymph node dissection: the ARTIST trial. *Journal of Clinical Oncology* 2012; **30**(3): 268–73.

but otherwise no definite evidence of distant metastatic spread. At ERCP, a short-segment stricture was identified in the lower common bile duct and a stent was inserted. Biliary brushings yielded dysplastic cells only. The specialist MDT recommended an EUS, which confirmed a 3 cm mass in the head of pancreas appearing to invade into the SMV. Peripancreatic lymphadenopathy measuring 11 mm was noted. EUS-guided fine-needle aspirate from the pancreatic mass confirmed an adenocarcinoma, staining positively for carbohydrate antigen 19-9 (CA19.9), CEA, and CK19 by IHC.

The patient's diagnosis was determined to be borderline operable pancreatic ductal adenocarcinoma (PDAC), by virtue of impingement on the SMV, stage T3N1M0. The patient was reviewed in the surgical outpatient clinic when he was feeling a little better with resolving jaundice, but he was still losing weight. He was informed of the cancer diagnosis and that laparoscopic exploration of his cancer was needed to determine whether surgery was possible. In view of ongoing steatorrhoea, a faecal elastase test was requested, and the patient was started on pancreatic enzyme replacement therapy for nutrient malabsorption secondary to pancreatic insufficiency.

⊕ Clinical tip Obstructive jaundice as a common presentation of PDAC

At least two-thirds of patients ultimately diagnosed with PDAC present with obstructive jaundice, and endoscopic biliary stenting with a plastic or metallic stent is frequently the initial treatment for symptom relief. Plastic stents block more easily; metallic stents are wider and remain patent for longer. Where endoscopic insertion is technically impossible, percutaneous drainage of bile may be appropriate, with subsequent internalisation when feasible. Oral drugs, such as antihistamines and bile acid sequestrants, may relieve symptoms, whilst waiting for the bilirubin level to fall. The decision to pursue initial drainage needs to take into account the likelihood of surgical resectability, since stents may impede the potential to resect the tumour and/or optimally achieve anastomoses.

✪ Learning point Resectability criteria for PDAC

Optimal imaging of PDAC may employ a 'pancreatic protocol' whereby the cross-sectional imaging includes a non-contrast phase, as well as arterial pancreatic parenchymal and portal venous phases of contrast enhancement, with thin slices through the abdomen. Multiplanar reconstruction can then be employed to determine resectability, which is determined by the relationship of the primary mass to adjacent structures, as well as evidence of distant spread.

Tumours considered *resectable* have the following features [18]:

- no distant metastases
- no radiographic evidence of SMV or portal vein distortion
- clear fat planes around the coeliac axis, hepatic artery, and superior mesenteric artery (SMA).

Borderline resectable pancreatic cancers include the following features:

- no distant metastases
- no extension to the coeliac axis
- distortion or narrowing of the SMV or PV, or occlusion of the vessels but with suitable vessels proximally and distally, allowing the possibility of resection and vessel grafting
- gastroduodenal artery encasement with abutment or short-segment encasement of the hepatic artery
- tumour abutment of the SMA not exceeding 180° of the vessel circumference.

❝ Expert comment

Less than 20% of PDAC patients present with clearly operable disease. Although adjuvant chemotherapy has been shown to improve survival after surgical resection of PDAC in randomized trials, the use chemotherapy or radiotherapy in downstaging inoperable primary tumours is currently under investigation. Recognition of borderline operable PDAC has led to neoadjuvant trials focussing on this subgroup as having the greatest promise for improving resectability rates.

Nutritional problems are common with PDAC, so all patients should have access to specialist dietetic advice.

- Cachexia, a syndrome of weight loss (>10%), anorexia, and systemic inflammation, is very common in advanced PDAC, but the evidence base for direct treatments is poor.
- Steatorrhoea and associated symptoms of bloating and abdominal discomfort secondary to pancreatic exocrine insufficiency (post-operative or disease-related) should be investigated with a faecal elastase test, and pancreatic enzyme replacement therapy can be commenced immediately, whilst awaiting confirmation.
- Secondary diabetes may cause weight loss.
- Nausea and vomiting may be managed medically, but more severe symptoms suggestive of gastric outlet or duodenal obstruction should be investigated with endoscopic examination and stent insertion, if appropriate. In some patients, gastrojejunostomy may be appropriate.

Whilst awaiting a date for surgery, the patient became acutely breathless, and he attended the ED. On arrival, he was tachypnoeic, hypotensive (BP 97/54 mmHg), and hypoxic (oxygen saturations 88% breathing room air). His calves were soft and non-tender. An ECG confirmed sinus tachycardia, with evidence of right heart strain. A CXR was unremarkable, but a CT pulmonary angiogram demonstrated a saddle PE, in addition to several new lung and liver metastases, which were not evident on his previous scan 3 weeks earlier (Figure 9.2). The patient was admitted to hospital, resuscitated, and treated with therapeutic dose of low-molecular-weight heparin (LMWH).

➕ **Clinical tip** Differential diagnosis of breathlessness in the cancer patient

- PE (associated with thrombus formed locally around malignant sites or through a generalized hypercoagulable state).
- Lower respiratory tract infection.
- Lung metastases.
- Pleural effusion (exudate from malignant deposits or transudate from hypoalbuminaemia).
- Anaemia.
- Cardiac ischaemia (smoking is common to the aetiology of both PDAC and cardiovascular disease).
- Consider co-morbidities and multifactorial causes.

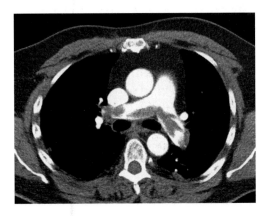

Figure 9.2 A CT image acquired at the level of the bifurcation of the pulmonary artery, demonstrating a low attenuation saddle embolus. Further emboli were identified within the peripheral pulmonary vasculature.

Image courtesy of Dr Ferdia Gallagher, University of Cambridge, UK.

❝ **Expert comment**

In retrospect, the lung nodules identified on the patient's initial staging CT scan probably did represent early metastases. However, modern CT scanners frequently identify subcentimetre lesions of uncertain significance, and often the best plan is to undertake surveillance imaging 2–3 months later. FDG-PET scans are sometimes used in high-risk patients to detect extra-pancreatic metastases, in an attempt to differentiate benign from malignant nodules, but the resolution of PET means lesions under 5 mm are difficult to assess. FDG-PET is not a good technology to evaluate the pancreas, since it does not differentiate between malignancy and inflammation, which may be a feature of PDAC as well as benign pancreatitis.

> **⊗ Learning point (Acute oncology)** Coagulation in PDAC
>
> **The problem**
>
> Up to 60% of patients with PDAC suffer VTE, reflecting a hypercoagulable state. Whilst these patients share prothrombotic risk factors associated with a cancer diagnosis, tumour-specific factors, including the retroperitoneal location of the tumour, increased circulating levels of prothrombotic agents (including tissue factor, fibrinogen, and thrombin), and decreased levels of antithrombotic agents (including antithrombin III, proteins C and S, and thrombomodulin) mean the VTE risk is particularly high in PDAC patients.
>
> **The evidence**
>
> Subcutaneous LMWHs allow anticoagulation without the need for monitoring and have become the standard treatment for VTE, and they appear to offer clinical benefit as prophylaxis in PDAC patients. The CONKO-004 trial demonstrated that concurrent administration of chemotherapy with LMWH (1 mg/kg of enoxaparin od for 3 months, then 40 mg od) prophylaxis led to a reduced incidence of symptomatic VTE at 3 months (1.25% versus 9.87%) and 12 months (5% versus 15.13%), with no significant increase in bleeding risk [4]. In the FRAGEM trial, advanced PDAC patients were randomized to gemcitabine alone or with daily dalteparin for 12 weeks [10]. The incidence of VTE was reduced both during the treatment period (23% versus 3.4%; $p = 0.002$) and beyond (28% versus 12%; $p = 0.039$). Despite these compelling data, LMWH is not routinely offered to this high-risk population. Reasons cited are that evidence is based on small, underpowered trials, patient reluctance to self-administer daily injections, and potential increased risk of bleeding in end-stage cancer. Further research to evaluate the role of LMWH and newer oral anticoagulants in palliating advanced PDAC is warranted.

The patient was informed of the new scan findings confirming metastatic disease. Surgical resection was therefore no longer an option, and his condition was now incurable. He was discharged home and reviewed in the oncology clinic the following week. At this appointment, he was no longer breathless at rest, was fatigued, but otherwise asymptomatic, with ECOG PS of 1. The oncologist explained that his life expectancy was now under 1 year, but palliative chemotherapy could be offered to maintain disease stabilization, possibly with modest survival benefits. In view of his general good level of fitness, combination chemotherapy with FOLFIRINOX (bolus and infusional 5-FU, folinic acid, irinotecan, and oxaliplatin) was offered as his best potential to extend his life. Owing to elevated liver enzymes, the irinotecan starting dose was reduced from 180 mg/m^2 to 135 mg/m^2 (Table 9.1).

Table 9.1 Chemotherapy prescribing in hepatic impairment

Regimen and cytotoxic	Dosing in normal hepatic function	Dosing in hepatic impairment	
		Bilirubin 1.5–3 times ULN or ALP >5 times ULN	Bilirubin >3 times ULN
FOLFIRINOX			
Oxaliplatin	85 mg/m^2	Continue 100% dose	Reduce dose by 50%
Irinotecan	180 mg/m^2	Reduce dose by 50%	Omit dose
5-FU	400 mg/m^2 bolus 2400 mg/m^2 over 46 hours	Continue 100% dose	Reduce dose by 50%
GEMCITABINE			
Gemcitabine	1000 mg/m^2	Limited information available—if bilirubin >1.5 times ULN, consider reducing to 75% dose	

During the first week of his first cycle of chemotherapy, the patient experienced significant diarrhoea and abdominal cramps, despite using regular loperamide. The 5-FU bolus was omitted with subsequent cycles, and the chemotherapy was then much better tolerated, with only mild diarrhoea occurring on days 2 and 3 of each cycle. A restaging CT scan after six cycles of FOLFIRINOX showed a partial response, with a reduction in size of the lung and liver lesions. Chemotherapy was continued, but the patient began complaining of cold-induced tingling of the fingertips during cycles 7 and 8. By cycle 9, the peripheral neuropathy had worsened, so that there was ongoing pain and numbness of the fingertips on both hands throughout the cycle.

The dose of oxaliplatin was reduced by 25% for subsequent cycles. However, during cycle 10, the patient presented to the ED with right upper quadrant pain, worsening jaundice, and fevers with rigors (Charcot's triad). An infection screen was performed, and he was given IV piperacillin/tazobactam within 1 hour of arrival for presumed biliary sepsis. His blood tests confirmed neutropenia, an obstructive pattern of LFTs, and a prolonged prothrombin time. He was admitted for IV fluids and antibiotics, and LMWH was discontinued to minimize the bleeding risk. Blood cultures grew *Escherichia coli* sensitive to piperacillin/tazobactam. Ultrasound imaging revealed intrahepatic biliary duct dilatation, consistent with obstruction. Seven days later, when the patient was well and no longer septic, an ERCP was undertaken. This confirmed a blocked plastic stent (with intraluminal sludge), which was removed and replaced with a metallic stent. The patient was discharged with a 1-week supply of oral ciprofloxacin.

✓ Evidence base FOLFIRINOX, compared with gemcitabine, in metastatic PDAC [3]

- Randomized Phase II/III study.
- A total of 342 chemotherapy-naïve metastatic PDAC patients, PS 0 or 1, randomized to either the 2-weekly combination regimen FOLFIRINOX (oxaliplatin 85 mg/m^2, irinotecan 180 mg/m^2, leucovorin 400 mg/m^2, and 5-FU bolus 400 mg/m^2, followed by 46-hour 5-FU infusion 2400 mg/m^2) or standard gemcitabine.
- The trial met its primary endpoint, in terms of OS (median 11.1 months for FOLFIRINOX versus 6.8 months for gemcitabine; $p < 0.001$).
- In addition, 12-month survival (48.4% versus 20.6%) and objective response rates (31.6% versus 9.4%) favoured FOLFIRINOX.
- Toxicities were generally higher in the FOLFIRINOX arm, particularly neutropenia, diarrhoea, and neuropathy. G-CSF was administered to 43% of patients on trial to offset the haematological toxicity associated with the regimen.

Source: data from Conroy T et al., FOLFIRINOX versus gemcitabine for metastatic pancreatic cancer, *New England Journal of Medicine*, Volume 364, Number 19 pp. 1817–25, Copyright © 2011 Massachusetts Medical Society. All rights reserved.

The patient returned to the oncology clinic 1 week later, when his ECOG PS had deteriorated to 3. He was requiring help with ADLs, due to paraesthesiae of both hands and discomfort in the balls of his feet as a result of oxaliplatin. His cancer was stable radiologically, but a decision was made to defer chemotherapy, in view of his symptomatic deterioration. Two months later, he became increasingly breathless on mild exertion, with a persistent dry cough. Serum CA19.9 was elevated at 150, and a CT scan revealed multiple new lung metastases, with further and extensive subsegmental PEs. Therapeutic-dose LMWH was restarted. The patient's PS later improved to 2, and further treatment options were discussed at clinic. These included single-agent gemcitabine chemotherapy or best supportive care. The patient was keen to be managed actively and therefore was prescribed gemcitabine chemotherapy at a modified dose of 800 mg/m^2, in view of abnormal liver blood tests (bilirubin 30,

❝ Expert comment

With the median survival of advanced PDAC being under 12 months, even with optimal chemotherapy, maintaining the QoL by avoiding drug-induced toxicity is really important. Oxaliplatin-induced peripheral neuropathy is insidious but needs to be acted upon promptly. Although reported to be reversible on stopping treatment, many patients may not recover sensation and function for many months, so a more prompt dose reduction would probably have been sensible for this patient.

ALP 189, aspartate aminotransferase (AST) 84). He tolerated this chemotherapy well, and, after cycle 3, reassessment by CT imaging demonstrated stable disease, with CA19.9 remaining stable at around 130. However, during cycle 4, he complained of increasing epigastric pain, anorexia, and further weight loss, suggesting clinical progression. On discussion with the patient, it was agreed to stop chemotherapy and concentrate on symptom control.

Over the next month, the patient experienced worsening epigastric pain, necessitating increasing levels of analgesia. He became increasingly troubled by early satiety and abdominal distension due to ascites. Arrangements were made for elective paracentesis, but the patient's condition deteriorated before admission, and he died at home, supported by the community nursing team.

Discussion

This case demonstrates several of the challenges associated with the management of PDAC and its complications. The diagnosis of PDAC is difficult and often delayed, as patients generally present with non-specific symptoms. Evidence suggests that patients diagnosed with PDAC have attended their GP on several occasions in the previous year, complaining of symptoms attributable to GI disturbance. Persistent, unexplained symptoms, especially epigastric pain and weight loss, warrant investigation, and people presenting with clinical or biochemical features suggestive of PDAC should be referred under the 2-week wait in the UK (or an appropriate local alternative scheme) to ensure rapid assessment and definitive diagnosis. Clinical prognostic factors suggesting poor outcome include advanced disease at diagnosis, poor PS, and high serum CA19.9 tumour marker (>59 times the ULN). For those patients undergoing surgical resection, the 5-year survival rate is around 20% at best. Poor prognostic features include incomplete (R1) resection (tumour at the surgical margin), perineural or vascular invasion, and lymph node involvement.

Decisions regarding diagnosis and treatment should involve multidisciplinary specialist groups, offering a regional service where surgery is centralized. Curative surgery involves Whipple resection (pancreatico-duodenectomy) or distal pancreatectomy. Involvement of major vessels adjacent to the pancreas frequently prohibits surgery. However, some locally advanced tumours are now classified as 'borderline resectable', due to increasing employment of vascular resection and grafts, and neoadjuvant strategies are now being tested to try to downstage these tumours and improve resection rates. Adjuvant chemotherapy after resection of PDAC has been shown to improve survival rates [13,14]. The role of radiotherapy is controversial, however, and European trials do not support the use of radiotherapy in the adjuvant setting [13]. There is conflicting evidence on its utility in locally advanced disease, although, when used, generally it is recommended that it is administered following a period of induction chemotherapy, during which time occult metastatic disease may become clinically apparent [7,15].

In the presence of locally advanced disease or distant metastases, treatment is palliative, with consideration given to the patient's QoL as well as the potential for longevity. PDAC patients are frequently highly symptomatic from their disease, and their management can be complex, with palliative care clinicians and dieticians playing a major role in patient support. For many years, the standard chemotherapy for advanced PDAC has been gemcitabine monotherapy, due to a favourable 1-year survival rate (18% versus 2%) and objective improvement of clinical benefit response when compared with bolus 5-FU [1]. The addition of other cytotoxics or molecularly targeted biological agents to gemcitabine have generally proved disappointing. A single trial combining the EGFR TKI erlotonib with gemcitabine reported a statistically significant survival gain [11], but the modest duration of benefit—10 days—is generally not thought to be clinically meaningful.

⊘ Evidence base Weekly gemcitabine chemotherapy in 5-FU-refractory PDAC [17]

- This phase II trial examined the effect of weekly gemcitabine in patients with advanced PDAC who had progressed on 5-FU (then the standard of care).
- A total of 63 patients deemed 5-FU-refractory were treated with gemcitabine, with 17 patients (23%) experiencing a clinical benefit response (a composite outcome taking into account pain scores, weight, and PS) and a median survival for all patients of 3.85 months.
- This trial demonstrated significant activity of gemcitabine in 5-FU-refractory patients, who previously had no established treatment options.

Source: data from Rothenberg M L et al., A phase II trial of gemcitabine in patients with 5-FU-refractory pancreas cancer, *Annals of Oncology*, Volume 7, Issue 4, pp. 347–53, Copyright © 1996 European Society for Medical Oncology.

⊘ Evidence base Gemcitabine, compared with 5-FU, in PDAC [1]

- This single-blinded phase III trial was performed in parallel with the study by Rothenberg *et al.* [17], and it randomized 126 patients with inoperable locally advanced or metastatic PDAC to receive either 1 g/m^2 of weekly gemcitabine or weekly 5-FU boluses.
- This trial demonstrated the superiority of gemcitabine over 5-FU in this setting, meeting its primary objective, in terms of clinical benefit response (23.8% versus 4.8%), and also demonstrating a difference in the 12-month survival rate (18% versus 2%) and median OS benefit (5.65 months versus 4.41 months).
- Following the publication of this trial, gemcitabine became the international standard of care in the treatment of inoperable PDAC and has since been the comparator for most PDAC therapy trials.

Source: data from Burris H A et al., Improvements in survival and clinical benefit with gemcitabine as first-line therapy for patients with advanced pancreas cancer: a randomized trial, *Journal of Clincial Oncology*, Volume 15, Number 6, pp. 2403–13, Copyright © 1997 American Society of Clinical Oncology.

Recently, however, two new combination chemotherapy regimens have reported convincing survival gains in a randomized controlled setting when compared with gemcitabine. The patient discussed here received the first of these combination regimens FOLFIRINOX which was tested by a French consortium in fit (PS 0 or 1) metastatic PDAC patients [3]. This trial demonstrated a dramatic improvement in OS, PFS, and response rate with FOLFIRINOX, compared with gemcitabine alone. However, associated significant toxicity means this regimen is unlikely to be suitable for a high proportion of PDAC patients. More recently, the international phase III MPACT study compared the nanoparticle albumin-bound (nab)-paclitaxel, combined with gemcitabine, with gemcitabine alone and reported a significant improvement in OS [19]. This combination is arguably less toxic than FOLFIRINOX, although these two regimens have not been compared directly.

Evidence base   Gemcitabine, with or without nab-paclitaxel, in metastatic PDAC [19]

- In this international multicentre trial, 861 metastatic PDAC patients, with ECOG PS 0–2, were randomized to either nab-paclitaxel plus gemcitabine or gemcitabine alone.
- Authors reported a median OS of 8.5 months versus 6.7 months, in favour of the combination regimen (HR 0.72; $p < 0.001$). The addition of nab-paclitaxel also improved the median PFS (5.5 months versus 3.7 months; HR 0.69; $p < 0.001$) and response rate (23% versus 7%; $p < 0.001$).
- The most frequently occurring toxicities were neutropenia, fatigue, and neuropathy.

Source: data from Von Hoff DD *et al.,* Increased survival in pancreatic cancer with nab-paclitaxel plus gemcitabine, *New England Journal of Medicine,* Volume 369, Number 18, pp. 1691–703, Copyright © 2013 Massachusetts Medical Society. All rights reserved.

Historically, few patients with PDAC remained well enough after progression post-first-line chemotherapy for consideration of further therapy for advanced disease. However, with improvements in early diagnosis of the disease and with potentially more active first-line chemotherapy becoming standard, there is likely to be an increasing demand for second-line treatment. Few second-line advanced PDAC trials have been conducted to date. Limited data with FOLFOX and single-agent capecitabine may justify their use in selected patients. Given the poor outcomes with even the most effective palliative chemotherapy regimens to date, there is great interest in interrogating the biology of PDAC further to identify novel targets for therapy.

Learning point   Understanding PDAC biology and new directions in systemic therapy

The commonest genetic abnormalities in PDAC include mutations in the notoriously 'undruggable' *K-ras* (over 95% of cases), as well as *TP53*, and deletions of *SMAD4* (*DPC3*) and *CDKN2A* (*p16*). Mutations in DNA repair genes, such as *BRCA2* and *PALB2*, and amplifications in *ERBB2* (*HER2/neu*) can also be observed [5]. Novel susceptibility targets in PDAC include stromal proteins [9], as the contribution of the dense, desmoplastic stroma with associated high interstitial fluid pressure is hypothesized to reduce the sensitivity of PDAC to cytotoxics. One such extracellular matrix target is secreted protein acidic and rich in cysteine (SPARC), of which the putative albumin-binding capacity has been proposed as a reason for selective targeting by nab-paclitaxel [20], although this has not been borne out in practice [12]. Other stromal targets being investigated to improve cytotoxic drug delivery include macromolecular components such as hyaluronan [8].

Signalling pathways implicated in pancreatic tumour biology include those regulated by transforming growth factor (TGF)-beta, NOTCH, and Hedgehog. Upregulation of inflammatory proteins by NF-kappa B, interleukin (IL)-6, and cyclo-oxygenase (COX)-2 are also proposed to contribute to PDAC progression. Immune strategies are therefore being evaluated, including targeting of immune tolerance observed in PDAC using T-cell activation checkpoint inhibitor antibodies such as anti-CTLA-4, anti-PD1, and anti-PDL1. The search for more informative PDAC models has led to the increasing use of genetically engineered mouse models [16], including the KPC mouse that is a *TP53* mutant with constitutively active *K-ras* within pancreatic progenitor cells [6], as well as primary patient-derived tumour xenografts (such as PancXenoBank) [20]. It is hoped that these models may allow novel target and biomarker discovery and provide a relevant platform for therapeutic preclinical studies, with the ultimate aims of developing new and individualized treatments.

A final word from the expert

PDAC carries an extremely poor prognosis; in the UK, it is the fourth commonest cause of death from cancer, and there are as many deaths recorded annually as new diagnoses, suggesting current treatment is woefully inadequate. PDAC is generally considered to be both chemo- and radioresistant, so early detection is critical to improving outcomes from this disease. However, the diagnosis is not straightforward, and robust screening tools are not currently available. Thus, surgical resection rates remain below 20% worldwide.

Patients with inoperable PDAC fall into two camps: locally advanced (stage III) tumours without evidence of distant spread (accounting for around 20% of cases) and distantly metastatic (stage IV) PDAC. It is not entirely clear whether these groups are biologically different. There are some data to suggest genetic differences exist (e.g. differences in *SMAD4* and *DPC4* expression), but any significance, in terms of disease behaviour and response to treatment, is not clear. In the past, interventional clinical trials recruited both groups of patients, but nowadays trials are being designed to target specifically either stage III or IV disease.

For stage IV PDAC, two combination regimens—FOLFIRINOX and nab-paclitaxel plus gemcitabine—have now been shown to be more active than gemcitabine monotherapy, the previous international standard of care. Due to treatment-related toxicities, these regimens are suitable for fit patients only, who constitute around one-third of patients at best. More effective ways of managing less fit patients are urgently needed. Understanding the molecular biology of this disease may help to identify novel targeted approaches in the future. Alongside, and after, systemic therapy, supportive interventions, including pain control, nutrition, and psychosocial care, are essential to improve PDAC patient and carer QoL.

References

1. Burris HA, 3rd, Moore MJ, Andersen J *et al.* Improvements in survival and clinical benefit with gemcitabine as first-line therapy for patients with advanced pancreas cancer: a randomized trial. *Journal of Clinical Oncology* 1997; **15**(6): 2403–13.
2. Caraceni A, Portenoy RK. Pain management in patients with pancreatic carcinoma. *Cancer* 1996; **78**(3 Suppl): 639–53.
3. Conroy T, Desseigne F, Ychou M *et al.* FOLFIRINOX versus gemcitabine for metastatic pancreatic cancer *The New England Journal of Medicine* 2011; **364**(19): 1817–25.
4. Riess H, Pelzer U, Deutschinoff G *et al.* A prospective, randomized trial of chemotherapy with or without the low molecular weight heparin (LMWH) enoxaparin in patients (pts) with advanced pancreatic cancer (APC): Results of the CONKO 004 trial. *Journal of Clinical Oncology* 2009; **27**(18S): LBA4506.
5. Han H, Von Hoff DD. SnapShot: pancreatic cancer. *Cancer Cell* 2013; **23**(3): 424–e1.
6. Hingorani SR, Wang L, Multani AS *et al.* Trp53R172H and KrasG12D cooperate to promote chromosomal instability and widely metastatic pancreatic ductal adenocarcinoma in mice. *Cancer Cell* 2005; **7**(5): 469–83.
7. Huguet F, Andre T, Hammel P *et al.* Impact of chemoradiotherapy after disease control with chemotherapy in locally advanced pancreatic adenocarcinoma in GERCOR phase II and III studies. *Journal of Clinical Oncology* 2007; **25**(3): 326–31.
8. Jacobetz MA, Chan DS, Neesse A *et al.* Hyaluronan impairs vascular function and drug delivery in a mouse model of pancreatic cancer. *Gut* 2013; **62**(1): 112–20.

9. Lunardi S, Muschel RJ, Brunner TB. The stromal compartments in pancreatic cancer: are there any therapeutic targets? *Cancer Letters* 2014; **343**(2): 147–55.

10. Maraveyas A, Waters J, Roy R *et al.* Gemcitabine versus gemcitabine plus dalteparin thromboprophylaxis in pancreatic cancer. *European Journal of Cancer* 2012; **48**(9); 1283–92.

11. Moore MJ, Goldstein D, Hamm J *et al.* Erlotinib plus gemcitabine compared with gemcitabine alone in patients with advanced pancreatic cancer: a phase III trial of the National Cancer Institute of Canada Clinical Trials Group. *Journal of Clinical Oncology* 2007; **25**(15): 1960–6.

12. Hidalgo M, Plaza C, Illei P *et al.* SPARC analysis in the phase III MPACT trial of nab-paclitaxel (nab-p) plus gemcitabine (gem) vs gem alone for patients with metastatic pancreatic cancer. *Ann Oncol* 2014; 25 (suppl 2): ii105-ii117.

13. Neoptolemos JP, Stocken DD, Friess H *et al.* A randomized trial of chemoradiotherapy and chemotherapy after resection of pancreatic cancer. *The New England Journal of Medicine* 2004; **350**(12): 1200–10.

14. Oettle H, Post S, Neuhaus P *et al.* Adjuvant chemotherapy with gemcitabine vs observation in patients undergoing curative-intent resection of pancreatic cancer: a randomized controlled trial. *JAMA* 2007; **297**(3): 267–77.

15. Hammel P, Huguet F, Van Laethem J-L *et al.* Comparison of chemoradiotherapy (CRT) and chemotherapy (CT) in patients with a locally advanced pancreatic cancer (LAPC) controlled after 4 months of gemcitabine with or without erlotinib: Final results of the international phase III LAP 07 study. *Journal of Clinical Oncology* 2013; **31**(Suppl): LBA4003.

16. Perez-Mancera PA, Guerra C, Barbacid M, Tuveson DA. What we have learned about pancreatic cancer from mouse models. *Gastroenterology* 2012; **142**(5): 1079–92.

17. Rothenberg ML, Moore MJ, Cripps MC *et al.* A phase II trial of gemcitabine in patients with 5-FU-refractory pancreas cancer. *Annals of Oncology* 1996; **7**(4): 347–53.

18. Varadhachary GR, Tamm EP, Abbruzzese JL *et al.* Borderline resectable pancreatic cancer: definitions, management, and role of preoperative therapy. *Annals of Surgical Oncology* 2006; **13**(8): 1035–46.

19. Von Hoff DD, Ervin T, Arena FP *et al.* Increased survival in pancreatic cancer with nab-paclitaxel plus gemcitabine. *The New England Journal of Medicine* 2013; **369**(18): 1691–703.

20. Von Hoff DD, Ramanathan RK, Borad MJ *et al.* Gemcitabine plus nab-paclitaxel is an active regimen in patients with advanced pancreatic cancer: a phase I/II trial. *Journal of Clinical Oncology* 2011; **29**(34): 4548–54.

21. Ziske C, Schlie C, Gorschluter M *et al.* Prognostic value of CA 19-9 levels in patients with inoperable adenocarcinoma of the pancreas treated with gemcitabine. *British Journal of Cancer* 2003; **89**(8): 1413–17.

10 Hepatocellular cancer and venous thromboembolism

Hannah Taylor

✦ **Expert commentary** Paul Kooner

Case history

A 45-year-old lady with known alcohol dependency and liver cirrhosis was under regular review with her local gastroenterology clinic. Due to her cirrhosis, she was deemed to be in a high-risk group for developing hepatocellular carcinoma (HCC), and surveillance with 6-monthly liver ultrasonography and AFP was recommended. On her most recent USS, two well-circumscribed hypoechoic masses were demonstrated, measuring 4 cm × 3 cm and 2 cm × 2.5 cm.

She was recalled to the clinic and was asymptomatic. She reported that she had been abstinent from alcohol for 9 months. A review of her past medical history revealed generalized anxiety disorder and depression. She had one previous admission with alcoholic hepatitis and ascites, which was now diuretic-controlled. Her medication history included thiamine, vitamin B Co-strong, spironolactone, and sertraline. On clinical examination, there was a palpable liver edge, but no ascites or encephalopathy. Her Child–Pugh score was B.

> ✪ **Learning point** HCC—setting the scene
>
> In the UK, HCC is the eighteenth commonest malignancy, accounting for 1% of cancers. In 2009, there were 3960 new cases, with a male to female ratio of 17:10 [1]. Incidence in the UK is increasing, due to rising alcohol consumption and an increase in hepatitis B and C infection. Worldwide, HCC is the sixth commonest malignancy, being most prevalent in areas of endemic hepatitis B infection such as South East Asia.
>
> Prognosis in untreated HCC is poor, with a 5-year survival of 3% and a median survival of 1–8 months. At presentation, only 20% of patients qualify for surgery, with the remainder of patients having advanced disease or inadequate hepatic function that renders them ineligible for radical treatment. In these cases, when the disease is still confined to the liver, palliative locoregional therapies focus on disease control, with 5-year survival rates of between 35% and 75% in selected patients. For patients with disease that has spread beyond the liver, outcomes are poor. Despite treatment with systemic therapies, the median OS in these patients is in the range of 8–10 months.

> ⊕ **Clinical tip** Role of AFP in HCC
>
> - AFP is the most commonly used tumour marker in the diagnosis and surveillance of HCC, although dynamic imaging is now the favoured approach.
> - It is a plasma protein produced by the fetal liver and yolk sac during development.
> - It can be elevated in normal pregnancy, liver cirrhosis, and certain malignancies (HCCs, non-seminomatous germ cell tumours, and some upper GI cancers).
> - The normal range for AFP is 10–20 ng/mL.
> - Steadily rising AFP levels, or an AFP level above 400 ng/mL, are usually considered diagnostic for HCC in patients with a suspicious liver lesion.
> - Up to 20% of HCCs do not produce AFP.
> - 60% of HCC of <4 cm in diameter are associated with an AFP level of under 200 ng/mL [2].

ⓖ Expert comment

AFP is the most widely used biomarker for HCC; however, it has been removed from the most recent surveillance guidelines, due to its variability and poor negative predictive value. It is more useful as a diagnostic test in the presence of a nodule. When combined with USS surveillance, AFP testing is only likely to detect an additional 6–8%. Only a small proportion of early HCCs of between 10 and 20% will secrete AFP. In addition, elevations in serum AFP levels are recognized during biochemical flares of viral hepatitis B and C.

✪ Learning point Diagnosis of HCC

Early detection is vital, as only 20% of new cases are amenable to curative treatment. The need for early detection, along with the identification of a high-risk group of patients, has led to the development of screening in this high-risk population with 6-monthly liver ultrasonography [3].

In a patient with cirrhosis, the presence of a focal lesion of >1 cm has a high chance of being HCC. Patients should be referred to a regional hepatobiliary MDT and should have specialist imaging with 4-phase multidetector CT or dynamic contrast-enhanced MRI with liver-specific contrast (Primovist®) to assess local disease, and a CT of the chest to look for metastatic spread.

The radiological hallmark of HCC is a lesion which is hypervascular in the arterial phase, with washout in the portal venous or delayed phases [3] (Figure 10.1). Single-modality dynamic imaging is sufficient to diagnose HCC in the majority of cases, with no further diagnostic investigations being required. Contrast-enhanced USS is gaining popularity in Europe and is useful for characterizing single nodules.

Biopsy of the lesion is rarely required. Biopsy is associated with the risk of cancer seeding and should only be performed in selected inoperable cases where there is a high degree of diagnostic uncertainty, and only at the request of a specialized hepatobiliary MDT.

One area where uncertainty is often encountered is in patients with cirrhosis and a nodule under 1 cm. Nodules under 1 cm rarely represent HCCs; however, they are known to progress from a regenerative phenotype, through a dysplastic phenotype, to a malignant phenotype, and so surveillance is required. The European Association for the Study of the Liver (EASL) surveillance guidelines recommend liver ultrasonography every 3 months in these cases, proceeding to further investigations if the lesion is enlarging [3].

ⓖ Expert comment

When patients present with symptoms of HCC, it is usually at an advanced stage and not amenable to active treatment. Many patients therefore present with their cirrhosis at the time of presentation with their HCC. All patients with cirrhosis should be considered for HCC surveillance, with USS surveillance at least 6-monthly, as the annual incidence is between 1% and 8% per year. In contrast to the UK, in Japan, 80% of HCCs are detected during surveillance, which offers a greater opportunity for curative treatments and longer survival.

In this patient's case, it was unfortunate that, despite 6-monthly surveillance, her HCC was not detected at an early stage and that further investigations were triggered by a rising AFP.

A serum AFP measurement taken in the clinic was 150 ng/mL. An urgent out-patient 4-phase CT CAP scan was requested and showed a 4 cm × 3.5 cm mass in the left lobe of the liver and a 2.4 cm × 2 cm mass in the right lobe of the liver. The masses were of low attenuation on non-contrast images and enhanced with IV contrast. On 4-phase multidetector CT, both lesions were hypervascular in the arterial phase. In the later portal phase, the hypervascularity 'washed out', relative to the background liver. There was no evidence of distant spread. Given her liver cirrhosis, the CT appearances were considered diagnostic of HCC. A biopsy of the lesion was not required.

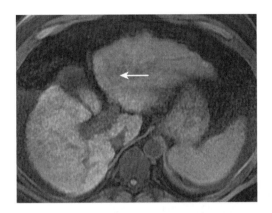

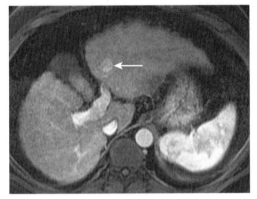

Figure 10.1 Gradient echo T1-weighted fat saturation pre-gadolinium axial image (top image) shows a faint mass (arrow) in a cirrhotic liver. This mass shows hyperenhancement on the late arterial phase (middle image) and hypoenhancement relative to liver parenchyma on the delayed phase (bottom image). The finding of a mass with arterial phase hyperenhancement and either later-phase hypoenhancement relative to liver (washout) or growth more than 1 cm in one year is sufficiently specific to be generally considered diagnostic for hepatocelluar carcinoma without biopsy for lesions larger than 2 cm. Additional features that suggest malignancy include a pseudocapsule surrounding the mass; mild to moderate hyperintensity on T2-ighted images; and reduced diffusion on diffusion weighted images.

Reproduced from Angela D. Levy et al. (Ed), *Gastrointestinal Imaging Cases*, Case 96, pp. 205–206, Oxford University Press, New York, USA, Copyright © 2013, by permission of Oxford University Press USA.

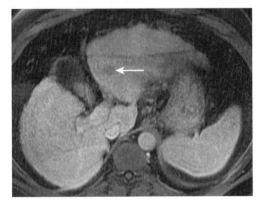

> ⭐ **Learning point** Staging of HCC
>
> HCCs are staged using the Barcelona-Clinic Liver Cancer (BCLC) classification (Figure 10.2). The classification separates patients into five groups that determine both the prognosis and treatment, taking into account the size and number of lesions, the presence of vascular invasion, and the presence of nodal involvement or distant metastatic spread. The liver function (assessed using the Child–Pugh scoring system), the presence of portal hypertension, and the performance status test are also taken into consideration.

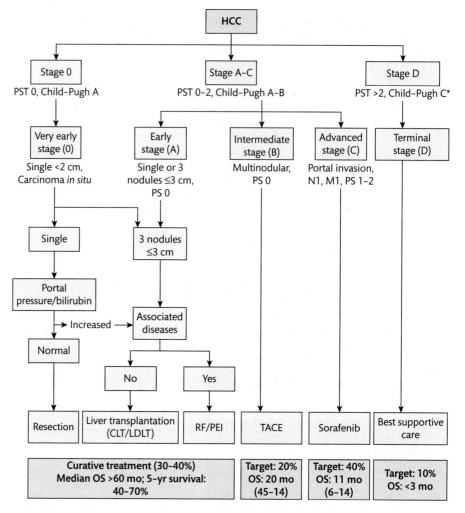

Figure 10.2 The BCLC classification.

Reproduced with permission from Llovet, J.M. *et al.*, The Barcelona Approach: Diagnosis, Staging, and Treatment of Hepatocellular Carcinoma, *Liver Transplantation*, Volume 10, Issue S2, pp. S115–120, Copyright © Wiley and Sons, Ltd.

⭐ **Learning point** Surgical management of HCC

Surgery, through liver transplantation or liver resection, is considered the only curative treatment approach in HCC. Studies have demonstrated 5-year survival rates of over 70% with surgical treatments [4].

Resection is appropriate if the tumour can be completely excised, with sufficient liver parenchyma remaining to sustain hepatic function. Resection can be an option for patients with cirrhosis and well-preserved liver function (Child–Pugh A), although the procedure carries an increased risk of post-operative hepatic decompensation. Absolute contraindications for resection are poor hepatic function of the liver remnant, extra-hepatic spread, and tumour thrombus extending into the major vessels.

Patients deemed inappropriate for resection should be considered for transplantation, provided they are felt to be suitable candidates. This was originally defined through the Milan criteria but has been superseded in the UK by the 2008 UK Transplant Criteria [5]. The criteria are set in order to identify

(continued)

patients who have a >50% chance of being alive at 5 years post-transplantation. Patients must not be considered suitable for resection and must fulfil one of the following criteria:

- a single lesion of <5 cm
- up to five tumours with diameters less than, or equal to, 3 cm
- a single tumour of 5–7 cm which shows no significant progression over 6 months (progression is defined as volume increase of >20%, extra-hepatic spread, or new nodule formation).

The last criterion recognizes that some larger lesions may progress slowly, reflecting biologically favourable disease. Absolute contraindications to transplantation include AFP >10 000, tumour rupture, macrovascular invasion, and extra-hepatic spread. Transplantation will be considered for patients with alcoholic liver disease if they have been abstinent from alcohol for at least 3 months.

Patients who are candidates for transplantation go through a lengthy work-up process, before they are placed on the UK liver transplantation waiting list. It has been shown that a wait of >6–12 months can result in increased dropout rates due to tumour progression; there is therefore a role for locoregional bridging therapies. In the UK, patients receive trans-arterial embolization, if their liver function allows, in order to reduce the risk of progression and dropout. Some patients may fail to meet the transplant criteria by a small margin; in these cases, downsizing of the tumour through locoregional treatment is not recommended, except in the context of clinical trials [3].

Her case was discussed at the hepatobiliary MDT meeting. Using the BCLC staging classification, the patient had intermediate-stage disease. The recommendation of the MDT was therefore palliative treatment with trans-arterial chemo-embolization (TACE). The patient was quoted a complication rate of 5%, with a mortality rate of 1%; she elected to proceed with treatment.

⊗ **Learning point** Locoregional therapies in the management of HCC

For patients not considered surgical candidates, management is aimed at disease control, using locoregional therapies such as chemo-embolization or ablative therapies. For patients with early-stage disease (BCLC A), this should be through ablative therapies; for patients with intermediate disease (BCLC B), this should be through TACE [3].

The most commonly used ablative techniques are percutaneous ethanol injection (PEI) and radiofrequency ablation (RFA). Ablative techniques are best suited for tumours of <3 cm which are located peripherally. In a study of cirrhotic patients (Child–Pugh A), the 3-year survival rates were 79% with transplantation, 71% with PEI, and 26% untreated [6]. With regard to long-term outcomes, RFA is felt to be at least as comparable as, but in all likelihood more effective than, PEI. RCTs comparing PEI and RFA are required; however, a non-randomized prospective study in small HCCs (<3 cm) found that PEI had a complete tumour necrosis rate of 80%, as opposed to 90% with RFA [7]. In addition, PEI required more treatment sessions (4.8 versus 1.2). On the basis of these and other similar results, RFA is now generally considered the primary ablative therapy. PEI remains a useful option for small lesions in locations that are difficult to treat with RFA, e.g. close to the heart or high in the liver under the dome of the diaphragm.

When treating small tumours with either RFA or PEI, some patients may be cured; this is not the case with larger tumours. When tumours of over 3 cm are treated with PEI, recurrence occurs in over half of cases, and only 10% of lesions are able to be completely ablated [8]. Using multi-tipped probes, RFA is able to treat tumours of up to 6 cm. Long-term follow-up data are absent, but studies have shown complete ablation rates of 47% in larger tumours [9]. Microwave ablation is a more recent ablative technique that is gaining popularity, although, in the UK, it is still considered to be under investigation and is not recommended as standard of care [3]. It has the advantage of not being affected by vessels in the vicinity of the tumour.

TACE is the primary therapy in intermediate-stage HCC, i.e. multifocal disease contained within the liver. It has been shown to cause tumour shrinkage as well as improve liver pain and bleeding; however, no OS benefit has been demonstrated. Studies comparing TACE and RFA in patients with inoperable HCC, when both treatments are considered appropriate, have found them to be comparable, in terms of time to progression and OS. The combination of TACE and RFA for lesions of between 3 and 5 cm has been shown to improve local control and increase survival [10].

The patient was admitted to the gastroenterology ward for chemo-embolization. On admission, she remained clinically stable, with a PS of 1 and liver function of Child–Pugh class B. Chemo-embolization was performed in the interventional radiology department, without complication, and the patient returned to the ward. She had an overnight stay, with minimal post-embolectomy syndrome.

> ### ✪ Learning point What is TACE?
>
> - Normal liver parenchyma has a dual blood supply, being supplied by the PV and the hepatic artery. TACE exploits the preference of HCCs to be supplied by the hepatic artery, allowing the arterial supply of the tumour to be targeted, whilst minimizing the effect on normal liver tissue.
> - Prior to TACE, patients should be adequately hydrated and receive antibiotic prophylaxis.
> - For the procedure, the patient is conscious. A catheter is inserted into the femoral artery and passed up into the hepatic artery under image guidance. Contrast is injected to identify the tumour vasculature and enable the catheter to be placed in the branch of the hepatic artery that supplies the tumour. A chemotherapeutic agent is then injected, followed by an embolization agent to block the artery.
> - The effects of TACE on the tumour are 2-fold. There is the direct anti-tumour activity of the chemotherapy, enhanced by the increased contact time with the tumour also due to reduced chemotherapy washout post-embolization. The embolization itself results in an ischaemic insult to the tumour due to the interruption of the tumour blood supply.
> - The current standard of care is embolization with drug-eluting 'DC beads' where the chemotherapeutic agent is doxorubicin. Fewer adverse systemic effects are seen with drug-eluting beads, compared with traditional TACE [11].
> - Repeat embolizations are commonly performed at 2- to 3-monthly intervals.
> - TACE has a low morbidity, but complications, when they occur, can be serious. The risk of death is approximately 1%, with a 3–5% risk of major complications which include thrombosis or perforation of the hepatic artery, non-target embolization resulting in gastric ulceration, pancreatitis, or cholecystitis, hepatic and non-hepatic abscesses, sepsis, and hepatic decompensation [12].
> - Post-embolization syndrome can occur in up to 90% of patients and is characterized by fever, right upper quadrant pain, malaise, nausea, and vomiting. The severity is variable, and the duration can be anything from 24 hours to over 7 days.
> - Systemic side effects of the chemotherapeutic agent, such as myelosuppression and alopecia, can be seen.
> - Future standards of care may include the combination of chemo-embolization with anti-angiogenic factors such as bevacizumab [13].
> - Trials are under way to see if the addition of sorafenib to embolization offers benefit [14].

> ### ✪ Learning point What is RFA?
>
> - RFA uses high-frequency alternating current to create heat within the tumour and cause coagulation necrosis.
> - A needle probe, with an insulated shaft and non-insulated tip, is inserted percutaneously into the tumour under image guidance.
> - Probes can be single-tipped for ablation of small lesions or multi-tipped for use in larger lesions.
> - Using grounding pads, placed onto the patient's back or thigh muscles, an electrical circuit is created.
> - RFA can be administered on an outpatient basis, without the need for a general anaesthetic. An average session takes 10–30 min; local anaesthetic is administered, along with a sedating agent such as midazolam.
> - The major complication rate for RFA is 2–3%, with a mortality rate of 0.1–0.5% [15].
> - Complications include sepsis, hepatic decompensation, intraperitoneal bleeding, hepatic abscess, bile duct injury, and grounding pad burns.

A CT scan 4 weeks post-treatment showed a good response to chemo-embolization, with partial devascularization in both lesions. The patient underwent TACE at 3-monthly intervals for a further three treatments. She was kept under regular review in the gastroenterology clinic and with 3-monthly CT imaging.

At her 18-month follow-up, the surveillance CT scan unfortunately showed progression of the cancer beyond the liver with multiple lung metastases. Despite this, she remained PS 1, with a Child–Pugh score B. She was commenced on the small molecule multikinase inhibitor sorafenib. Sorafenib is an oral tablet where two tablets are taken twice daily until progression. The patients tolerated the medication well, with only a grade 1 hand–foot skin reaction. Her 21-month scan showed stable disease.

> **✪ Learning point** Systemic therapies in advanced HCC
>
> Systemic chemotherapy has a very limited role in the treatment of advanced HCC. The most commonly used drug is single-agent doxorubicin. Response rates are low (in the order of 10%), and, despite multiple studies, no survival benefit has been demonstrated [16]. Combination regimes, such as PIAF (cisplatin, interferon (IFN)-alpha, doxorubicin, and 5-FU), have shown response rates in the range of 20%; however, even in good PS patients, toxicity rates are higher, and any gain in median OS has not been shown to be statistically significant [16].
>
> Sorafenib is a small molecule multikinase inhibitor, of which targets include the Raf kinase cascade, the VEGFR, and the platelet-derived growth factor receptor (PDGFR). It was licensed in the UK for use in advanced HCC in 2007, after studies demonstrated a 3-month increase in median survival and time to radiological progression with sorafenib, compared to placebo [17]. The cost of sorafenib is approximately £3000 per month; in 2009, NICE decided not to approve sorafenib for patients with advanced HCC, on the grounds that it was not a cost-effective use of National Health Service (NHS) resources. As a result, sorafenib is only available in the UK on an individually funded basis.

> **⊘ Evidence base** The SHARP trial: sorafenib in advanced HCC [17]
>
> - A total of 602 patients with advanced HCC randomized to sorafenib or placebo until progression; cross-over was not permitted in this randomized, double-blind, placebo-controlled phase III trial.
> - Planned interim analysis found a median OS of 10.7 months in the sorafenib group, compared to 7.9 months in the placebo group (HR in the sorafenib group 0.69, 95% CI 0.55–0.87; $p <0.001$).
> - No difference in time to symptomatic progression between the two groups.
> - Time to radiological progression 5.5 months in the sorafenib arm, and 2.8 months in the placebo arm ($p <0.001$).
> - Radiological response rates were low, with no complete responses in either group, and only 2% and 1% of patients having a partial response in the sorafenib and placebo groups, respectively.
> - Adverse events were more frequent in the sorafenib group but were generally mild to moderate in severity, and discontinuation rates were comparable between the two arms.
> - The commonest grade 3 events were hand–foot skin reaction and diarrhoea, both of which occurred in 8% of patients in the sorafenib group.
> - The findings of the SHARP trial were reproduced in 2009 in an Asia-Pacific population. This randomized phase III study found a median OS of 6.5 months with sorafenib versus 4.2 months with placebo [18].
> - Taken together, these trials are the strongest evidence yet seen for any treatment in advanced HCC.
>
> *Source:* data from Josep M. Llovet *et al.*, Sorafenib in Advanced Hepatocellular Carcinoma, *New England Medical Journal*, Volume 359, Number 4, pp. 378–390, Copyright © 2008 Massachusetts Medical Society. All rights reserved.

At her 2-year follow-up, she reported malaise, fevers, and upper abdominal pain. Observations revealed oxygen saturations of 92% on air, a temperature of 37.8°C, and a pulse rate of 120 bpm. On examination, she had jaundiced sclerae and was tender in the right upper quadrant, with shifting dullness. She was admitted to the gastroenterology ward for further investigation. Her LFTs on admission showed bilirubin 70, ALT 220, international normalized ratio (INR) 2.1, and albumin 29. A contrast-enhanced CT CAP scan was arranged which showed multiple new liver lesions, moderate ascites, progression of the lung nodules, and thrombosis of the portal vein. Serum AFP levels had increased to 18 000 ng/mL.

Expert comment

As cirrhosis advances, the production of clotting factors may decrease, leading to coagulopathy. Prothrombotic states are also recognized in cirrhotics. Thrombosis of the portal vasculature in the context of HCC may occur with vascular involvement. Anticoagulation must be considered with caution and using a multidisciplinary approach. Advanced cirrhotics may be sensitive to anticoagulants, including LMWH, and already may be auto-anticoagulating. Gastroscopy is recommended to survey for varices and assess the bleeding risk before anticoagulation.

⭐ Learning Point (Acute Oncology) VTE in malignancy

The annual incidence of VTE in cancer patients has been estimated at 1 in 200 [19]. Studies have suggested a 4-fold increase in the rate of VTE in cancer patients above that of the general population [19]. After adjusting for prevalence of cancers in the population, the neoplasms most commonly associated with VTE include advanced lung, brain, GU, and pancreatic cancers. A more advanced stage is associated with higher rates of VTE. Chemotherapy further increases the risk of VTE to 6.5-fold that of the non-cancer population [20], with the highest incidence seen with gemcitabine and platinum-containing regimes; the effect appears to be additive with gemcitabine plus cisplatin or carboplatin, resulting in the highest rates of VTE [21]. The mechanisms through which chemotherapy increases VTE risks are thought to include platelet activation, endothelial damage, and a reduction in coagulation inhibitors. Newer targeted anti-angiogenic agents carry their own risk of VTE; the use of the VEGF inhibitor bevacizumab is associated with a 33% increase in the incidence of VTE [21]. VTE prophylaxis for cancer patients receiving chemotherapy is not recommended [19].

The presence of VTE in a patient with cancer carries a worse prognosis. Studies have suggested that this cannot be attributed to fatal complications of VTE alone, as there also appears to be poorer prognosis with regard to the cancer [19]. Patients with symptomatic VTE have a lower response rate to chemotherapy and reduced PFS and OS; it seems likely that this reflects a more aggressive tumour biology.

✔ Evidence base The CLOT trial: treatment of symptomatic venous thromboembolism (VTE) in malignancy, assessing the role of warfarin versus dalteparin [22]

- A total of 676 patients were randomized to the traditional treatment of initial bridging with the LMWH dalteparin followed by conversion to the oral anticoagulant warfarin versus treatment with dalteparin alone.
- Results favoured dalteparin alone, with a RR reduction in recurrent VTE of 52% (HR 0.48; p = 0.002). The incidence of recurrent VTE was 17% in the oral anticoagulation arm, and 9% in the LMWH arm.
- No difference in bleeding events or mortality at 6 months between the two arms.
- The trial changed practice worldwide, with at least 6 months of LMWH becoming the new treatment standard for symptomatic VTE in patients with malignancy.
- HCC patients were not specifically excluded; however, the exclusion criteria of 'a platelet count less than 75 'and 'conditions associated with a high risk of serious bleeding 'would have led to many cirrhotic patients being ineligible.

⭐ Learning Point (Acute Oncology) Management of pulmonary embolic disease in cancer patients

Symptomatic PE in patients with cancer should be treated with full anticoagulation, as would be the case in the non-cancer patient. The CLOT trial suggests that the first 6 months of treatment should be with dalteparin (although this is often extrapolated to include any LMWH) [22]. Certainly, if patients are receiving chemotherapy, dalteparin is preferable to warfarin, due to the effects of chemotherapy on the INR. In the acute setting, patients should be considered for thrombolysis if they meet certain criteria, e.g. those with large PEs who are haemodynamically unstable or those with severe right heart strain. A vena cava filter should be considered for patients with recurrent VTE, despite adequate anticoagulation, or for those patients in whom anticoagulation is contraindicated.

(continued)

Anticoagulation should be continued whilst there is evidence of active malignant disease; this will mean indefinitely for patients with metastatic disease [19]. In patients on lifelong anticoagulation, dalteparin is preferred, although for those not receiving chemotherapy, a case can be made for the use of warfarin with respect to QoL.

The incidental detection of PE on CT imaging is commoner in patients with cancer than in the non-cancer population, due not only to the higher incidence of VTE in cancer patients, but also to the more frequent use of CT scans in these patients. Whether these patients benefit from full anticoagulation is a question that is under discussion. At present, guidelines recommend that incidental PEs should be treated with full anticoagulation.

Patients with HCC commonly have an underlying cirrhosis and therefore require special consideration with regard to anticoagulation. Patients often have low platelet counts, and the effect of LMWH can be potentiated. Haematology guidance is generally required, along with anti-factor Xa activity monitoring. As a result, LMWH is rarely used in patients with HCC and an underlying cirrhosis.

Due to her underlying liver dysfunction, the patient was not commenced on anticoagulation for her portal venous thrombosis. Her consultant arranged a time to meet with the patient and her family to go through the results of her CT scan. The consultant told them that the patient's cancer had progressed. She explained that further active treatment was likely to cause more harm than benefit and that the best course of action was to focus on controlling any symptoms the patient developed. The patient reported increasing abdominal discomfort, so her ascites was drained, with albumin replacement, and she was discharged to the care of her GP and the community palliative care team.

> ⊕ **Clinical tip** Colloid replacement in cirrhotic patients, following paracentesis
> - In patients with an underlying cirrhosis, the infusion of albumin, following paracentesis, remains controversial.
> - Current guidelines [23] recommend colloid replacement, only if the total amount of ascites drained is >5 L.
> - Replacement should be with 6–8 g of 20% human albumin solution, per litre of ascites drained.

Over the next 8 weeks, she was admitted electively to the ambulatory care unit for drainage of her ascites, with albumin replacement on three occasions. She remained in the community, with her symptoms well controlled, until her family reported that she had become drowsy and confused. Her GP visited her at home and found her to be encephalopathic and obtunded. It was not considered in her best interests to be admitted to hospital, as she had previously expressed a wish to die at home. Provision for end-of-life care was put in place, and she died 3 days later.

Discussion

Despite recent advances, HCC remains a disease where the majority of patients present with advanced unresectable disease. The key to improving outcomes lies in prevention and earlier diagnosis. Options for prevention include the treatment of active viral hepatitis. Earlier diagnosis may be achieved through the use of surveillance USS in high-risk patients. Advances in radiology, surgery, and oncology mean that patients are living longer and may experience multiple treatment modalities during the course of their disease. Now more than ever, the treatment of HCC requires a multidisciplinary approach.

A final word from the expert

This example highlights that the management of HCC necessitates the management of the complications of cirrhosis by each specialist. It also reflects the rising incidence and mortality from HCC, in addition to chronic liver disease, in the UK, due to rising levels of alcohol-related liver disease, viral hepatitis, and non-alcoholic fatty liver disease. Important lessons can be learned from programmes, such as the Japanese programme where the best survival is achieved by a national strategy, resulting in high engagement in surveillance and leading to early detection and the best chance of curative treatments.

References

1. Cancer Research UK. *Liver cancer incidence statistics.* Available at: <http://www.cancerresearchuk.org/cancer-info/cancerstats/types/liver/incidence/uk-liver-cancer-incidence-statistics>.
2. Alpert E. Human alpha-1 fetoprotein. In: Okuda K, Peters RL, eds. *Hepatocellular carcinoma.* New York: Wiley, 1976; pp. 353–67.
3. European Association For The Study Of The Liver, European Organisation for Research and Treatment of Cancer. EASL–EORTC clinical practice guidelines: management of hepatocellular carcinoma. *Journal of Hepatology* 2012; **56**(4): 908–43.
4. Llovet JM, Schwartz M, Mazzaferro V. Resection and liver transplantation for hepatocellular carcinoma. *Seminars in Liver Disease* 2005; **25**(2): 181–200.
5. Liver Advisory Group; on behalf of NHS Blood and Transplant. *Policy POL196/3. Deceased donor liver distribution and allocation.* Available at: <http://www.odt.nhs.uk/pdf/liver_allocation_policy.pdf>.
6. Livraghi T, Bolondi L, Buscarini L *et al.* No treatment, resection and ethanol injection in hepatocellular carcinoma: a retrospective analysis of survival in 391 patients with cirrhosis. Italian Cooperative HCC Study Group. *Journal of Hepatology* 1995; **22**(5): 522–6.
7. Livraghi T, Goldberg SN, Lazzaroni S, Meloni F, Solbiati L, Gazelle GS. Small hepatocellular carcinoma: treatment with radio-frequency ablation versus ethanol injection. *Radiology* 1999; **210**(3): 655–61.
8. Vilana R, Bruix J, Bru C, Ayuso C, Solé M, Rodés J. Tumor size determines the efficacy of percutaneous ethanol injection for the treatment of small hepatocellular carcinoma. *Hepatology* 1992; **16**(2): 353–7.
9. Livraghi T, Goldberg SN, Lazzaroni S *et al.* Hepatocellular carcinoma: radio-frequency ablation of medium and large lesions. *Radiology* 2000; **214**(3): 761–8.
10. Cheng BQ, Jia CQ, Liu CT *et al.* Chemoembolization combined with radiofrequency ablation for patients with hepatocellular carcinoma larger than 3 cm: a randomized controlled trial. *JAMA* 2008; **299**(14):1669–77.
11. Lammer J, Malagari K, Vogl T *et al.* Prospective randomized study of doxorubicin-eluting-bead embolization in the treatment of hepatocellular carcinoma: results of the PRECISION V study. *CardioVascular and Interventional Radiology* 2010; **33**(1): 41–52.
12. Clark TW. Complications of hepatic chemoembolization. *Seminars in Interventional Radiology* 2006; **23**(2): 119–25.
13. Buijs M, Reyes DK, Pawlik TM *et al.* Phase 2 trial of concurrent bevacizumab and transhepatic arterial chemoembolization in patients with unresectable hepatocellular carcinoma. *Cancer* 2013; **119**(5): 1042–9.
14. Lencioni R, Zou J, Leberre M *et al.* Sorafenib (SOR) or placebo (PL) in combination with transarterial chemoembolization (TACE) for intermediate-stage hepatocellular carcinoma (SPACE). *Journal of Clinical Oncology* 2010; **28**(15 Suppl): TPS178.

15. Rhim H. Complications of radiofrequency ablation in hepatocellular carcinoma. *Abdominal Imaging* 2005; **30**(4): 409–18.

16. Zhu AX. Systemic therapy of advanced hepatocellular carcinoma: how hopeful should we be? *The Oncologist* 2006; **11**(7): 790–800.

17. Llovet JM, Ricci S, Mazzaferro V *et al.* Sorafenib in advanced hepatocellular carcinoma. *The New England Journal of Medicine* 2008; **359**(4): 378–90.

18. Cheng AL, Kang YK, Chen Z *et al.* Efficacy and safety of sorafenib in patients in the Asia-Pacific region with advanced hepatocellular carcinoma: a phase III randomised, double-blind, placebo-controlled trial. *The Lancet Oncology* 2009; **10**(1): 25–34.

19. Mandalà M, Falanga A, Roila F; ESMO Guidelines Working Group. Management of venous thromboembolism (VTE) in cancer patients: ESMO Clinical Practice Guidelines. *Annals of Oncology* 2011; **22**(Suppl 6): vi85–92.

20. Lee AYY, Levine MN. Four topics in venous thromboembolism. Venous thromboembolism and cancer: risks and outcomes. *Circulation* 2003; **107**: I-17–I-21.

21. Barni S, Labianca R, Agnelli G *et al.* Chemotherapy-associated thromboembolic risk in cancer outpatients and effect of nadroparin thromboprophylaxis: results of a retrospective analysis of the PROTECHT study. *Journal of Translational Medicine* 2011; **9**: 179.

22. Lee AY, Levine MN, Baker RI *et al.* Low-molecular–weight heparin versus a coumarin for the prevention of recurrent venous thromboembolism in patients with cancer. *The New England Journal of Medicine* 2003; **349**(2): 146–53.

23. Runyon BA; AASLD. Introduction to the revised American Association for the Study of Liver Diseases Practice Guideline management of adult patients with ascites due to cirrhosis 2012. *Hepatology* 2013; **57**(4): 1651–3.

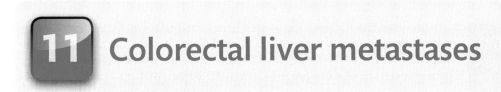

11 Colorectal liver metastases

Khurum Khan

Expert commentary Nick Maisey

Case history

A 63-year-old gentleman presented in August 2007 with a pT2N1M0 adenocarcinoma of the sigmoid colon and underwent an anterior resection, followed by eight cycles of adjuvant capecitabine and oxaliplatin. Following the completion of adjuvant treatment, a CT CAP scan confirmed that there was no evidence of residual disease, and the CEA was within the normal range. He was followed up with 6-monthly clinical reviews and measurements of CEA, as well as annual restaging CT CAP scans.

⊗ Learning point Classification of colorectal carcinoma

The TNM classification has superseded the older Dukes classification and is the current accepted standard system for clinical and pathological staging of colorectal carcinoma (CRC).

The prefix 'c' or 'p' is added to denote whether the staging is based on clinical or pathological criteria, and the prefix 'y' is added for those cancers that have undergone neoadjuvant treatment. For example, patients who achieve a complete pathologic response (CR) to neoadjuvant treatment are classified as ypT0N0cM0. The prefix 'r' can be used for those cancers that have recurred after a disease-free interval.

For patients with resectable CRC, site-specific prognostic markers include pretreatment CEA levels, the presence of perforation or obstruction, the status of the circumferential margin (CRM), the presence or absence of perineural and lymphovascular invasion, microsatellite instability (MSI) (prognostic as well as predictive), *BRAF* gene analysis, and tumour regression grade (for tumours undergoing neoadjuvant therapy). For patients with metastatic CRC (mCRC), *BRAF* mutation appears to confer a poor survival, whilst *K-ras* is predictive of the response to anti-EGFR therapy but does not appear to have any prognostic value.

⊕ Clinical tip Presentation of colon cancer

CRC typically remains asymptomatic in the majority of patients during early-stage disease. Symptoms depend on the location of the tumour and its growth into the lumen of the bowel or adjacent structures. Typical presenting symptoms include:

- abdominal pain
- change in bowel habit
- melaena
- weakness
- weight loss
- anaemia and related symptoms.

Occasionally, patients can present with bowel obstruction, peritoneal infiltration, and intestinal perforation [1]. Patients with distant metastatic disease can present with symptoms related to their site. Unusual presentations include malignant fistulae into the adjacent organs such as the bladder or small bowel, pyrexia of unknown origin due to intra-abdominal, retroperitoneal, or abdominal wall abscesses, or as a carcinoma of unknown primary (CUP). The presence of symptoms raising the clinical suspicion of CRC should prompt appropriate investigations, particularly colonoscopy and subsequent discussion by the MDT.

⊕ Expert comment

MSI is thought to be associated with the underlying pathogenesis of approximately 15% of sporadic colon cancers. The typical phenotype includes right-sided tumours, mucinous pathology, and female sex. Large retrospective reviews have demonstrated that fluoropyrimidine therapy is ineffective as adjuvant therapy and indeed may lead to a worse outcome in these patients, particularly in those with stage II disease. When considering the use of adjuvant therapy in patients with node-negative disease, it is therefore vital to assess the MSI status to inform the treatment decision.

Twenty-six months later, the patient complained of a 4-week history of loss of appetite, lethargy, and weight loss. Routine blood tests, including LFTs, were unremarkable. A CT CAP, however, identified extensive metastatic disease of the liver, with no evidence of extra-hepatic disease. Following MDT discussion, it was felt that the hepatic metastases were not amenable to upfront surgical resection, and the patient was offered four cycles of neoadjuvant chemotherapy with capecitabine, oxaliplatin (CAPOX), and cetuximab, following the molecular characterization of the original tumour which did not identify a *K-ras or N-ras activating* mutation.

The first cycle of treatment was delivered without complication. Four days after the second cycle, the patient developed severe diarrhoea and skin rash and attended the local ED. Initial examination was unremarkable, except for a maculopapular

---

★ Learning point Cetuximab molecular biology

Cetuximab is a chimeric mAb which competitively binds to the extracellular domain of EGFR. It works by blocking the phosphorylation and activation of the receptor tyrosine kinases and by inhibiting cell growth and proliferation [2].

EGFR is a glycoprotein, which belongs to the ErbB family, and remains in a state of inhibition in the absence of specific ligands, including epidermal growth factor (EGF) and TGF-alpha. Binding of these proteins leads to a cascade of events which then leads to the activation of downstream signalling pathways by the phosphorylation of tyrosine kinases in the EGFR intracellular domain (Figure 11.1) [3]. Cetuximab theoretically blocks these downstream events; mutations in downstream proteins (most notably *K-ras*) can, however, cause the constitutive activation of these pathways and resistance to EGFR blockade.

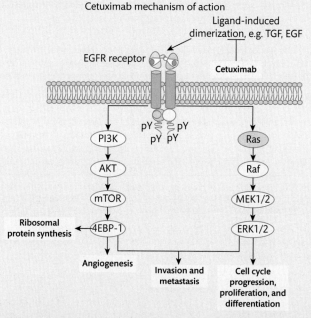

Figure 11.1 Schematic diagram of cetuximab-induced blockade of the EGFR signal transduction pathway. The EGFR belongs to one of the four members of ErbB family of receptor tyrosine kinases. It consists of an extracellular ligand-binding domain, a transmembrane domain, and an intracellular tyrosine kinase domain. Binding of a ligand-like TGF-alpha or EGF to EGFR causes receptor dimerization. This leads to receptor autophosphorylation, which results in the activation of downstream pathways by the signal transduction cascade involved in cell proliferation and survival. The two distinct pathways include the RAS–RAF–MEK–ERK pathway and the phosphoinositide 3-kinase–serine/threonine kinase (PI3K–AKT) pathway. Cetuximab blocks the binding of ligands to EGFR, thereby inhibiting the receptor phosphorylation and downstream events. mTOR, mammalian target of rapamycin; 4EBP-1, 4E-binding protein; MAPK, mitogen-activated protein kinase; TGF, transforming growth factor.

rash over the anterior chest and arms. The only abnormal blood tests were slightly deranged LFTs. Following discussion with the acute oncology team, it was agreed that the patient's presentation was secondary to treatment and that he did not require immediate hospital admission. Capecitabine was withheld, and the patient was advised to contact his oncology team the next day to discuss restarting the medication. He was given loperamide and was told to maintain a good fluid intake.

⊗ Learning point (Acute Oncology) Management of chemotherapy-induced diarrhoea

Diarrhoea is a common chemotherapy-induced complication, particularly associated with fluoropyrimidines, irinotecan, and raltitrexed, in the context of CRC treatment.

Prompt treatment of diarrhoea is required. Patients should be instructed to use loperamide when they experience:

- poorly formed or loose stool
- occurrence of more bowel movements than usual in 1 day, or
- unusually high volume of stool.

Loperamide should be deferred if blood or mucus is present in the stool or if diarrhoea is accompanied by fever. In this case, diagnostic microbiological specimens should be obtained to exclude an infectious aetiology.

Adequately controlled diarrhoea without complications, does not necessarily require dose modification. Diarrhoea, with complications, (moderate or severe abdominal pain, sepsis, neutropenia, dehydration, or frank bleeding), patients may require hospital admission, further investigations, intravenous fluids, antibiotics (such as oral ciprofloxacin) and consideration of s/c octreotide according to the severity of the symptoms [4].

❝ Expert comment

Prior to starting chemotherapy treatment, patients should always be asked whether they have a stoma and, if so what type. The faecal content of an ileostomy is significantly looser than that of a colostomy, and patients are therefore at increased risk of a high-output stoma, with subsequent pre-renal impairment and electrolyte imbalance. Due to the higher rate of grade 3/4 diarrhoea with capecitabine, infused 5-FU is the fluoropyrimidine of choice for a patients with an ileostomy. If diarrhoea is a problem, loperamide tablets should be used, in preference to loperamide capsules.

⊗ Learning point (Acute Oncology) Skin rash with cetuximab

Acne or acneiform eruptions are commonly seen with cetuximab. Dermatological complications are cosmetically distressing and may affect compliance. It is therefore important they are managed effectively.

Management

General measures include hydration of the skin using bath oil instead of gel or soap. Emollient creams can prevent dry skin. Effective sun barrier preparations are also important.

Grade 1 reactions can be treated with topical anti-acne agents such as clindamycin gel or lotion . Grade 2 reactions can additionally be managed with oral anti-histamines and oral tetracycline. If a patient experiences grade 3 skin toxicity (rash affecting >30% of the BSA), cetuximab can be interrupted for up to two consecutive infusions, with no change in the dose level. If the toxicity resolves to grade 2 or less (10–30% of the BSA), treatment is generally resumed.

With the second and/or third occurrence of grade 3 skin toxicity, cetuximab can again be interrupted for up to 2 consecutive weeks, with concomitant dose reductions. Dose reductions should be permanent.

With the fourth occurrence of grade 3 or 4 skin toxicity (>30% of the BSA associated with fluid or electrolyte abnormalities), the treatment should be discontinued.

Two days later, the patient called the cancer centre helpline, as the diarrhoea had worsened. He had also developed severe odynophagia and dysphagia, which was significantly limiting the oral intake of solids and liquids. The patient was advised to attend the emergency department where he was noted to be severely dehydrated. His BP was 90/60 mmHg, and clinical examination revealed grade 3 oral mucositis with grade 2 PPE. He was also found to have grade 2 peripheral neuropathy.

> **Expert comment**
>
> Long-term oxaliplatin-related peripheral neuropathy can be a cause of significant morbidity. Clinicians should pay very careful attention to the degree and duration of neuropathic symptoms during treatment and also be aware that, on some occasions, neuropathy may only become apparent, following the end of treatment. A low threshold should be adopted for oxaliplatin dose reduction or even cessation. This is particularly true in elderly patients receiving adjuvant oxaliplatin-based therapy where there are conflicting data regarding the benefit over single-agent fluoropyrimidine therapy and in whom peripheral neuropathy could have a very significant impact.

> **★ Learning point** Oxaliplatin-induced neuropathy
>
> Oxaliplatin is often associated with the development of peripheral neuropathy, which can be acute or chronic.
>
> *Acute neuropathy*: can present either as cold-related dysaesthesia or acute laryngeal dysaesthesia. The patients are advised to use preventative measures, including wearing gloves and a scarf when exposed to cold.
>
> *Chronic neuropathy*: is believed to be dose-dependent and appears to be associated with cumulative doses of oxaliplatin, generally appearing after approximately 3 months of oxaliplatin treatment. A number of international studies (including the UK-based SCOT study) are examining the optimal duration of adjuvant oxaliplatin-based chemotherapy, in an attempt to reduce the cumulative dose but maintain efficacy. A trial conducted by de Gramont and colleagues demonstrated that a dosing schedule, termed STOP and GO (OPTIMOX), could potentially reduce the risk of chronic peripheral neuropathy, whilst maintaining efficacy [5].
>
> Early dose reduction or discontinuation should be considered, depending upon the severity of neuropathy.
>
> *Prevention*: calcium/magnesium infusions were initially felt to be effective in preventing peripheral neuropathy in a retrospective study, but a recent phase III study unfortunately failed to validate these findings [6].
>
> *Treatment of established neuropathy*: drug treatment is largely ineffective, and management strategy includes early intervention with dose reduction or discontinuation.
>
> | Non-haematological toxicity | Grade 1 or 2 persisting <7 days | Grade 2 persisting >7 days | Grade 3 | Grade 4 |
> | --- | --- | --- | --- | --- |
> | Oxaliplatin-induced neurosensory toxicity | Full-dose oxaliplatin | Discontinue treatment until resolved to ≤ grade 1, and reduce dose by 25% for subsequent cycles | Discontinue oxaliplatin | Discontinue oxaliplatin |
>
> *Source*: data from David Brighton and Miriam Wood, *The Royal Marsden Hospital Handbook of Cancer Chemotherapy: A Guide for the Multidisciplinary Team*, Churchill Livingston, Copyright © 2005 Elsevier.

> **⊕ Clinical tip** Chemotherapy-induced peripheral neuropathy
>
> Chemotherapy-induced peripheral neuropathy can affect an estimated 30–40% of patients. The drugs which are common culprits are the platinum agents, taxanes, and vinca alkaloids. Other drugs include thalidomide, bortezomib, and IFN-alpha.

Initially, the gentleman was given intravenous hydration, along with anti-diarrhoeal therapy, mouthwashes, oral fluconazole, and topical moisturizers. Despite this, he continued to clinically deteriorate, ultimately requiring inotropic support to maintain his BP on the intensive care unit (ICU). He eventually recovered and was discharged from the ICU on day 10.

Despite his previous tolerance of capecitabine in the adjuvant setting, it was decided to test for dihydropyrimidine dehydrogenase deficiency (DPD) which was not found to be present. Following a full recovery, a decision was made to continue neoadjuvant therapy with a 25% dose reduction of capecitabine.

Reassessment scans after completion of chemotherapy showed a partial response to the treatment, with almost complete resolution of the hepatic metastatic disease

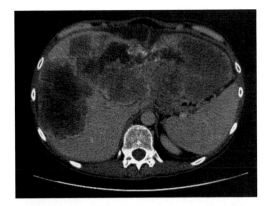

Figure 11.2 CT scan of the patient prior to treatment.

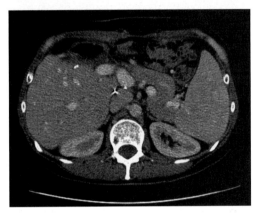

Figure 11.3 CT scan after resection of the liver metastases.

> ⊕ **Clinical tip** DPD deficiency
>
> DPD deficiency is an autosomal recessive metabolic condition, with an absent or decreased activity of the DPD enzyme, which is involved in the metabolism of uracil and thymine. It is also a critical enzyme in the metabolism of fluoropyrimidines (including 5-FU, capecitabine, and tegafur), and thus a deficiency can cause significant toxicities. DPD deficiency can be associated with neurological, mucosal, and cardiac toxicities. Screening of DPD deficiency is not performed routinely but should be considered in patients experiencing severe toxicities [7].

(Figure 11.2 and Figure 11.3). He underwent successful resection of the metastatic disease with clear margins and remains on high risk follow-up, with no evidence of recurrence of his disease 3 years after the second surgery.

Discussion

This case highlights some of the commonly identified management problems associated with patients presenting with mCRC. Despite significant improvements in the screening and management of CRC, the 5-year survival rate for mCRC remains below 10%, and about 40–50% of patients develop mCRC during the course of their illness. Liver metastases are present in half of the patients with mCRC and contribute to two-thirds of the deaths in these patients [8].

When patients present with liver metastases, the two commonest scenarios include [10]:

- R0 resectable disease, and
- borderline or unresectable disease.

Clinical tip Criteria for operability

The optimal selection of patients for hepatic resection is evolving, and the criteria for resectability differ amongst individual liver surgeons. Absolute unresectability is defined as non-treatable extra-hepatic disease, unfitness for surgery, or involvement of >70% of the liver or six segments. For resection to be considered, there needs to be an absence of radiographic involvement of the hepatic artery, major bile ducts, main portal vein, or coeliac/para-aortic lymph nodes, and an adequate predicted functional hepatic reserve post-resection. Preoperative liver MRI and intraoperative ultrasound offer the optimal assessment of the number, size, and proximity of tumours to key vascular and biliary structures. Complete (R0) resection must be feasible. The primary tumour also needs to be resected for cure.

Evidence base Clinical risk scoring for adjuvant chemotherapy following hepatic resection [11]

- Retrospective review of 1001 patients after hepatic resection for mCRC.
- The 5-year and 10-year survival rates were 37% and 22%, respectively.
- Seven independent factors, including positive margins, extra-hepatic disease, node-positive primary, disease free survival (DFS) from primary to metastatic disease, number of hepatic tumours >1, largest tumour >5 cm, and CEA >200 ng/mL, were found to be predictors of poor survival.
- Patients with three, four, or five criteria (out of the last five factors) were recommended to be considered for adjuvant chemotherapy trials.

Source: data from Fong, Y. *et al.*, Clinical score for predicting recurrence after hepatic resection for metastatic colorectal cancer: analysis of 1001 consecutive cases, *Annals of Surgery*, Volume 230, Issue 3, pp. 309–18, Copyright © 1999 Lippincott Williams & Wilkins, Inc.

Role of chemotherapy in R0 resectable disease: neoadjuvant chemotherapy

Surgical resection is regarded as the standard of care for patients, but relapse is common. These patients can therefore be considered for neoadjuvant chemotherapy. Recent data, however, suggest that the initial advantage seen in progression free survival (PFS) for patients receiving additional systemic treatment may not actually translate into a meaningful overall survival (OS) advantage [12]. Its benefit for these patients therefore remains controversial.

Evidence base EORTC 40983: perioperative chemotherapy, compared with upfront surgery, for colorectal liver metastases [13]

- Randomized phase III trial.
- FOLFOX4 (5-FU/LV and oxaliplatin) six cycles before and six cycles after surgery (n = 182) versus upfront surgery alone (n = 182).
- Patients assigned to the chemotherapy arm had an overall response rate of 36%.
- 83% patients were resected after a median of six cycles of preoperative chemotherapy, compared to 84% in the surgery group.
- The improvement in PFS at 3 years for patients receiving neoadjuvant chemotherapy, in addition to surgery, was 9.2%.
- Reversible complications occurred more frequently in the chemotherapy group (25% versus 16%).
- No statistically significant difference was found in the OS between the two groups at 8.5 years of median follow-up.

Source: data from *The Lancet*, Volume 371, Issue 9617, Nordlinger, B. *et al.*, Perioperative chemotherapy with FOLFOX4 and surgery versus surgery alone for resectable liver metastases from colorectal cancer (EORTC Intergroup trial 40983): a randomised controlled trial, pp. 1007–16, Copyright © 2008 Elsevier Ltd. All rights reserved.

Adjuvant chemotherapy

Post-operative adjuvant chemotherapy has a well-defined role in high-risk patients with CRC; the data for adjuvant therapy in resected stage IV disease are limited. Two randomized phase III studies evaluated the role of adjuvant treatment in this setting, and their pooled analysis is summarized.

> ✪ **Learning point** Pooled analysis of adjuvant therapy trials in resected stage IV disease [14]
>
> - Pooled analysis of French FFCD [15] and EORTC trials ($n = 278$ patients).
> - Both trials used the 5-FU and leucovorin chemotherapy, administered for 5 days consecutively in a 4-week cycle for 6 months; both closed prematurely due to poor accrual.
> - Median DFS of 28 months versus 19 months ($p = 0.058$) and OS of 62 months versus 47 months were noted, in favour of chemotherapy ($p = 0.095$).
> - The improvement in DFS and OS was deemed statistically insignificant but could represent a clinically meaningful advantage.

> ✪ **Learning point** Management of unresectable hepatic metastatic disease using neoadjuvant chemotherapy (conversion chemotherapy)
>
> Only a minor subgroup of patients with colorectal liver metastases are able to undergo primary surgical resection. Induction chemotherapy has been used to downsize tumours, in an attempt to make the metastatic disease resectable. Earlier reports suggested that, with oxaliplatin-based chemotherapy, 13% of patients with initially unresectable liver metastases could have resection of their disease, following chemotherapy [16]. The 5- and 10-year OS rates of 33% and 27%, respectively, were observed in this cohort of patients [17]. Moreover, approximately 15% of patients never developed recurrent disease and could be considered 'cured' [18].
>
> The liver resection rate after chemotherapy correlates strongly with the radiological response, and patients with R0 resected disease have significantly longer survival, compared to those who did not undergo resection [19]. One of the major aims of conversion chemotherapy therefore is to achieve the highest possible response. The combination of 5-FU with oxaliplatin and irinotecan in a triple-drug regimen has demonstrated very high response rates of between 60% and 70%, with higher rates of R0 resections, compared to FOLFIRI, in patients with resectable liver metastases (36% versus 12%; $p = 0.017$) [20].

Targeted therapies, along with more effective chemotherapy regimens such as the triplet regimen, have thus been combined together to optimize the response to treatment.

> ✪ **Learning point** Role of biologics in colorectal liver metastases
>
> **Anti-VEGF therapy in combination with chemotherapy**
>
> The observational phase IV MO18024 'First Beat' study highlighted the safety profile of bevacizumab, a humanized mAb targeting VEGF, in combination with various chemotherapy regimens like FOLFOX, XELOX, FOLFIRI, or capecitabine [21]. This study enrolled 1914 unselected patients, all with mCRC. In patients with the liver as the only site of disease ($n = 704$), curative liver metastasectomies were performed in 11.9% of patients, and 9.8% had R0 resection post-operatively. The R0 resection rate was higher in patients who received oxaliplatin-based chemotherapy (13%). Overall, the data from this study show that a large percentage of patients underwent curative resections when bevacizumab was added to the chemotherapy; however, these results should be interpreted as hypothesis-generating only, as the trial was designed as a feasibility study and had no control arms for comparisons.
>
> A more recent trial assessing neoadjuvant CAPOX plus bevacizumab resulted in a high response rate for patients with liver metastases with poor-risk features, not selected for upfront resection, and converted 40% of patients to resectability

⊕ **Clinical tip** Bevacizumab toxicities

- High BP—which needs to be checked regularly.
- Bleeding problems, including post-surgical bleeding.
- Slow wound healing, requiring a break in treatment of 4 weeks before and after major surgery.
- Thromboembolic events.
- Proteinuria.
- Bowel perforation.
- Infusion reactions—usually within hours of treatment and only with the first or second infusion.

⊘ **Evidence base** BOXER: bevacizumab with chemotherapy in mCRC [22]

- Poor-risk patients with colorectal liver metastases were prospectively offered CAPOX with bevacizumab within this phase II study.
- Poor risk was defined by one or more of the following risk factors: >4 metastases confined to the liver, diameter of >5 cm, unlikely R0 resection, inadequate viable liver function if undergoing resection, inability to retain the liver vascular supply, or synchronous colorectal primary presentation.
- A total of 46 patients were recruited. Following CAPOX and bevacizumab, the overall response rate was 78%, allowing 12/20 (40%) patients with non-synchronous unresectable colorectal liver metastases to be converted to resectability. Additionally, 10/15 (67%) patients with synchronous resectable colorectal liver metastases underwent liver resection.

Source: data from Wong, R. *et al.*, A multicentre study of capecitabine, oxaliplatin plus bevacizumab as perioperative treatment of patients with poor-risk colorectal liver-only metastases not selected for upfront resection, *Annals of Oncology*, Volume 22, Issue 9 pp. 2042–8, Copyright © 2011 European Society for Medical Oncology.

Anti-EGFR therapy in management of unresectable disease

Anti-EGFR therapy has shown clinical efficacy in mCRC patients in first, second, or later lines, as single agents or as combination therapy. However, not all patients with CRC respond, and a variety of molecular characteristics have been evaluated to define predictive biomarkers. So far, multiple preclinical studies and clinical trials have demonstrated that anti-EGFR therapy is ineffective in the presence of a *K-ras* mutation. Although it has been suggested that patients with *K-ras G13D* mutations may benefit from anti-EGFR treatment [23], further retrospective analysis of three phase III studies failed to demonstrate the same clinical efficacy in patients with *K-ras G13D* mutations [23].

Anti-EGFR therapy should only be offered to patients with *K-ras* wild-type tumours. The potential for cetuximab to downsize liver metastases has also been evaluated, with mixed results. The CELIM trial showed an improvement in the resectability rate with cetuximab, compared to historical controls [25], and the CRYSTAL and OPUS trials also showed an improvement in the R0 resection rate [26,27]. However, this was not confirmed subsequently by the COIN trial [28].

The addition of panitumumab to first-line treatment in the phase III PRIME study resulted in an improvement in the PFS of 1.6 months (HR 0.8; $p = 0.02$) [29]. The efficacy of cetuximab and panitumumab is broadly similar, although cetuximab is more widely used.

⊘ **Evidence base** FIRE-3 study: cetuximab or bevacizumab with FOLFIRI in K-ras wild-type mCRC [30]

Randomized phase III study, comparing FOLFIRI plus cetuximab (A) versus FOLFIRI plus bevacizumab (B) as first-line treatment of *K-ras* wild-type mCRC.

- A total of 592 patients with *K-ras* wild-type disease.
- Overall response rate of 62% and 58%, with median PFS of 10.0 months and 10.3 months in arms A and B, respectively.
- OS of 28.7 months in arm A, compared to 25.0 months in arm B (HR 0.77; $p = 0.017$).
- The final results of this trial are currently awaited and, when available, may help us understand the lack of correlation between the PFS and OS.
- Importantly, this study did not treat patients with colorectal liver metastases alone and thus was not powered to answer the question about the management of liver-only metastases which were initially deemed inoperable.

Source: data from V. Heinemann, *et al.*, *Randomized comparison of FOLFIRI plus cetuximab versus FOLFIRI plus bevacizumab as first-line treatment of KRAS wilytype metasticic colorectal cancer, Germain AIO study KRK_03606 (FIRE 3)*, American Society of Clinical Oncology (ASCO), Copyright © 2013.

Loco-ablative techniques can also be used to manage hepatic metastases from CRC, with or without systemic therapy, when there is macroscopically incomplete resection or lesions that are not amenable to surgical excision.

⊗ **Learning point** Other localized therapies

Radiofrequency ablation (RFA)

RFA can be carried out, using open, laparoscopic, or percutaneous techniques, to ablate the incompletely resected or inoperable metastases. The choice of procedure is often operator-dependent, as there is no evidence to support a superior approach.

Lesions located close to large vessels (>1 cm), along the inferior edge of the liver, and multiple lesions are difficult to treat with RFA. It is a relatively well-tolerated procedure; the reported complications range from 6% to 9%, with mortality of 0–2%. These include liver abscess, pleural effusions, pneumothorax, acute renal insufficiency, and hypoxaemia.

Hepatic intra-arterial (HIA) chemotherapy

HIA chemotherapy, with or without systemic therapy, can be used to downstage the tumour size. Some studies have shown encouraging results with this approach; sample sizes have often been small.

✓ **Evidence base** CLOCC study: randomized phase II study of RFA, in addition to chemotherapy, in unresectable liver metastases [31]

- Patients with liver metastases, but no extra-hepatic disease, showed results as below ($n = 119$).
- A total of 59 patients had chemotherapy (CT) alone; 60 had RFA plus CT.
- The median PFS was 16.8 months in the RFA plus CT arm, compared to 9.9 months in the CT arm ($p = 0.025$).
- The 30-month OS was 61.7% in the RFA plus CT arm, and 57.6% in the CT arm.

Source: data from Ruers, T. *et al.*, Final results of the EORTC intergroup randomized study 40004 (CLOCC) evaluating the benefit of radiofrequency ablation (RFA) combined with chemotherapy for unresectable colorectal liver metastases (CRC LM), *Journal of Clinical Oncology*, Volume 28, Number 15 Suppl, abstract 3526, Copyright © 2010 by American Society of Clinical Oncology.[JC6]

✓ **Evidence base** Phase I trial of HIA with systemic chemotherapy [32, 31]

- Phase I clinical study ($n = 49$).
- Patients were treated with HIA plus systemic oxaliplatin and irinotecan.
- The overall response rate was 92%, with 8% CR and 84% PR.
- A total of 23 (47%) of the patients were able to undergo resection of the tumour; of those, 19 (82%) achieved free resection margins.
- The median OS for the entire cohort was 40 months.

HIA has not been evaluated in large randomized clinical trials and is rarely undertaken in the UK.

Source: data from Kemeny, N.E. *et al.*, Conversion to resectability using hepatic artery infusion plus systemic chemotherapy for the treatment of unresectable liver metastases from colorectal carcinoma, *Journal of Clinical Oncology*, Volume 27, Number 21, pp. 3465–71, Copyright © 2009 by American Society of Clinical Oncology.

Selective internal radiation therapy

Selective internal radiation therapy (SIRT) can be used, with or without chemo-therapy, to treat patients unsuitable for surgery or ablation, including those with low-volume extra-hepatic disease. Localized high-dose radiation is delivered to the metastases by the infusion of radioisotope-coated microspheres. SIRT treatment can be repeated [32, 33].

Only small RCTs have been performed to date, and some have shown an improved median survival when SIRT was used with systemic chemotherapy, compared to systemic chemotherapy alone [33, 34].

SIRT may be potentially beneficial for the treatment of unresectable colorectal liver metastases, but more research is required to demonstrate its efficacy and to establish the potential use of SIRT in treatment-naïve liver metastases [33, 32].

A final word from the expert

The prognosis for patients with mCRC has changed dramatically over the past 10-15 years. A large driver for this improved survival has been the introduction of a number of active anti-cancer drugs, both conventional cytotoxics as well as targeted biological agents. Equally important has been the recognition that a small subgroup of patients whose metastatic disease is confined to the liver have potentially curable disease. This recognition has necessitated the formation of specialized MDTs and, for selected patients, has led to curative treatments that were unthinkable only a few years ago.

References

1. Speights VO, Johnson MW, Stoltenberg PH, Rappaport ES, Helbert B, Riggs M. Colorectal cancer: current trends in initial clinical manifestations. *Southern Medical Journal* 1991; **84**(5): 575–8.
2. Mendelsohn J, Baselga J. Epidermal growth factor receptor targeting in cancer. *Seminars in Oncology* 2006; **33**(4): 369–85.
3. Lemmon MA, Schlessinger J. Regulation of signal transduction and signal diversity by receptor oligomerization. *Trends in Biochemical Sciences* 1994; **19**(11): 459–63.
4. Benson AB, 3rd, Ajani JA, Catalano RB *et al.* Recommended guidelines for the treatment of cancer treatment-induced diarrhea. *Journal of Clinical Oncology* 2004; **22**(14): 2918–26.
5. Tournigand C, Cervantes A, Figer A *et al.* OPTIMOX1: a randomized study of FOLFOX4 or FOLFOX7 with oxaliplatin in a stop-and-Go fashion in advanced colorectal cancer—a GERCOR study. *Journal of Clinical Oncology* 2006; **24**(3): 394–400.
6. Loprinzi CL, Qin R, Dakhil SR *et al.* Phase III randomized, placebo (PL)-controlled, double-blind study of intravenous calcium/magnesium (CaMg) to prevent oxaliplatin-induced sensory neurotoxicity (sNT), N08CB: An alliance for clinical trials in oncology study. *Journal of Clinical Oncology* 2013; **31**(Suppl): 3501.
7. Deenen MJ, Cats A, Mandigers CM *et al.* [Prevention of severe toxicity from capecitabine, 5-fluorouracil and tegafur by screening for DPD-deficiency]. *Nederlands Tijdschrift voor Geneeskunde* 2012; **156**(48): A4934.
8. Stangl R, Altendorf-Hofmann A, Charnley RM, Scheele J. Factors influencing the natural history of colorectal liver metastases. *The Lancet* 1994; **343**(8910): 1405–10.
9. Tomlinson JS, Jarnagin WR, DeMatteo RP *et al.* Actual 10-year survival after resection of colorectal liver metastases defines cure. *Journal of Clinical Oncology* 2007; **25**(29): 4575–80.
10. Khan K.H, Wale A, Brown G, Chau I. Colorectal cancer with liver metastases: chemo-therapy, surgical resection first or palliation alone? World journal of gastroenterology. **21**, 12391–12406, 2014
11. Fong Y, Fortner J, Sun RL, Brennan MF, Blumgart LH. Clinical score for predicting recur-rence after hepatic resection for metastatic colorectal cancer: analysis of 1001 consecu-tive cases. *Annals of Surgery* 1999; **230**(3): 309–18; discussion 318–21.

12. Jones RP, Malik HZ, Fenwick SW, Poston GJ. Perioperative chemotherapy for resectable colorectal liver metastases: where now? *European Journal of Surgical Oncology* 2013; **39**(8): 807–11.

13. Nordlinger B, Sorbye H, Glimelius B *et al*. Perioperative chemotherapy with FOLFOX4 and surgery versus surgery alone for resectable liver metastases from colorectal cancer (EORTC Intergroup trial 40983): a randomised controlled trial. *The Lancet* 2008; **371**(9617): 1007–16.

14. Mitry E, Fields AL, Bleiberg H *et al*. Adjuvant chemotherapy after potentially curative resection of metastases from colorectal cancer: a pooled analysis of two randomized trials. *Journal of Clinical Oncology* 2008; **26**(30): 4906–11.

15. Portier G, Elias D, Bouche O *et al*. Multicenter randomized trial of adjuvant fluorouracil and folinic acid compared with surgery alone after resection of colorectal liver metastases: FFCD ACHBTH AURC 9002 trial. *Journal of Clinical Oncology* 2006; **24**(31): 4976–82.

16. Adam R, Delvart V, Pascal G *et al*. Rescue surgery for unresectable colorectal liver metastases downstaged by chemotherapy: a model to predict long-term survival. *Annals of Surgery* 2004; **240**(4): 644–57; discussion 657–8.

17. Adam R, Wicherts DA, de Haas RJ *et al*. Patients with initially unresectable colorectal liver metastases: is there a possibility of cure? *Journal of Clinical Oncology* 2009; **27**(11): 1829–35.

18. Adam R, Aloia TA. Is hepatic resection justified after chemotherapy in patients with colorectal liver metastases and lymph node involvement? *Journal of Clinical Oncology* 2009; **27**(8): 1343–5; author reply 1345.

19. Folprecht G, Bechstein WO. [Neoadjuvant therapy concepts for liver metastases]. *Der Chirurg* 2011; **82**(11): 989–94.

20. Falcone A, Ricci S, Brunetti I *et al*. Phase III trial of infusional fluorouracil, leucovorin, oxaliplatin, and irinotecan (FOLFOXIRI) compared with infusional fluorouracil, leucovorin, and irinotecan (FOLFIRI) as first-line treatment for metastatic colorectal cancer: the Gruppo Oncologico Nord Ovest. *Journal of Clinical Oncology* 2007; **25**(13): 1670–6.

21. Van Cutsem E, Rivera F, Berry S *et al*. Safety and efficacy of first-line bevacizumab with FOLFOX, XELOX, FOLFIRI and fluoropyrimidines in metastatic colorectal cancer: the BEAT study. *Annals of Oncology* 2009; **20**(11): 1842–7.

22. Wong R, Cunningham D, Barbachano Y *et al*. A multicentre study of capecitabine, oxaliplatin plus bevacizumab as perioperative treatment of patients with poor-risk colorectal liver-only metastases not selected for upfront resection. *Annals of Oncology* 2011; **22**(9): 2042–8.

23. Tejpar S, Celik I, Schlichting M, Sartorius U, Bokemeyer C, Van Cutsem E. Association of KRAS G13D tumor mutations with outcome in patients with metastatic colorectal cancer treated with first-line chemotherapy with or without cetuximab. *Journal of Clinical Oncology* 2012; **30**(29): 3570–7.

24. Peeters M, Douillard JY, Van Cutsem E *et al*. Mutant KRAS codon 12 and 13 alleles in patients with metastatic colorectal cancer: assessment as prognostic and predictive biomarkers of response to panitumumab. *Journal of Clinical Oncology* 2013; **31**(6): 759–65.

25. Folprecht G, Gruenberger T, Bechstein WO *et al*. Tumour response and secondary resectability of colorectal liver metastases following neoadjuvant chemotherapy with cetuximab: the CELIM randomised phase 2 trial. *The Lancet Oncology* 2010; **11**(1): 38–47.

26. Bokemeyer C, Van Cutsem E, Rougier P *et al*. Addition of cetuximab to chemotherapy as first-line treatment for KRAS wild-type metastatic colorectal cancer: pooled analysis of the CRYSTAL and OPUS randomised clinical trials. *European Journal of Cancer* 2012; **48**(10): 1466–75.

27. Van Cutsem E, Köhne CH, Hitre E *et al*. Cetuximab and chemotherapy as initial treatment for metastatic colorectal cancer. *The New England Journal of Medicine* 2009; **360**(14): 1408–17.

28. Maughan TS, Adams RA, Smith CG *et al*. Addition of cetuximab to oxaliplatin-based first-line combination chemotherapy for treatment of advanced colorectal cancer: results of the randomised phase 3 MRC COIN trial. *The Lancet* 2011; **377**(9783): 2103–14.

29. Douillard JY, Siena S, Cassidy J *et al.* Randomized, phase III trial of panitumumab with infusional fluorouracil, leucovorin, and oxaliplatin (FOLFOX4) versus FOLFOX4 alone as first-line treatment in patients with previously untreated metastatic colorectal cancer: the PRIME study. *Journal of Clinical Oncology* 2010; **28**(31): 4697–705.

30. Heinemann V, Fischer von Weikersthal L, Decker T et al. Randomized comparison of FOLFIRI plus cetuximab versus FOLFIRI plus bevacizumab as first-line treatment of KRAS wild-type metastatic colorectal cancer: German AIO study KRK-0306 (FIRE-3). *Journal of Clinical Oncology* 2013; **31**(Suppl): LBA3506.

31. Ruers T, Punt CJ, van Coevorden F *et al.* Final results of the EORTC intergroup randomized study 40004 (CLOCC) evaluating the benefit of radiofrequency ablation (RFA) combined with chemotherapy for unresectable colorectal liver metastases (CRC LM). *Journal of Clinical Oncology* 2010; **28**(15 Suppl): abstr 3526.

32. Kemeny NE, Melendez FD, Capanu M *et al.* Conversion to resectability using hepatic artery infusion plus systemic chemotherapy for the treatment of unresectable liver metastases from colorectal carcinoma. *Journal of Clinical Oncology* 2009; **27**(21): 3465–71.

33. National Institute for Health and Care Excellence. *Selective internal radiation therapy for non-resectable colorectal metastases in the liver.* 2011. Available at: < http://www.nice.org.uk/guidance/ipg401 >.

34. Van Hazel G, Blackwell A, Anderson J *et al.* Randomised phase 2 trial of SIR-spheres plus fluorouracil/leucovorin chemotherapy versus fluorouracil/leucovorin chemotherapy alone in advanced colorectal cancer. *Journal of Surgical Oncology* 2004; **88**(2): 78–85.

12 Muscle-invasive transitional cell carcinoma of the bladder

Shanthini Crusz

🎙 **Expert commentary** John Chester

Case history

A 65-year-old man presented to his GP with a first occurrence of painless haematuria, with no other lower urinary tract symptoms. His only significant past medical history was that of hypertension, treated with 5 mg of ramipril daily. There was no family history of malignancy. He was a lifelong smoker. He was a retired plumber, with no history of chemical exposure, and remained fully active. Systems examination was unremarkable, and his performance status (PS) was assessed as 0.

Urine dipstick analysis revealed macroscopic haematuria, with 3+ blood and no leucocytes or nitrites. The patient was immediately referred for an urgent 2-week appointment with the urology team for suspected cancer.

The patient was assessed in a 'one-stop' urology clinic, 10 days later. Urine culture sent by the GP showed no bacterial growth, but urine cytology revealed abnormal epithelial cells, suspicious for malignancy. Flexible cystoscopy showed a tumour in the bladder, close to the left ureteric orifice.

Urgent formal cystoscopy with transurethral resection of bladder tumour (TURBT) took place 7 days later. This confirmed a large, abnormally raised lesion on the anterior bladder wall, extending to the left ureteric orifice. A post-operative staging CT of the thorax, abdomen, and pelvis was also performed.

The patient's case and results of the investigations were presented at the next urology MDT meeting, 7 days following TURBT. Histology showed a grade 3 transitional cell carcinoma (TCC) of the bladder, with invasion of the underlying detrusor muscle (pT2, at least). Staging CT showed no obvious involvement of perivesical fat, or pelvic or retroperitoneal nodes, and the chest was clear of metastatic disease. An atrophic right kidney was noted. The patient was thus staged as T2N0M0. The MDT meeting concluded that the patient was fit enough for radical treatment, either with cystectomy or chemo-radiotherapy (CRT).

The options of surgery versus bladder-conserving treatment were discussed with the patient by the urologist and a non-surgical oncologist in the outpatient clinic later the same day. The patient was not keen to undergo cystectomy at this stage. It was felt that he would be a good candidate for neoadjuvant chemotherapy. The potentially curable, but life-threatening, nature of his disease was discussed, and the potential benefits of neoadjuvant chemotherapy were conveyed to the patient and his wife. A provisional plan for three cycles of neoadjuvant gemcitabine/cisplatin (GC) chemotherapy, followed by CRT, was agreed, and the patient was given relevant information sheets to take home and discuss with his family and GP.

➕ **Clinical tip** Symptoms and risk factors in suspected bladder cancer

- Symptoms at presentation can include painless haematuria, dysuria, recurrent urinary infections, and rarely symptoms of metastases.
- Any episode of haematuria should never be ignored and should be promptly investigated.
- Always remember to assess for risk factors, including exposure to aromatic amines and cigarette smoking.
- Remember that cigarette smoking alone can triple the risk of developing bladder cancer and has been shown to be related to a higher mortality rate during long-term follow-up.

➕ **Clinical tip** Appropriate communication and information giving

Effective communication between the MDT and patient is essential when making treatment decisions in the outpatient oncology setting. Ideally, clinical information, as in this scenario, should be conveyed at one time point with the presence of a clinical nurse specialist, surgeon, and oncologist. Joint discussion is always ideal, but not always practical; therefore, appropriate timing of conversations between different disciplines requires thoughtful planning. Providing patients with clinical information sheets to go away and read, prior to further consultation, is important and assists in a patient-informed decision.

Baseline blood tests, taken in clinic, noted a decline in the renal function, compared with blood tests taken by the GP several weeks earlier, with serum creatinine significantly above the upper limit of normal (ULN) and a calculated glomerular filtration rate (GFR) of 49 mL/min (previously normal at 67 mL/min). An urgent ultrasound of the kidney, ureters, and bladder showed a new left-sided hydroureter and hydronephrosis, which had developed since the preceding CT scan. Ramipril was discontinued, and consideration was given to whether adequate renal function could be restored to permit cisplatin-based neoadjuvant chemotherapy, as had been planned. Following discussion with the interventional radiology team, a left-sided nephrostomy, with immediate antegrade ureteric stent insertion, took place the following day. Several days later, his urine output was good and clear of blood, and his serum creatinine had returned within normal limits, with a calculated GFR of 65 mL/min.

⭐ **Learning point** Epidemiology and classification of bladder cancer

Bladder cancer is the commonest malignancy of the urinary tract. In 2012, an estimated 151,000 new cases were diagnosed in Europe, and it was the cause of 52,400 cancer deaths. Over 70% of patients are >65 years of age at diagnosis.

The AJCC TNM classification is currently used for the staging of bladder cancer [1]. This is summarized in Figure 12.1. Treatment of localized disease is based on the extent of disease infiltration—whether the disease is muscle-invasive (MIBC) or non-muscle-invasive (NMIBC).

NMIBC (defined as stage Ta, Tis, or T1) is a disease which commonly recurs and requires intensive cystoscopic surveillance, thereby imposing a major health economic burden. It accounts for approximately 75–85% of cases, and treatment options are based on the calculated risk of recurrence and prognosis.

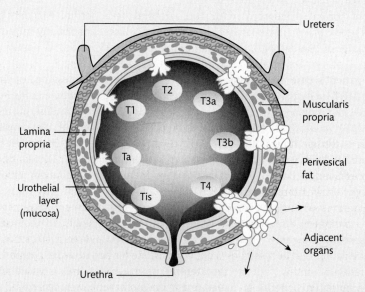

Figure 12.1 Bladder cancer staging, adapted from Pomerantz *et al.*, based on the AJCC classification of bladder cancer [1].

Reproduced from Mark M. Pomerantz *et al.*, Genitourinary Cancers: Prostate, Kidney, Bladder, and Testis, Figure 13.2, pp. 120, in Ajay K. Singh and Joseph Loscalzo (Ed), *The Brigham Intensive Review of Internal Medicine*, Oxford University Press, New York, USA, Copyright © 2012, by permission of Oxford University Press, USA.

> **❝ Expert comment**
>
> As in the systemic treatment of other cancers, chemotherapy regimens tested in the advanced disease setting have been brought forward into the potentially curative perioperative setting (neoadjuvant or adjuvant chemotherapy).
>
> There are three commonly accepted standards of care for first-line chemotherapy in advanced bladder cancer patients with good PS, good renal function, and manageable co-morbidities: GC, MVAC (methotrexate/vinblastine/adriamycin/cisplatin), and 'accelerated' MVAC. Two large RCTs comparing the long-standing, but toxic, 'gold standard' chemotherapy MVAC with GC or with accelerated MVAC have demonstrated that all three regimens have similar outcomes. However, lesser toxicity and better QoL outcomes with the other two regimens mean that 'classical' MVAC is now little used.
>
> In the neoadjuvant setting, such as this case, a meta-analysis clearly demonstrates the value of cisplatin-based combinations for advanced disease. Although there is a relative paucity of comparative data on which is the best regimen, GC is possibly the most widely used.

> **✔ Evidence base** ABC meta-analysis collaboration: neoadjuvant chemotherapy in MIBC [2]
>
> - A meta-analysis of 3005 patients from 11 randomized trials.
> - Comparison between neoadjuvant chemotherapy (NC) in conjunction with local treatment (radical cystectomy (RC) alone/radiotherapy alone/radiotherapy in combination with RC) versus local treatment alone.
> - NC included combination platinum-based regimens, such as MVAC, dose-dense MVAC, and GC, and also single-agent platinum treatment.
> - Absolute 5-year OS benefit of 5% (HR 0.86, 95% CI 0.77–0.95; $p = 0.003$), favouring platinum-based combination NC.
> - Absolute DFS at 5 years of 9% using platinum-based combination treatment (HR 0.78, 95% CI 0.71–0.86; $p < 0.0001$).
> - Platinum combination therapy was found to be superior to platinum monotherapy; single-agent platinum did not yield significantly better outcomes.
> - Benefits were irrespective of the T stage and were seen in (smaller numbers of) radical radiotherapy patients, as well as in RC patients.
>
> *Source*: data from *European Urology*, Volume 48, Issue 2, Vale CL, Neoadjuvant chemotherapy in invasive bladder cancer: update of a systematic review and meta-analysis of individual patient data advanced bladder cancer (ABC) meta-analysis collaboration, pp. 202–5, Copyright © 2005 Elsevier B.V. All rights reserved.

At clinic review, a few days after discharge, the patient was felt to be fit to go ahead with full-dose cisplatin-based neoadjuvant chemotherapy, as planned. He was treated as an outpatient on the chemotherapy day unit, with gemcitabine (1000 mg/m^2) and cisplatin (70 mg/m^2) on day 1, followed by a second dose of gemcitabine alone on day 8. Two further cycles of chemotherapy were performed at 21-day intervals, with careful monitoring of the FBC, renal and liver function, bone profile, and magnesium levels. All were well tolerated, with no decline in PS or significant weight loss, although there was some low-grade lethargy and nausea, successfully controlled with oral anti-emetics. The patient denied hearing loss, tinnitus, or peripheral neuropathy. After the third cycle, a cystoscopy showed a complete response in the bladder tumour, and a radiotherapy planning CT scan showed no evidence of significant change since the pre-chemotherapy scan.

The patient underwent radiotherapy with concomitant 5-FU/mitomycin C. He received 64 Gy in 32 fractions over 6.5 weeks. He was treated as an outpatient, with a continuous infusion of 5-FU (500 mg/m^2 per day) given with fractions

1–5 and 16–20 of radiotherapy and an IV bolus of mitomycin C (12 mg/m^2) on day 1 of therapy. Following completion of radiotherapy, he was monitored with a repeat cystoscopy every 3 months and regular outpatient appointments.

> ✪ **Learning point** Chemoradiation
>
> CRT (a combination of chemotherapy and radiotherapy) is an accepted treatment regime for many solid tumours, including rectal, cervical, and head and neck cancers. By combining treatment modalities, inherent tumour cell resistance can be overcome, 'spatial cooperation' takes place (i.e. radiotherapy to treat the primary tumour and chemotherapy for any occult 'micrometastatic' disease), decreased tumour cell repopulation between fractionation occurs, and 'sensitization' takes place, i.e. the systemic drug enhances the activity of radiation within the radiotherapy field. In bladder cancer, this combination is offering further therapy options in bladder-conserving treatment.

> ⊘ **Evidence base** Major trials assessing CRT as potentially curative bladder-conserving therapy in localized MIBC muscle-invasive bladder cancer
>
> **The BC2001 trial [3]: radiotherapy with or without synchronous chemotherapy**
>
> - A phase III RCT in patients with MIBC.
> - Compared radiotherapy with or without synchronous chemotherapy (5-FU during fractions 1–5 and 16–20 of radiotherapy and mitomycin C on day 1).
> - The 2-year DFS was improved in the chemotherapy arm, compared to radiotherapy alone (67% (95% CI 59–74) versus 54% (95% CI 46–62), respectively).
> - HR was 0.68 with CRT (95% CI 0.48–0.96; $p = 0.03$).
> - The 5-year OS was 48% (95% CI 40–55), compared to 35% in the radiotherapy alone (95% CI 28–43).
> - Approximately a third of patients in this trial received neoadjuvant chemotherapy prior to treatment, and the concomitant treatment effect did not vary significantly when adjusting for this.
>
> **The Bladder Carbogen Nicotinamide (BCON) study [4]: assessing the issue of targeting tumour hypoxia in synchronous therapy with radiosensitization**
>
> - Phase III randomized controlled study using carbogen and nicotinamide with radiotherapy, compared to radiotherapy alone, in MIBC.
> - Improvement seen in the estimated OS, risk of death, and local relapse rates, compared to radiotherapy alone.
> - This study further supports the use of chemotherapy in bladder cancer and offers a potential new choice of drug regime to be considered.
>
> Source data from James ND *et al.*, Radiotherapy with or without chemotherapy in muscle-invasive bladder cancer, *New England Journal of Medicine*, Volume 336, Number 16, pp. 1477–88, Copyright © 2012 Massachusetts Medical Society; and Hoskin PJ *et al.*, Radiotherapy with concurrent carbogen and nicotinamide in bladder carcinoma, *Journal of Clinical Oncology*, Volume 28, Number 33, pp. 4912–18, Copyright © 2010 by American Society of Clinical Oncology.

Twelve months after completion of treatment, a surveillance cystoscopy showed local tumour recurrence within the bladder. TURBT biopsy revealed recurrent grade 3 muscle-invasive TCC. CT again showed no visible metastatic spread, and thus the MDT decision was to offer salvage cystectomy, in view of the localized muscle-invasive recurrence (Figure 12.2). After discussion with the consultant urologist and the urology clinical nurse specialist regarding the implications of surgery, the patient agreed to undergo cystectomy, with bilateral pelvic lymphadenectomy and bladder diversion with an ileal conduit. He had elective surgery 3 weeks later, with no early post-operative complications, and was discharged from

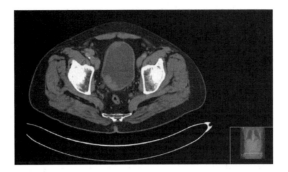

Figure 12.2 CT demonstrating a polypoid mass projecting from the left bladder wall.

hospital 9 days after surgery, having had stoma nurse input for advice on stoma care. The post-operative histology, discussed in the MDT, confirmed a multifocal grade 3 TCC with clear surgical resection margins. Fifteen nodes had been resected, of which one contained micrometastatic disease. He continued on regular outpatient follow-up, with a plan for regular 3-monthly imaging by CT of the thorax, abdomen, and pelvis.

> ⓚ **Expert comment**
>
> Tumour involvement of pelvic lymph nodes at cystectomy, as here, has long been recognized as a poor prognostic indicator, leading to the consideration of post-operative 'adjuvant' chemotherapy, in an attempt to improve survival outcomes in this situation.
>
> The value of adjuvant chemotherapy for localized MIBC remains a hotly debated topic. A variety of small trials have been performed, most of which have had associated methodological flaws, prompting a meta-analysis. The ABC Meta-analysis Collaboration on adjuvant chemotherapy in invasive bladder cancer assessed 491 patients from six trials [5], but the results have provided insufficient evidence to advocate the routine use of adjuvant chemotherapy, other than in an appropriate clinical trial. There is therefore a lingering paradox that there is firm level 1 evidence for the use of preoperative, but not post-operative, chemotherapy. Thus, in the absence of reliable level 1 data, a post-operative surveillance option, as in this case, seems entirely reasonable, particularly in view of previous neoadjuvant chemotherapy.

Unfortunately, a follow-up scan at 6 months after cystectomy showed borderline retroperitoneal lymphadenopathy and 2 subcentimetre lung nodules. The next scan, 9 months after cystectomy, showed multiple lung metastases, ranging in size from 0.7 cm to 1.6 cm in diameter, plus retroperitoneal lymphadenopathy of 3 cm in maximum dimension. The potential benefits of palliative chemotherapy were discussed with the patient and his family, and he accepted.

Assessment in clinic concluded the patient's renal function had declined, and his PS was now 1. His renal biochemistry blood tests showed a calculated GFR of 58 mL/min, with no reversible cause found. Following extensive discussion, a decision was made to re-treat with GC chemotherapy, in view of the time interval between the initial treatment and metastatic recurrence. The patient was consented for another six cycles of GC chemotherapy, but a split dose of cisplatin was given (35 mg/m^2 on days 1 and 8), in view of his renal impairment and PS.

⊕ Clinical tip Radiological interpretation of progression

The radiological appearances seen in this case at 6 months following cystectomy would not normally be regarded as definitive evidence of recurrent disease. A policy of an early repeat assessment at 3 months to assess whether radiological lesions have progressed, consistent with metastatic disease, is common practice, as a short delay in starting palliative chemotherapy is unlikely to affect the overall outcomes in an asymptomatic patient.

Stable or improved radiological appearances on a repeat scan at a short interval would not normally be considered an adequate justification for exposing a patient to potentially toxic chemotherapy in the absence of clearly progressive disease. Significantly worse appearances however (as here) shift cost-benefit analysis towards chemotherapy given the proven survival benefits of first-line palliative chemotherapy.

⓰ Expert comment

The treatment of metastatic bladder cancer, following adjuvant treatment, with a cisplatin-based regime remains an inexact clinical science, lacking in solid published data to guide the clinician. As in other chemotherapy indications, recurrence within 6 months of completion of the first course of chemotherapy is often considered to represent primary platinum-resistant disease. In that case, alternative chemotherapy regimens can be employed. These may still be cisplatin-based, but combined with other agents known to have activity in this disease to which the tumour cells have not yet been exposed (e.g. MVAC or 'accelerated' MVAC), or may involve other platinum agents and/or taxanes, e.g. carboplatin/paclitaxel or single-agent paclitaxel. However, if (as here) recurrence occurs after >12 months, it is generally accepted that a rechallenge with the same regimen can be offered, with a non-zero possibility of response.

✪ Learning point Chemotherapy in the 'cisplatin-unfit' patient

Renal impairment, PS, and co-morbidity play a large part in decisions on how best to treat an individual patient. Data from two retrospective analyses of large cohorts of patients show that 30–60% of bladder cancer patients can be considered ineligible for cisplatin-based chemotherapy [6].

Renal impairment (based on the calculated GFR of the Cockcroft–Gault equation) is common in bladder cancer, due to the nature of the disease and co-morbidities. Thus, clinicians are frequently confronted with decisions on how best to treat a patient who is fit enough to receive chemotherapy, aside from renal impairment.

- It is widely accepted that a calculated (or measured) GFR of >60 mL/min is adequate to use cisplatin-based combinations in patients who are otherwise suitable for systemic therapy.
- In patients with advanced disease and a calculated GFR of 50–60 mL/min, many non-surgical oncologists opt to use cisplatin at full dose, but 'split' between days 1 and 2 or 1 and 8.
- For patients with GFR of 30–50 mL/min, there is consensus that the use of a carboplatin-based, rather than cisplatin-based, regimen is appropriate (e.g. carboplatin/gemcitabine, rather than cisplatin/gemcitabine). There are no published RCTs comparing regimens which differ only in cisplatin versus carboplatin, but it is widely accepted that outcomes with carboplatin-based combinations are meaningful, but inferior to those with cisplatin.
- For patients with GFR of <30 mL/min, it is widely regarded as inappropriate to use platinum-based regimens, but agents which are not dependent on the renal clearance, such as single-agent taxanes, may be appropriate.

It should be noted that, in the neoadjuvant setting, there are insufficient data to suggest a survival benefit from the use of carboplatin-based regimens; a meta-analysis supports only the use of cisplatin-based combinations [2].

Source data from James ND et al., Radiotherapy with or without chemotherapy in muscle-invasive bladder cancer, New England Journal of Medicine, Volume 336, Number 16, pp. 1477-88, Copyright © 2012 Massachusetts Medical Society; and Hoskin PJ et al., Radiotherapy with concurrent carbogen and nicotinamide in bladder carcinoma, Journal of Clinical Oncology, Volume 28, Number 33, pp. 4912-8, Copyright © © 2010 by American Society of Clinical Oncology.

After cycle 3, the patient had obtained a good radiological response to palliative chemotherapy in both his retroperitoneal lymphadenopathy and his lung metastases, felt to amount to a partial response by RECIST v1.1 criteria. Subjective toxicities included low-grade lethargy, peripheral neuropathy, and nausea. Chemotherapy was therefore continued for a further three cycles, with an end-of-treatment restaging scan showing response was maintained. The patient had residual mild tinnitus and grade 2 peripheral neuropathy on completion of treatment. In the absence of a trial of maintenance therapy, it was decided that he should be closely monitored in the non-surgical oncology clinic.

Seven months after completion of his chemotherapy, he experienced symptoms of lumbar back pain and mild breathlessness on exertion. A restaging scan revealed progressive disease with worsening of his nodal and pulmonary metastases and a new liver metastasis. The patient remained with PS of 1, with stable blood tests, and was felt to be fit enough to consider second-line chemotherapy. After discussion with the patient and his family regarding further systemic therapy, he declined further active treatment.

The patient gradually became more symptomatic from his metastatic disease, with worsening shortness of breath. His PS further declined. He was referred to the community palliative care team for symptom control as an outpatient. After regular input by the community team, he was eventually commenced on home oxygen and oral modified-release morphine for symptomatic relief. After further deterioration and discussions between the patient and his family, he opted for admission to his local hospice for end-of-life care and died, pain-free, 40 months after diagnosis.

Discussion

This case highlights some of the major challenges faced in treating both localized muscle-invasive and metastatic bladder cancer.

Muscle invasive bladder cancer (MIBC) (defined as stage T2 and beyond) is a life-threatening disease, but potentially curable. Surgery with Radical cystectomy is the current standard of care. Radical cystectomy with pelvic node dissection is offered to patients with non-metastatic MIBC who are fit enough to undergo radical surgery. The decision to proceed is based on discussions within the MDT and with the patient and family/carers.

Organ-preserving therapy, employing radiotherapy, with or without concomitant systemic therapy, is emerging as an effective option for those who are not fit enough for radical surgery or who express a preference for avoiding cystectomy and/or a stoma. Full discussion, counselling, and support should be offered to patients when explaining the options of surgery versus bladder preservation. Where appropriate, the outcomes of surgery, including the use of urinary diversion procedures or orthotopic bladder reconstruction, and their impact on the QoL should also be clearly explained.

Despite potentially curative treatments, approximately 50% of patients with muscle-invasive disease develop metastases within 2 years. There is therefore an urgent need to improve outcomes by investigating additional therapeutic interventions. Perioperative systemic chemotherapy (either neoadjuvant or adjuvant) offers the possibility of improved outcomes via the elimination of micrometastatic disease. There are level 1 data to support the use of chemotherapy in the neoadjuvant setting, resulting in better 5-year OS and DFS [2]. Despite the strong evidence for neoadjuvant chemotherapy, it has not been universally accepted as an essential component of routine clinical treatment pathways; for example, a study in 2011 demonstrated that only 12% of T2–T4aN0M0 bladder carcinoma patients received neoadjuvant chemotherapy, and only 22% received adjuvant chemotherapy [7].

Organ-preserving radical radiotherapy is associated with a relatively high rate of incomplete response and local recurrence (up to 50%), although recurrence is frequently non-muscle-invasive bladder cancer [8]. Meaningful comparisons of outcomes from radical surgery versus radical radiotherapy are difficult to make, due to differing case mixes (with older and less fit patients tending to receive radiotherapy rather than undergo surgery), and, although there are published retrospective series, e.g. the ABC Meta-analysis Collaboration [2], there are no definitive published RCT data.

Recent data showing improved outcomes with the use of synchronous CRT offer patients further choice in radical treatment. A small RCT of 99 patients comparing CRT with a cisplatin-based regimen versus radiotherapy alone demonstrated improved locoregional control of locally advanced disease but showed no benefit in OS [9]. However, cisplatin in combination with radiotherapy may not be ideal for all bladder cancer patients, many of whom have impaired renal function and in whom the side effects of chemotherapy and/or radiotherapy may be more severe due to co-morbidities. The BC2001 trial, using non-platinum-based chemotherapy, has shown that 5-FU and mitomycin C in combination with radiotherapy significantly improves the locoregional control of bladder cancer compared to radiotherapy alone [3]. Similarly, the use of hypoxia radiosensitizers have been explored, and the BCON trial, using inhaled carbogen and oral nicotinamide with radiotherapy, has shown improvement in estimated OS, death, and local relapse rates, compared to radiotherapy alone [4]. Following all bladder preservation protocols, close surveillance is indicated, and salvage cystectomy is recommended for local recurrence as the only remaining possibility of cure.

Once disease has advanced beyond the bladder, the long-term survival for metastatic bladder cancer is poor and has not improved dramatically in recent decades, despite the widespread use of palliative chemotherapy. The three commonest regimes used are GC, MVAC, and 'accelerated' MVAC. In a phase III trial comparison of GC with MVAC, both had similar efficacy, with similar median survival and 5-year PFS, but GC had a better safety and tolerability profile when directly compared to MVAC. GC had more thrombocytopenia requiring transfusion, but lower toxic death rates, neutropenic events, severe mucositis, and alopecia. Reflecting this, more patients completed six cycles of GC with less dose adjustments, compared to MVAC [10]. High dose-intensity, 'accelerated' MVAC, with G-CSF support, can also be considered as this has been shown to achieve higher rates of complete response and improved median PFS, compared to standard MVAC [11]. Lesser toxicity and better QoL outcomes with the other two regimens mean that 'classical' MVAC is now little used, although these two regimens have never been compared directly.

In the event of relapse following first-line palliative chemotherapy, one must be careful in the selection of patients to whom further second-line chemotherapy should be offered. Adverse prognostic factors for survival in second-line advanced disease include PS of ≥1, liver metastasis, and Hb s<10 g/dL. The only validated RCT in patients who have relapsed after platinum-based combination therapy showed a favourable survival benefit with vinflunine (a novel third-generation vinca alkaloid agent), compared to best supportive care alone. However, the survival benefit reported was only seen in a per-protocol analysis, rather than on an intention-to-treat

(ITT) basis, and there were some significant toxicities. Therefore, although this trial represents the best data currently available, single-agent vinflunine has not been universally accepted as standard of care for second-line therapy of metastatic bladder cancer.

> **ⓕ Expert comment**
>
> There has been one phase III RCT of 370 patients, comparing vinflunine plus best supportive care with best supportive care alone following failure of platinum-based chemotherapy [12]. Primary analysis of the ITT population showed a significant difference in the objective response, but the survival difference between both arms was not found to be significant (6.9 months versus 4.6 months; HR 0.88, 95% CI 0.69–1.12; $p = 0.287$). The authors hypothesized that this was due to an imbalance in prognostic factors and the presence of patients who should not have been included, according to the original protocol. Thus, a per-protocol analysis was carried out, removing 13 'non-eligible' patients. This unplanned analysis showed an improved median OS in the treatment arm by 2.6 months ($p = 0.0227$). The treatment was not without toxicity, and, although caution must be used in interpreting the results of unplanned analyses, this study is as yet the only published RCT to date which examines the second-line treatment of metastatic bladder cancer.

A final word from the expert

There have been significant recent improvements in the management of localized muscle-invasive bladder cancer, i.e. neoadjuvant chemotherapy and concomitant CRT for localized disease, and in both first- and second-line chemotherapy for metastatic disease. However, there is still considerable scope for further improvements in outcomes, and novel well-designed clinical trials remain a priority. As in other cancers, the use of targeted agents may be beneficial, but their use, concurrently or sequentially with current standard therapies, is yet to show a meaningful clinical impact. An exciting recent Phase I trial shows efficacy of immune check-point blockade (anti-PDL-1) in the metastatic setting for bladder cancer [13]. Future treatment options for metastatic and/or locally-advanced bladder cancer, and data from further clinical trials with this and similar agents, are eagerly awaited.

References

1. Edge S, Byrd DR, Compton CC, Fritz AJ, Greene FL, Trotti A, eds. *AJCC cancer staging manual*, 7th edn. New York: Springer, 2010; p. 497.
2. Advanced Bladder Cancer (ABC) Meta-analysis Collaboration. Neoadjuvant chemotherapy in invasive bladder cancer: update of a systematic review and meta-analysis of individual patient data advanced bladder cancer (ABC) meta-analysis collaboration. *European Urology* 2005; **48**(2): 202–5; discussion 205–6.
3. James ND, Hussain SA, Hall E *et al.* Radiotherapy with or without chemotherapy in muscle-invasive bladder cancer. *The New England Journal of Medicine* 2012; **366**(16): 1477–88.
4. Hoskin PJ, Rojas AM, Bentzen SM, Saunders MI. Radiotherapy with concurrent carbogen and nicotinamide in bladder carcinoma. *Journal of Clinical Oncology* 2010; **28**(33): 4912–18.
5. Advanced Bladder Cancer (ABC) Meta-analysis Collaboration. Adjuvant chemotherapy in invasive bladder cancer: a systematic review and meta-analysis of individual patient data Advanced Bladder Cancer (ABC) Meta-analysis Collaboration. *European Urology* 2005; **48**(2): 189–99; discussion 199–201.

6. Dash A, Galsky MD, Vickers AJ *et al.* Impact of renal impairment on eligibility for adjuvant cisplatin-based chemotherapy in patients with urothelial carcinoma of the bladder. *Cancer* 2006; **107**(3): 506–13.

7. Bajorin DF, Herr HW. Kuhn's paradigms: are those closest to treating bladder cancer the last to appreciate the paradigm shift? *Journal of Clinical Oncology* 2011; **29**(16): 2135–7.

8. Cooke PW, Dunn JA, Latief T, Bathers S, James ND, Wallace DM. Long-term risk of salvage cystectomy after radiotherapy for muscle-invasive bladder cancer. *European Urology* 2000; **38**(3): 279–86.

9. Coppin CM, Gospodarowicz MK, James K *et al.* Improved local control of invasive bladder cancer by concurrent cisplatin and preoperative or definitive radiation. The National Cancer Institute of Canada Clinical Trials Group. *Journal of Clinical Oncology* 1996; **14**(11): 2901–7.

10. von der Maase H, Hansen SW, Roberts JT *et al.* Gemcitabine and cisplatin versus methotrexate, vinblastine, doxorubicin, and cisplatin in advanced or metastatic bladder cancer: results of a large, randomized, multinational, multicenter, phase III study. *Journal of Clinical Oncology* 2000; **18**(17): 3068–77.

11. Sternberg CN, de Mulder P, Schornagel JH *et al.* Seven year update of an EORTC phase III trial of high-dose intensity M-VAC chemotherapy and G-CSF versus classic M-VAC in advanced urothelial tract tumours. *European Journal of Cancer* 2006; **42**(1): 50–4.

12. Bellmunt J, Fougeray R, Rosenberg JE *et al.* Long-term survival results of a randomized phase III trial of vinflunine plus best supportive care versus best supportive care alone in advanced urothelial carcinoma patients after failure of platinum-based chemotherapy. *Annals of Oncology* 2013; **24**(6): 1466–72.

13. Powles T, Eder JP, Fine GD *et al* MPDL3280A (anti-PD-L1) treatment leads to clinical activity in metastatic bladder cancer. *Nature* 2014; **515**(7528): 558–62.

13 Metastatic renal cell cancer and hypercalcaemia

Meenali Chitnis

Ⓔ **Expert commentary** Matthew Wheater

Case history

A 63-year-old man presented to his GP with a 2-week history of new-onset lower back pain and lethargy. The pain was present at all times, including at rest, and was inadequately controlled by simple analgesia. In the week prior to presentation, the patient's wife had noticed him to be intermittently confused. On further questioning, the patient had urinary frequency and nocturia, which was new. He had not opened his bowels for 2 days. His appetite was good, but he had lost 1 kg in weight over the last 2 months and had experienced mild nausea.

He had a history of hypertension, diagnosed at the age of 54 and controlled on amlodipine 5 mg daily. He was a retired maths teacher and had continued to keep active with hobbies, including cycling, reading, and fishing, but had been struggling with these over the preceding 2–3 weeks.

On examination, he was apyrexial, and his BP was 150/85. Routine examination of the cardiovascular, respiratory, and abdominal systems was normal. There was no neurological deficit, but the patient did have percussion tenderness over the area corresponding to T12/L1. The GP arranged for the patient to be reviewed by the on-call medical team at the local hospital.

He underwent routine blood tests and had plain X-ray films of the thoracic and lumbar spine. Biochemistry (Table 13.1) showed the patient to have renal impairment and hypercalcaemia. A plain X-ray of the thoracolumbar spine revealed a compression fracture of the T12 vertebral body. The patient was admitted to the medical ward for treatment of his hypercalcaemia, analgesia for his back pain, and for further investigations.

He received 3 L of fluid over the course of the evening and overnight. Blood results the following day revealed a minor improvement in hypercalcaemia, with the corrected calcium now measuring 2.9 mmol/L. His renal function had normalized, with urea of 5.3 mmol/L and serum creatinine of 110 µmol/L. He received an infusion of 90 mg of pamidronate in saline over an hour, with subsequent normalization

Table 13.1 Routine blood tests carried out on initial hospital admission

FBC	Biochemistry	Biochemistry
Hb 13.7	Na 135 mmol/L	Bilirubin 9 µmol/L
WCC 4.67	K 3.7 mmol/L	ALT 57 IU/L
Neutrophils 2.23	Urea 8.9 mmol/L	ALP 920 IU/L
Platelets 163	Creatinine 150 µmol/L	Albumin 37 g/L
	LDH 250 IU/L	Corrected calcium 3.06 mmol/L

Expert comment

In patients with extensive bone involvement, bisphosphonates have also been shown to reduce the risk of skeletal-related events, including pathological fracture, and the requirement for palliative radiotherapy to bone [1].

of his serum calcium levels within the next 48 hours. His prostate-specific antigen (PSA) level had been checked and was normal.

Overall, he felt much better, and his pain was well controlled with regular paracetamol and ibuprofen, with occasional breakthrough oral morphine sulfate.

⊕ Clinical tip Hypercalcaemia of malignancy

Aetiology

Hypercalcaemia of malignancy is often associated with bone metastases but can also occur in the absence of bone disease, secondary to the secretion of cytokines such as parathyroid hormone-related peptide.

Clinical features

Headache, nausea and vomiting, confusion, polyuria, polydipsia, constipation, and patients may be markedly dehydrated on presentation both clinically and biochemically.

Management

- Mild hypercalcaemia (corrected serum calcium <3 mmol/L) may respond to IV rehydration and treatment of the underlying cancer. In the majority of cases, however, further treatment of hypercalcaemia with bisphosphonates is required.
- Moderate to severe hypercalcaemia (corrected serum calcium >3 mmol/L) requires aggressive IV rehydration, often 3–6 L in the first 24 hours, to improve symptoms and normalize the renal function, thus allowing treatment with bisphosphonates.
- Bisphosphonates inhibit osteoclastic activity, and, in hypercalcaemia of malignancy, pamidronate is often used. A dose of between 30 and 90 mg is given IV, depending on the initial serum calcium levels, and the rate of infusion depending on the renal function and creatinine clearance following rehydration. A decrease in serum calcium is often observed within 48 hours of bisphosphonate infusion, with maximum effect seen within 7 days. Infusions may need to be repeated monthly, or oral bisphosphonates commenced. In cases resistant to pamidronate, zoledronate, a more potent inhibitor of osteoclastic activity, can be employed. Steroids, calcitonin, and diuretics have a selective role to play in certain cases of hypercalcaemia.

A staging whole-body MRI scan and CT CAP were requested to exclude any risk to the spinal cord from the probable bony metastatic disease and to try and establish a diagnosis. The MRI scan showed metastatic bone deposits within the T12 vertebral body, causing collapse and compression of the spinal cord at that level (Figure 13.1). Further small metastatic deposits were present in the mid-thoracic and upper lumbar spine. The CT scan showed a large tumour arising from the left kidney, with enlarged abdominal lymph nodes and bilateral small-volume pulmonary metastases (Figure 13.2 and Figure 13.3).

The patient was commenced on oral steroids, and his case discussed with the spinal surgical team, in view of the single level of cord compression from a probable renal carcinoma and good PS. He was transferred for spinal decompression and stabilization, followed by post-operative radiotherapy. The patient recovered well, and the histology from the resected bone metastasis confirmed metastatic clear cell renal cell carcinoma (ccRCC). At the urology multidisciplinary meeting, the option of cytoreductive nephrectomy was considered. In the absence of significant symptoms from the primary, and multiple sites of metastatic disease,

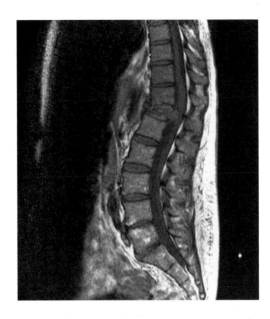

Figure 13.1 MRI of the spine revealing metastatic cord compression at T12.

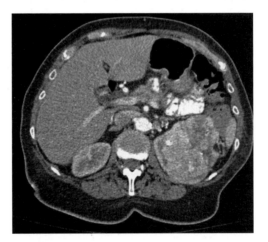

Figure 13.2 CT of the abdomen demonstrating a large tumour arising from the left kidney.

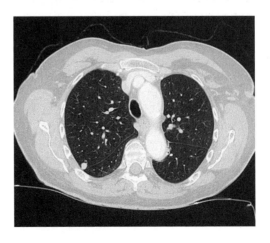

Figure 13.3 CT of the chest demonstrating small-volume pulmonary metastases.

a decision was made to proceed with systemic therapy, retaining the option of palliative nephrectomy, if indicated in the future. He was discharged home, with an urgent oncology outpatient appointment to discuss further management of his metastatic disease.

✪ Learning point Classification of renal cell cancer

Renal cell carcinoma (RCC) represents 90% of renal cancers. These are classified histopathologically, with 75% of these being ccRCCs and the remaining 25% comprising papillary carcinomas (types I and II), chromophobe carcinomas, and oncocytomas.

Oncocytomas are generally regarded as benign tumours, with only rare reports of metastatic spread. Both clear cell and papillary tumours, however, may have areas of sarcomatoid change, portending a more aggressive disease course. There are conflicting data on the prognostic significance of histological subtype. Non-clear cell tumours tend to present at an earlier stage; however, when stage-matched, although some studies have shown non-clear cell histology to be significant on univariate analysis, this has not proved to hold true on multivariate analysis.

❝ Expert comment

The genetic abnormalities underlying the different histological subtypes of RCC provide some insight into their different behaviour. Sixty to 90% of ccRCCs have impaired function of von Hippel–Lindau protein (VHL) due to somatic gene mutation, promoter hypermethylation, or germline genetic mutation. The resultant increase in hypoxia-inducible factor (HIF) drives the transcriptional activation of target genes, including VEGF and platelet-derived growth factor (PDGF), the target of many of the TKIs now in clinical use.

Signalling through the MET receptor via HGF has been implicated in hereditary and some sporadic papillary RCCs and may explain why these tumours are often less sensitive to VEGF-targeted TKIs.

✪ Learning point Cytoreductive nephrectomy in metastatic RCC

Nephrectomy prior to systemic immunotherapy with IFN-alpha has been shown to improve PFS and OS, compared with immunotherapy alone, in two randomized phase III trials (SWOG 8949 and EORTC 30947) in patients with good PS and limited metastatic disease [2,3].

With the advent of newer targeted agents, the role of cytoreductive surgery and its relationship to treatment initiation have been questioned. Some groups favour reserving surgery for those who respond to targeted therapies. Others favour a role for initial nephrectomy in selected patients, with targeted agents commenced in patients in whom surgery is less suitable.

Ongoing phase III trials are addressing these questions, looking at sunitinib alone versus the combination of nephrectomy followed by sunitinib (CARMENA) and looking at the timing of nephrectomy, immediate or deferred (SURTIME). Ultimately, the goal is to clarify the potential benefit conferred by nephrectomy in the era of molecular targeted therapies.

Box 13.1 Motzer or Memorial Sloan Kettering Cancer Center (MSKCC) criteria

The MSKCC criteria are the most widely used criteria to define the risk level of survival from renal cancer, based on 463 patients with metastatic RCC enrolled in clinical trials and treated with IFN-alpha [4].

The following five pretreatment risk factors were associated with a poorer survival:

- Karnofsky PS score of <80
- absence of prior nephrectomy
- Hb < the lower limit of normal
- LDH >1.5 times the ULN
- corrected serum calcium >10 mg/dL (equivalent to >2.5 mmol/L).

Risk was classified as:

- favourable: absence of risk factors; median survival of 20 months
- intermediate: 1–2 risk factors; median survival of 10 months
- poor: three or more risk factors; median survival of 4 months.

Source: data from Motzer RJ *et al*., Survival and prognostic stratification of 670 patients with advanced renal cell carcinoma, *Journal of Clinical Oncology*, Volume 17, Number 8, pp. 2530–40, Copyright © 1999 by the American Society of Clinical Oncology.

Box 13.2 Heng criteria for defining risk level for survival in metastatic RCC

The Heng criteria are based on 645 patients with metastatic RCC treated with anti-VEGF targeted therapies, thus being relevant in the era of targeted agents [5].

Poor survival was associated with:

- a low Hb
- Karnofsky PS score of <80
- diagnosis to treatment time of <1 year
- high corrected serum calcium
- platelets > ULN
- Neutrophil count > ULN.

Risk was classified as:

- favourable: absence of risk factors; median survival not reached; 2-year OS of 75%
- intermediate: 1–2 risk factors; median survival of 27 months; 2-year OS of 53%
- poor: 3–6 risk factors; median survival of 8.8 months; 2-year OS of 7%.

Unlike the Motzer criteria, elevated LDH and the nephrectomy status were not informative.

Source: data from Heng DY *et al*., Prognostic factors for overall survival in patients with metastatic renal cell carcinoma treated with vascular endothelial growth factor-targeted agents: results from a large, multicenter study, *Journal of Clinical Oncology*, Volume 27, Number 34, pp. 5794–9, Copyright © 2009 by the American Society of Clinical Oncology.

The patient was reviewed in the oncology clinic to discuss his diagnosis, prognosis, and treatment options. His survival risk was determined, according to both the Motzer criteria (Box 13.1) and Heng criteria (Box 13.2), which placed him in an intermediate-risk category.

The patient commenced treatment with the multi-targeted TKI sunitinib at the full dose of 50 mg daily for 28 days on and 14 days off. During the first month of treatment, his hypertension was less well controlled, necessitating an increase in his amlodipine dose from 5 mg to 10 mg daily. Following 7 weeks of treatment, he also developed altered taste, soreness of the mouth, lethargy, and grade 3 palmar–plantar syndrome, requiring a 25% dose reduction in subsequent cycles of sunitinib. With this dose reduction, the treatment was well tolerated, and, at first restaging, following 3 months of treatment, his CT scan showed a partial response within his pulmonary metastases, with stability in the bone disease. He went on to receive a further 8 months of treatment, with overall radiological disease stability.

> ⊕ **Clinical tip** Toxicity of VEGF-targeted TKIs
>
> Proactive management of the toxicity of VEGF-targeted TKIs allows the optimization of the dose, and hence clinical benefit. The commonest toxicities of sunitinib are diarrhoea, lethargy, stomatitis, hand–foot syndrome, and hypertension. Hypothyroidism is common in patients treated for long periods, and thyroid function tests should be monitored regularly, and thyroxine initiated if required. Standard anti-diarrhoeal medication is usually sufficient to control diarrhoea, and the hand–foot syndrome can be managed with regular emollients, together with soft footwear. The BP should be monitored regularly, and standard antihypertensives used when required.

> ✪ **Learning point** Small molecule inhibitors in the management of ccRCC
>
> Prior to the emergence of targeted therapies, the standard of care was cytokine therapy with agents such as IFN-alpha and IL-2. Toxicity was often marked, and response rates were poor, with modest benefits to OS.
>
> Treatment options have dramatically improved through an understanding of the biology of ccRCC. Mutations in the VHL gene occur in up to 75% of sporadic ccRCC tumours, leading to the constitutive expression of HIFs, which upregulate pro-angiogenic factors, including VEGF and PDGF. These findings have led to the development of small molecule inhibitors targeting the HIF/VEGF/PDGF pathway (Figure 13.4).
>
> Since 2005, five multi-targeted TKIs have been approved for use in advanced or metastatic ccRCC, following evaluation in phase III clinical trials. Positive results in the landmark TARGET trial of sorafenib versus placebo led to its approval by the FDA in 2005 for advanced RCC [6]. In 2006, first-line treatment of patients with the multikinase inhibitor sunitinib clearly demonstrated the superiority of sunitinib over IFN-alpha, thus changing the standard of care in ccRCC. An improvement of 6 months in PFS, and a significant improvement in the response rate and QoL, was observed in the sunitinib-treated group [7]. Pazopanib, a TKI targeting VEGF, PDGF, and c-kit, was also approved for use in advanced or metastatic ccRCC in the first-line setting [8]. Bevacizumab, in combination with IFN-alpha, has shown a superior PFS of 4.8 months, compared with IFN-alpha alone, in the AVOREN phase III trial, also establishing a role for this combination in the first-line treatment of advanced RCC [9].

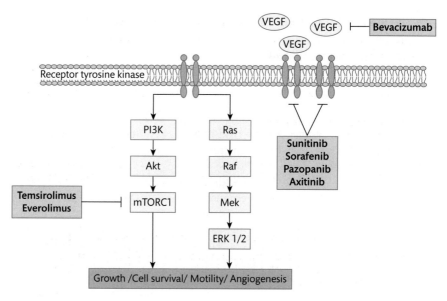

Figure 13.4 Molecular pathways targeted in renal cancer therapy.

❻ Expert comment

Both sunitinib and pazopanib are treatment options for the first-line use of patients with metastatic RCC and good PS. Each has proven efficacy in first-line use, but with differing toxicity profiles. The PISCES trial compared the two agents in a blinded fashion, with patients exposed to each agent consecutively [10]. A larger number of patients expressed a preference for treatment with pazopanib; however, efficacy was not an endpoint in this study. The COMPARZ study demonstrated the non-inferiority of pazopanib, compared to sunitinib, with PFS as the primary endpoint [11].

More recently, axitinib, a more potent and selective second-generation inhibitor of VEGF receptors 1, 2, and 3, has been licensed for second-line treatment of ccRCC, following following use of a TKI or cytokines. Axitinib demonstrated a 2-month improvement in the PFS and superior objective response rates in comparison with sorafenib [12], although OS was no different between the two groups [13]. This result establishes a place for axitinib in the second-line treatment of metastatic RCC and demonstrates the efficacy of a TKI after prior use of an agent from the same class, although perhaps not as marked an effect as in first-line use.

⊘ Evidence base TARGET: Treatment Approaches in Renal Cancer Global Evaluation Trial [14]

- Established the safety and efficacy of sorafenib in advanced ccRCC.
- Phase III, multicentre, randomized, double-blind, placebo-controlled trial.
- Sorafenib 400 mg PO bd continuously ($n = 451$) versus placebo ($n = 452$) in patients with unresectable or metastatic ccRCC who had progressed after one prior systemic therapy. Low- or intermediate-risk MSKCC score.
- At interim analysis, median PFS: sorafenib versus placebo, 5.5 months versus 2.8 months (HR 0.44, 95% CI 0.35–0.55; $p < 0.01$).
- Results of interim analysis on PFS led to the termination of the trial, cross-over of patients on placebo to sorafenib, and FDA approval of sorafenib for advanced RCC.
- OS benefit was not observed with sorafenib versus placebo on an ITT analysis [6], 17.8 months versus 15.2 months (HR 0.88; $p = 0.146$).

⊘ Evidence base Sunitinib, compared with IFN-alpha, in the first-line setting [7]

- Established superiority of sunitinib over the existing treatment in the first line.
- Phase III, multicentre, randomized trial.
- Sunitinib 50 mg PO od for 4 weeks every 6 weeks ($n = 375$) versus IFN-alpha 9 MU s/c three times weekly ($n = 375$) in patients with metastatic ccRCC, no prior systemic therapy, and ECOG PS of 0–1.
- Median PFS: sunitinib versus IFN-alpha, 11 months versus 5 months (HR 0.42, 95% CI 0.32–0.54; $p < 0.001$).
- Objective response rate: sunitinib versus IFN-alpha, 31% versus 6% ($p < 0.001$).
- Diarrhoea more common in the sunitinib group ($p < 0.05$), but QoL better than in patients on IFN-alpha ($p < 0.001$).

⊘ Evidence base AXIS: axitinib, compared with sorafenib, in second-line treatment [12]

- First head-to-head comparison of two molecular targeted treatments in RCC. Suggests that metastatic RCC remains sensitive, although perhaps to a lesser degree, to repeat VEGFR inhibition.
- Phase III, multicentre, randomized, non-blinded trial; primary endpoint PFS.

(continued)

- Axitinib 5 mg PO bd increased up to 10 mg bd continuously ($n = 361$) versus sorafenib 400 mg PO bd continuously ($n = 362$) in patients with metastatic ccRCC after progression on first-line treatment; ECOG PS of 0–1.
- The RECORD-1 data were not available at the time of design. As a result, the standard agent for comparison used in this study was sorafenib.
- Median PFS: axitinib versus sorafenib, 6.7 months versus 4.7 months (HR 0.464, 95% CI 0.544–0.812; $p < 0.0001$).
- Axitinib caused grade 3 or greater hypertension, diarrhoea, and fatigue, whilst sorafenib caused PPE, hypophosphataemia, hypertension, and lipase elevation.
- Mature OS data [12] showed no difference between axitinib versus sorafenib, 20.1 months versus 19.2 months (HR 0.969, 95% CI 0.800–1.174; $p = 0.37$).

The patient subsequently presented to clinic with a 4-week history of worsening shortness of breath and reduced exercise tolerance, whilst still on treatment with sunitinib. A CT pulmonary angiogram showed no evidence of PE but was suggestive of disease progression within the lungs. A formal restaging scan confirmed progressive disease within the lungs, with mediastinal lymphadenopathy, and also a probable metastasis in the left adrenal gland. Sunitinib was stopped, and the patient was commenced on second-line treatment with the mTOR inhibitor everolimus.

> ✪ **Learning point** mTOR inhibitors in RCC
>
> Inhibitors of the mTOR have demonstrated activity in metastatic RCC.
>
> The phase III ARCC study demonstrated a median PFS advantage of 2.4 months and a median OS benefit of 3.6 months with temsirolimus over IFN-alpha in patients with poor prognostic features [15]. This trial included patients with non-clear cell histology, with subset analysis showing a survival advantage in this group.
>
> Following progression on first-line anti-VEGF targeted therapy, mTOR inhibitors show activity in the second-line setting. Everolimus established itself as the agent of choice, following the phase III RECORD-1 trial, comparing everolimus with placebo in the second- and third-line setting.[16]. An improvement in the median PFS of 2.1 months with everolimus, compared with best supportive care, was seen in patients already treated with TKIs and cytokine therapy, thus establishing its use in the second- and subsequent-line treatment of ccRCC [16].

> ✔ **Evidence base** Temsirolimus, IFN-alpha, or both (Global ARCC Trial) [15]
>
> - Phase III, multicentre, randomized trial.
> - Temsirolimus 25 mg IV weekly ($n = 209$) versus IFN-alpha 3 MU increasing to 18 MU s/c three times weekly ($n = 207$) versus a combination of temsirolimus 15 mg IV weekly and IFN-alpha 6 MU s/c three times weekly ($n = 210$) in patients with previously untreated poor-prognosis advanced RCC.
> - Poor prognosis was defined by the presence of at least three of the following features: <1 year from the original diagnosis to the development of metastatic disease, metastases in multiple organs, low Karnofsky score, anaemia, and elevated serum levels of LDH and calcium.
> - Longer OS was observed in the temsirolimus group versus IFN-alpha group, 10.9 months versus 7.3 months (HR 0.73, 95% CI 0.58–0.92; $p = 0.008$). No OS benefit in the combination arm versus IFN-alpha, 7.3 months versus 8.4 months (HR 0.96, 95% CI 0.76–1.20; $p = 0.70$).
> - Fewer serious adverse effects were observed in the temsirolimus group, compared with the IFN-alpha group ($p = 0.02$).
>

> ☑ **Evidence base** RECORD-1: everolimus, compared with placebo, following progression on TKIs [16]
>
> - Phase III, multicentre, randomized, double-blind, placebo-controlled trial; primary endpoint PFS.
> - Everolimus 10 mg PO od continuously ($n = 272$) versus placebo ($n = 138$) in patients with metastatic ccRCC which had progressed on sunitinib and sorafenib, or both. Previous cytokine treatment or bevacizumab was also permitted. Karnofsky PS of ≥70%.
> - Median PFS at second interim analysis: everolimus versus placebo, 4 months versus 1.9 months (HR 0.3, 95% CI 0.22–0.4; p <0.0001).
> - Trial halted early, based on the difference in efficacy seen at interim analysis.
> - Mild to moderate stomatitis, rash, and fatigue were the commonest side effects on everolimus, with grade 3 pneumonitis also observed.
>
> Source: data from The Lancet, Volume 372, Issue 9637, Motzer RJ et al., Efficacy of everolimus in advanced renal cell carcinoma: a double-blind, randomised, placebo-controlled phase III trial, pp. 449–56, Copyright © 2008 Elsevier Ltd All rights reserved.

The patient currently continues on everolimus, with disease response on imaging following 8 weeks of treatment, with a reduction in the size of the pulmonary lesions, and stability in other sites of disease. His breathlessness has improved, and he maintains a good QoL 14 months following his initial diagnosis of metastatic renal cancer.

> ✪ **Learning point** Future directions in RCC
>
> **Neoadjuvant and adjuvant therapy**
>
> Up to 25% of patients treated with nephrectomy with curative intent relapse from their disease was seen. The potential for use of targeted agents in the neoadjuvant and adjuvant settings is an attractive one which remains under investigation.
>
> **Biomarkers to predict response**
>
> With the majority of molecular targeted therapies, there is a subgroup of patients who will not respond to treatment and risk morbidity as a result of treatment-associated toxicity. Identification of biomarkers to predict the response to treatment would enable the identification of patient groups most likely to derive benefit from the treatment. This is the focus of the E-PREDICT and S-PREDICT trials, looking at identifying predictive biomarkers in response to everolimus and sunitinib, respectively. These studies compare paired pre- and post-treatment tumour tissue, to look for changes in the tumour molecular signature as a result of treatment, and aim to correlate these with clinical data on efficacy. However, a separate publication reported on the analysis of four paired samples from the E-PREDICT study and demonstrated intra-tumour heterogeneity within tumour samples from the same patient [17]. It highlights the potential problems that could impede the development of predictive biomarkers and approaches to individualized medicine, directly as a result of sampling bias.

> ✪ **Learning point** Overcoming resistance
>
> Resistance mechanisms to anti-VEGF and mTOR targeted agents need to be elucidated, and strategies to overcome resistance developed. One approach is the design of more selective and potent VEGF inhibitors, such as axitinib which has shown 40 times greater potency than sunitinib for VEGFR-2 [12] and appears to be effective in sunitinib-refractory patients. Tivozanib, another second-generation TKI, is also being developed in metastatic RCC. Another strategy is the use of combination therapies. Intra-tumour heterogeneity may allow for the development of drug resistance within the tumour. The continued effort to identify signalling pathways mediating resistance will allow for the development of inhibitors of these pathways, which can then be used in combination with TKIs or mTOR inhibitors. For example:
>
> - AKT or PI3K inhibitors may suppress the rebound activation of AKT signalling seen with mTOR complex 1 inhibition

(continued)

- activation of the FGFR pathway has been identified as a potential resistance mechanism to VEGFR-targeted therapies. A dual anti-VEGFR and anti-FGFR small molecule inhibitor dovitinib is currently undergoing evaluation in metastatic RCC (GOLD-RCC randomized phase III trial), in comparison with sorafenib after VEGF- and mTOR-targeted therapies)
- numerous other small molecule inhibitors and antibody treatments are currently in preclinical and early-phase trials and will undoubtedly be trialled in combination regimes in RCC.

Discussion

This case demonstrates a typical presentation of metastatic ccRCC and the treatment options available. The advent of newer agents has increased the survival of these patients.

What is far from established is the optimal first-line agent of choice from all the available options. This is partly due to the lack of head-to-head comparisons of molecular targeted therapies in the first-line setting. In this case, the patient was treated with a TKI, followed by an mTOR inhibitor, and the local MDT made a decision for the patient not to undergo a nephrectomy.

Many changes in the management of metastatic renal cancer can be expected, as we expand our knowledge and expertise on existing treatments and continue to explore newer targets in order to improve survival from this tumour. There has been a resurgence of interest in immunotherapy in renal cancer, with the anti-programmed death-1 (PD-1) blocking antibody BMS 936558 showing promising activity in RCC in early-phase trials. The antibody is now being evaluated in metastatic renal cancer in phase III trials, in comparison with targeted small molecule inhibitors.

A final word from the expert

The choice of treatment should be based on the strength of available evidence for each agent, together with patient-specific factors such as PS and risk group, based on the Motzer or Heng criteria. With an increasing range of agents available in the first-, second-, and even third-line setting, decisions on the sequencing of these agents have become increasingly complex. In the absence of definitive head-to-head trial data, choices may be dependent on discussion of the toxicity profiles of the available drugs with patients on an individual basis.

The median OS in metastatic RCC with molecular targeted therapies is over 24 months, with the advantage of many active agents being oral. With continuous treatment until progression, and the potential for multiple lines of treatment for metastatic disease, the cost implication alone of these advances is significant. There are other areas in relation to these treatments that remain to be clarified. Given the toxicity of these agents when used in the longer term, the potential for treatment breaks is being investigated, and also the potential for alternating agents prior to progression, to prevent the emergence of resistance and maximize efficacy. Additional novel treatment strategies are likely to emerge in the near future, with both an increased range of molecular targeted agents and increased emphasis on the role of immunotherapies.

References

1. Rosen LS, Gordon D, Tchekmedyian S *et al.* Zoledronic acid versus placebo in the treatment of skeletal metastases in patients with lung cancer and other solid tumors: a phase III, double-blind, randomized trial—the Zoledronic Acid Lung Cancer and Other Solid Tumors Study Group. *Journal of Clinical Oncology* 2003; **21**(16): 3150–7.

2. Mickisch GH, Garin A, van Poppel H, de Prijck L, Sylvester R. Radical nephrectomy plus interferon-alfa-based immunotherapy compared with interferon alfa alone in metastatic renal-cell carcinoma: a randomised trial. *The Lancet* 2001; **358**(9286): 966–70.

3. Flanigan RC, Salmon SE, Blumenstein BA *et al.* Nephrectomy followed by interferon alfa-2b compared with interferon alfa-2b alone for metastatic renal-cell cancer. *The New England Journal of Medicine* 2001; **345**(23): 1655–9.

4. Motzer RJ, Mazumdar M, Bacik J, Berg W, Amsterdam A, Ferrara J. Survival and prognostic stratification of 670 patients with advanced renal cell carcinoma. *Journal of Clinical Oncology* 1999; **17**(8): 2530–40.

5. Heng DY, Xie W, Regan MM *et al.* Prognostic factors for overall survival in patients with metastatic renal cell carcinoma treated with vascular endothelial growth factor-targeted agents: results from a large, multicenter study. *Journal of Clinical Oncology* 2009; **27**(34): 5794–9.

6. Escudier B, Eisen T, Stadler WM *et al.* Sorafenib for treatment of renal cell carcinoma: Final efficacy and safety results of the phase III treatment approaches in renal cancer global evaluation trial. *Journal of Clinical Oncology* 2009; **27**(20): 3312–18.

7. Motzer RJ, Hutson TE, Tomczak P *et al.* Sunitinib versus interferon alfa in metastatic renal-cell carcinoma. *The New England Journal of Medicine* 2007; **356**(2): 115–24.

8. Sternberg CN, Davis ID, Mardiak J *et al.* Pazopanib in locally advanced or metastatic renal cell carcinoma: results of a randomized phase III trial. *Journal of Clinical Oncology* 2010; **28**(6): 1061–8.

9. Escudier B, Pluzanska A, Koralewski P *et al.* Bevacizumab plus interferon alfa-2a for treatment of metastatic renal cell carcinoma: a randomised, double-blind phase III trial. *The Lancet* 2007; **370**(9605): 2103–11.

10. Escudier B1, Porta C, Bono P et al. Randomized, controlled, double-blind, cross-over trial assessing treatment preference for pazopanib versus sunitinib in patients with metastatic renal cell carcinoma: PISCES Study. *J Clin Oncol.* 2014; **32**(14):1412-8.

11. Motzer RJ, Hutson TE, Cella D *et al.* Pazopanib versus sunitinib in metastatic renal-cell carcinoma. *The New England Journal of Medicine* 2013; **369**(8): 722–31.

12. Rini BI, Escudier B, Tomczak P *et al.* Comparative effectiveness of axitinib versus sorafenib in advanced renal cell carcinoma (AXIS): a randomised phase 3 trial. *The Lancet* 2011; **378**(9807): 1931–9.

13. Motzer RJ, Escudier B, Tomczak P *et al.* Axitinib versus sorafenib as second-line treatment for advanced renal cell carcinoma: overall survival analysis and updated results from a randomised phase 3 trial. *The Lancet Oncology* 2013; **14**(6): 552–62.

14. Escudier B, Eisen T, Stadler WM *et al.* Sorafenib in advanced clear-cell renal-cell carcinoma. *The New England Journal of Medicine* 2007; **356**(2): 125–34.

15. Hudes G, Carducci M, Tomczak P *et al.* Temsirolimus, interferon alfa, or both for advanced renal-cell carcinoma. *The New England Journal of Medicine* 2007; **356**(22): 2271–81.

16. Motzer RJ, Escudier B, Oudard S *et al.* Efficacy of everolimus in advanced renal cell carcinoma: a double-blind, randomised, placebo-controlled phase III trial. *The Lancet* 2008; **372**(9637): 449–56.

17. Gerlinger M, Rowan AJ, Horswell S *et al.* Intratumor heterogeneity and branched evolution revealed by multiregion sequencing. *The New England Journal of Medicine* 2012; **366**(10): 883–92.

14 Metastatic prostate cancer and spinal cord compression

Indrani S Bhattacharya

Expert commentary Helen O'Donnell

Case history

A 65-year-old man attended his GP practice for a routine PSA check. He was completely asymptomatic and denied any urinary or bowel symptoms. He had a past medical history of hypertension, for which he was taking ramipril. He had no known drug allergies and was not on any other medication. He was fully independent, did not smoke, and drank minimal alcohol.

His PSA level was raised at 9.5 ng/ml. Following this, the GP performed a digital rectal examination (DRE), which was normal. He was referred to the urologists for further assessment. He underwent transrectal ultrasound (TRUS)-guided biopsies, which revealed that he had prostate cancer with a Gleason grade of 3 + 4 in five left-sided cores and 3 + 3 in three right-sided cores. In total, 8/13 cores were involved with a 15 mm maximum tumour length on the left. He went on to have an MRI scan of the prostate, which did not show any focal abnormalities or targetable lesions. His bone scan showed no evidence of metastases.

> **Clinical tip** Detection of prostate cancer
>
> Most prostate cancers are PSA-detected (stage T1c), and many of these patients are asymptomatic. Some patients complain of troublesome lower urinary tract symptoms, including urinary frequency, hesitancy, poor stream, dribbling, and incomplete bladder emptying. Prostate cancer may also be found in prostate chippings, following transurethral resection of the prostate (TURP) procedures performed for presumed benign prostatic hypertrophy (stages T1a/b).

> **Clinical tip** Diagnosis of prostate cancer [1]
>
> PSA level and DRE must be performed in the first instance. Generally, patients with a PSA level of >4ng/ml) or a positive DRE with any PSA level are offered TRUS biopsies. If prostate cancer is found, further investigations are guided by the Gleason grade and PSA. A pelvic MRI allows detection of extracapsular spread, seminal vesicle involvement and pelvic lymphadenopathy. A bone scan will exclude bone metastases.
>
> MRI and bone scan are usually performed in patients who have a gleason grade of 7 or above, or those with a PSA level of >20ng/ml where radical treatment is being considered. There has also been a recent move towards pre-biopsy MRI scans in order to reduce confusion with post-biopsy haemorrhage and utilize the functional MRI capacity.

> **Expert comment**
>
> In younger men, a lower PSA level may prompt a prostate biopsy, and there are suggested age-related maximum levels. The rate of rise of serial PSA levels may also prompt a biopsy. PSA levels can be elevated in the absence of malignancy, e.g. in prostatitis, benign prostate hyperplasia (BPH), or trauma to the prostate. The sensitivity of PSA testing can be improved by measuring both the free and bound fractions of PSA and calculating the free/total PSA ratio (FTR). A negative biopsy does not rule out the possibility of prostate cancer, and, if PSA remains elevated or is rising, then further biopsies (either transrectal or template) are recommended. The use of functional MRI pre-biopsy can aid targeted biopsies.

> ✪ **Learning point** Pathology and Gleason grade [1]
>
> Most cancers of the prostate are adenocarcinomas. These are often multifocal and most frequently affect the postero-lateral part of the gland, with approximately 70% affecting the peripheral zone. Rarely, mucinous, small cell, squamous cell, and adenoid cystic carcinoma may occur.
>
> The Gleason grade is an important prognostic factor in prostate cancer. It describes the degree of malignant differentiation. Each tumour is graded twice and given a score of 3–5. The first Gleason grade relates to the most commonly observed pattern, and the second to the next most common pattern.
>
> For example, if the most common tumour pattern were grade 3, but some cells were found to be grade 4, the Gleason score would be 3 + 4 = 7. The Gleason grade or Gleason pattern ranges from 3 to 5, with 5 having the worst prognosis. For Gleason score 7, a Gleason 4 + 3 is a more aggressive cancer than a Gleason 3 + 4.

His prostate cancer was staged as T2N0M0 adenocarcinoma of the prostate [2], and, given his PSA level and Gleason grade, he was felt to be at intermediate risk. His case was discussed at the urology MDT meeting where active treatment for his intermediate-risk prostate cancer was recommended. The proposed treatment options included surgery, low-dose rate (LDR) brachytherapy, hormones plus EBRT, or hormones plus EBRT with a high-dose rate (HDR) brachytherapy boost. The patient was reviewed in the combined clinic where there were both a consultant urologist and a consultant oncologist present to allow the patient to discuss both the surgical and radiotherapy options, going through the risks and benefits of each.

> ✪ **Learning point** Prostate cancer risk stratification
>
> | Risk group | Definition |
> | --- | --- |
> | Low risk | T1–T2a, Gleason score ≤6, PSA <10 ng/mL |
> | Intermediate risk | T2b and/or Gleason score 7 and/or PSA 10–20 ng/mL |
> | High risk | ≥T2c and/or Gleason score 8–10 and/or PSA >20 ng/mL |

> ✪ **Learning point** Management of Localized disease [1]
>
> The treatment options for localized disease include active surveillance, watchful waiting, and radical treatment with either surgery or radiotherapy.
>
> **Active surveillance and watchful waiting**
>
> Some prostate cancers are slow-growing and will not affect life expectancy. These patients can therefore avoid the side effects associated with radical treatment options. Active surveillance is an intensive monitoring process which typically consists of 3-monthly clinics for the first 2 years followed by 6-monthly clinics. Each clinic attendance should include a PSA and DRE and TRUS biopsies repeated at 18 months. If the PSA doubling time is <2 years, or suspicious DRE or the Gleason grade is upgraded on repeat biopsy, then patients should be offered radical treatment. It is mainly low risk patients who are suitable for active surveillance. Those patients who are not fit for radical treatment should be offered watchful waiting where endocrine therapy is offered on development of symptoms and the treatment intent is palliative.
>
> (continued)

Radical treatment options include radical prostatectomy, external beam radiotherapy (EBRT), and brachytherapy; low dose rate (LDR) or high dose rate (HDR).

Radical prostatectomy

Radical prostatectomy is usually reserved for those with low–intermediate-risk disease and a good performance status. In recent years this is mainly being performed by minimally invasive surgery, either robotic or laparoscopic. This has reduced post-operative recovery time and hospital stay. Surgery has a 5–15% risk of urinary dysfunction ranging from mild leakage to incontinence. Nerve-sparing techniques can be an option for those with small-volume disease and has better morbidity, with impotence rates of approximately 50%. Some surgical candidates may also have pelvic lymph node sampling preoperatively. At present, the RADICALS study is investigating the use of radiotherapy and hormones after surgery for early prostate cancer.

EBRT

EBRT is an option for low, intermediate or high-risk disease. There is now a drive to have Intensity Modulated Radiotherapy (IMRT) as standard for all patients, which improves dose distributions and spares normal tissues. Prostate cancer is thought to have a lower alpha/beta ratio than other tumours (1.2–1.5 Gy) and hypofractionated radiotherapy with a higher dose per fraction may achieve better local control with a similar side effect profile. Results from the CHHiP trial are awaited.

Brachytherapy (LDR and HDR)

In LDR brachytherapy, approximately 50-100 iodine-125 radioactive seeds are implanted in the prostate gland via ultrasound guided transperineal needles whilst the patient is under general anaesthetic to achieve a prescribed dose of 145–160Gy. Brachytherapy is most often offered to those who have low-risk disease and a small prostate volume (<50 cc); however, with the use of real-time brachytherapy, it is possible to implant larger glands. Patients with significant lower urinary tract symptoms are not suited to brachytherapy. Those who have had previous TURPs are also less suited to brachytherapy. HDR brachytherapy can be delivered as a monotherapy or as a boost following (a shortened course of) EBRT. Combined EBRT and HDR boost is reserved for those patients with intermediate and high-risk disease. Catheters are implanted into the prostate under ultrasound guidance whilst the patient under general anaesthetic. Following this, the HDR treatment is delivered via the catheters. There are various HDR brachytherapy boost schedules in use.

Endocrine treatment in localized prostate cancer

Patients receiving radical radiotherapy are routinely treated with adjuvant hormones. Those with intermediate-risk disease are given a total of 6 months of hormones, and those with high risk disease are given a total of 2–3 years. A luteinizing hormone-releasing hormone (LHRH) analogue is usually used, and the main side effects include weight gain, hot flushes, and impotence. Other side effects include fatigue, osteoporosis, mood changes, and poor concentration and memory.

Expert comment

The challenge is to identify those patients who will benefit from radical treatment and in whom the side effects of treatment are justifiable. Towards this end, cases are conventionally classified into risk groups, in terms of the PSA level, Gleason score, and clinical T stage. These risk groups have been shown to predict the probability of biochemical recurrence *after* radical treatment and are used as a guide to treatment decision making. In particular, patients with intermediate- and high-risk disease, localized prostate cancer are considered good candidates for immediate radical treatment, rather than observation. Patients with low-risk disease are faced with the difficult decision of whether or not to have treatment, needing to weigh up the potential survival benefit against the known morbidity.

Clinical tip Side effects of radiotherapy

Acute side effects:

- dysuria
- increase in urinary frequency
- diarrhoea
- lethargy

Late side effects:

- proctitis
- impotence
- urinary incontinence.

✔ Evidence base RTOG 92-02: phase III trial of long-term adjuvant androgen deprivation after neoadjuvant hormonal cytoreduction and radiotherapy in locally advanced carcinoma of the prostate [4]

- Randomized trial testing of long-term adjuvant androgen deprivation after initial androgen deprivation with EBRT in patients with locally advanced prostate cancer.
- The long-term androgen deprivation (LTAD) plus RT group showed significant improvement over the short-term androgen deprivation (STAD) plus RT group for all endpoints, except OS.
- Endpoints included disease free survival (DFS) (13.2% versus 22.5%; p <0.0001), disease-specific survival (83.9% versus 88.7%; p = 0.0042), local progression (22.2% versus 12.3%; p <0.0001), distant metastasis (22.8% versus 14.8%; p <0.0001), biochemical failure (68.1% versus 51.9%; p ≤0.0001), and OS (51.6% versus 53.9%; p = 0.36).
- A subset analysis of patients with Gleason scores 8–10 showed that long-term adjuvant androgen deprivation resulted in a survival advantage (31.9% versus 45.1%; p = 0.0061)* .

Source: data from Horwitz EM, Bae K, Hanks GE et al. Ten-year follow-up of radiation therapy oncology group protocol 92-02: a phase III trial of the duration of elective androgen deprivation in locally advanced prostate cancer. *J Clin Oncol*. 2008 May 20;26(15):2497–504 Copyright © 2008 by American Society of Clinical Oncology.

✔ Evidence base Duration of androgen suppression in the treatment of prostate cancer [5]

- Patients (n = 970) with locally advanced prostate cancer were randomly assigned to external beam radiotherapy (EBM) plus short-term androgen suppression (6 months) (n = 483) versus EBM plus 2.5 years of further treatment with an LHRH agonist (long-term suppression) (n = 487).
- The 5-year overall mortality for short-term and long-term suppression was 19.0% and 15.2%, respectively.
- The observed HR was 1.42 (upper 95.71% confidence limit 1.79; p = 0.65 for non-inferiority).
- Adverse events in both groups included fatigue, diminished sexual function, and hot flushes.
- Radiotherapy plus 6 months of androgen suppression was associated with inferior survival, compared with radiotherapy plus long-term androgen suppression.

Source: data from Bolla *et al.*, Duration of androgen suppression in the treatment of prostate cancer, *New England Medical Journal*, Volume 360, Number 24, pp. 2516–27, Copyright © 2009 Massachusetts Medical Society. All rights reserved.

The patient opted to have 6 months of hormones plus EBRT. He was initiated on Zoladex® 10.8 mg s/c every 12 weeks and was given bicalutamide for 1 month to prevent tumour flare. Three months after starting Zoladex®, the patient was planned for radiotherapy treatment. The first stage of the radiotherapy planning was the insertion of fiducial markers. Two weeks after this, the patient went on to have the radiotherapy planning CT scan. At the time of scanning and for each daily treatment, the patient was asked to drink water to ensure the bladder was comfortably full. This was in order to reduce variation in bladder and bowel filling and therefore reduce prostate movement. The organs at risk (OAR) that were contoured included the bladder, rectum, urethral bulb, and femoral heads.

The planned treatment schedule was 74 Gy in 37 fractions over 7 weeks, which is the dose fractionation of the standard treatment arm in the CHHiP trial. The patient tolerated the treatment well, with acute toxicities of mild dysuria and increased bowel frequency. Six months following treatment, his PSA was found to be undetectable at <0.01 ng/ml.

⊘ **Evidence base** CHHiP Trial: conventional versus hypofractionated high-dose IMRT for prostate cancer [6]

- Multicentre, randomized study which recruited patients with histologically confirmed, previously untreated localized adenocarcinoma of the prostate who were randomized in a 1:1:1 ratio between:
  ○ a conventional radiotherapy fractionation of 74 Gy in 37 fractions over 7.4 weeks using conformal and IMRT techniques ($n = 153$) versus
  ○ one of each of the hypofractionated experimental groups of 57 Gy in 19 fractions over 3.8 weeks ($n =151$) and 60 Gy in 20 fractions over 4 weeks ($n =153$).
- All patients received neoadjuvant androgen suppression.
- Efficacy outcome yet to be reported.
- Analysis of the therapeutic ratio of each arm suggests that hypofractionated high-dose radiotherapy seems equally well tolerated as conventionally fractionated treatment at 2 years.

Source: data from *The Lancet Oncology*, Volume 13, Issue 1, Dearnaley D *et al.*, Conventional versus hypofractionated high-dose intensity-modulated radiotherapy for prostate cancer: preliminary safety results from the CHHiP randomised controlled trial, pp. 43–54, Copyright © 2012 Elsevier Ltd.

Five years following radiotherapy, the patient presented to his GP, complaining of lower back pain. Plain film X-rays of the lumbar spine showed degenerative changes. His PSA level was 200 ng/ml. A bone scan went on to show multiple sclerotic lesions throughout the spine and hips. He had a staging CT CAP which confirmed multiple bone deposits throughout the spine and hips and low-volume pelvic lymphadenopathy. He was initiated on an LHRH analogue and given palliative radiotherapy to the sacro-iliac joints for his pain. He was also given monthly bisphosphonate infusions for his bone pain.

His PSA responded to hormones, and his PSA level went down to 20 ng/ml within 3 months of his first injection of the LHRH analogue. After 9 months, his PSA level began to rise. At this point, bicalutamide was added (total androgen blockade); however, his PSA did not respond to this. Despite having a rising PSA, he was relatively asymptomatic, and his bone pain was well controlled. His performance status (PS) was 1, and it was felt that he would be a candidate for single-agent docetaxel 75 mg/m^2 3-weekly and prednisolone 10 mg od. Baseline restaging with CT and bone scans were performed prior to initiation of chemotherapy. The patient tolerated the first three cycles well, with minimal side effects. His PSA responded, and disease response was confirmed on CT scanning after three cycles. The patient continued with a further three cycles, and then, due to increasing fatigue, the chemotherapy was stopped.

✪ **Learning point** Management of metastatic disease

Metastatic disease is managed in the first instance with hormones alone. Patients who become hormone-refractory are considered for other treatment options which include chemotherapy (docetaxel, cabazitaxel) or abiraterone. Cabazitaxel can also be used second line in those who have progressed with docetaxel.

(continued)

Clinical tip Abiraterone

Abiraterone acetate is an inhibitor of 17 alpha-hydroxylase. Until recently, it was only licensed for use in those patients who had progressed on chemotherapy; however, it can now be used prior to chemotherapy [8]. It is taken orally at a dose of 1 g daily, with a low dose of prednisolone. It is relatively well tolerated. Side effects can include hypertension, hypokalaemia, peripheral oedema, and liver impairment.

Clinical tip Docetaxel

Docetaxel is well established in the management of castrate-resistant prostate cancer. It is a member of the taxane family of tubulin-binding agents and acts as a microtubule destabilizer. Docetaxel is administered at a dose of 75 mg/m^2 3-weekly, with prednisolone (to reduce the risk of hypersensitivity [10]), for up to ten cycles in total. Adverse effects include nausea, vomiting, neutropenia, infection, peripheral neuropathy, and nail changes.

There are an increasing number of treatments available for advanced/metastatic castrate-resistant prostate cancer. The STAMPEDE study is currently assessing whether treating patients earlier with a multimodality approach will lead to a better outcome [7]. STAMPEDE originally included five arms:

- hormones plus zoledronic acid
- hormones plus chemotherapy (docetaxel)
- hormones plus celecoxib
- hormones plus abiraterone
- hormones plus prostate radiotherapy.

The celecoxib arm closed early, due to increased risk of cardiotoxicity. In 2012, the zoledronic acid and chemotherapy arms closed, as a sample size had been reached that provided a sufficient power for analysis. More recently, the abiraterone arm has closed and a new arm including hormones, abiraterone and enzalutamide has been opened.

Enzalutamide (formerly known as MDV3100) is another new androgen receptor (AR) antagonist drug, developed for the treatment of metastatic castration-resistant prostate cancer. It has an approximately 5-fold higher binding affinity for the AR, compared to the anti-androgen bicalutamide. The study AFFIRM [9] aimed to determine the effectiveness of enzalutamide in patients who progressed following chemotherapy treatment with docetaxel. In November 2011, this trial was halted, after an interim analysis revealed that patients given the drug lived for approximately 5 months longer than those taking placebo. FDA approval was granted in August 2012. At present, the PREVAIL study is investigating the effectiveness of enzalutamide in patients who are chemotherapy-naïve. Side effects include lethargy, arthralgia, headaches, peripheral neuropathy, hot flushes, diarrhoea, seizures, and peripheral oedema.

Evidence base TAX 327 study: docetaxel plus prednisone, or mitoxantrone plus prednisone, for advanced prostate cancer [10]

Randomized trial comparing docetaxel administered every 3 weeks, weekly docetaxel, and mitoxantrone, each with prednisone.

Median survival time was:

- 19.2 months (95% CI 17.5–21.3 months) in the 3-weekly docetaxel arm
- 17.8 months (95% CI 16.2–19.2 months) in the weekly docetaxel arm, and
- 16.3 months (95% CI 14.3–17.9 months) in the mitoxantrone arm.

Survival of men with metastatic hormone-resistant prostate cancer was significantly longer after treatment with 3-weekly docetaxel, compared with mitoxantrone. Consistent results were observed across subgroups of patients.

Source: data from Berthold DR *et al*., Docetaxel plus prednisone or mitoxantrone plus prednisone for advanced prostate cancer: updated survival in the TAX 327 study, *Journal of Clinical Oncology*, Volume 26, Issue 2, pp. 242–5, Copyright © 2008 by American Society of Clinical Oncology.

Clinical tip Cabazitaxel

Cabazitaxel, a taxane derivative, is approved for use, in combination with prednisone, for the treatment of patients with hormone-refractory metastatic prostate cancer previously treated with a docetaxel-containing regimen. In the TROPIC trial [11], OS was significantly prolonged with cabazitaxel plus prednisone versus mitoxantrone plus prednisone in patients with metastatic castrate-resistant prostate cancer who had progressed during or after docetaxel therapy. PFS, time to tumour progression, and PSA progression were improved with cabazitaxel plus prednisone. Side effects of cabazitaxel include neutropenia, anaemia, nausea, vomiting, diarrhoea, and risk of hypersensitivity.

Three months later, the patient was admitted with upper back pain and arm weakness. Clinical examination showed reduced power in both upper limbs. An MRI scan of the whole spine confirmed spinal cord compression at C3 and C4 (Figure 14.1). The patient was immobilized and started on high-dose dexamethasone

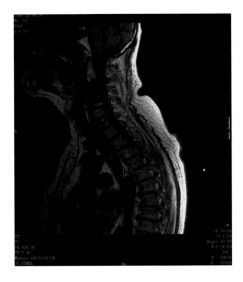

Figure 14.1 MRI of the spine demonstrating metastatic disease at C3, C4, C5, and C7, with spinal cord compression at C3 and C4.

with a proton pump inhibitor. The patient was discussed with the neurosurgical team; however, given the widespread metastases, it was felt that he would not be a neurosurgical candidate. The patient was given 20 Gy in five fractions to his cervical spine over 1 week. He was immobilized in a shell and treated, using lateral parallel opposed fields. The high-dose dexamethasone was then tapered down gradually after his last fraction of radiotherapy.

> ⊗ **Learning point** Diagnosis and management of malignant spinal cord compression [12]
>
> Spinal cord compression is a medical and oncological emergency. Clinical features include radicular back pain, lower limb sensory disturbance, bladder and/or bowel dysfunction and weakness of the legs. Symptoms and neurological signs will depend on the site of spinal cord compression and compression below L1 will result in the cauda equina syndrome. The symptoms of spinal cord compression may have an insidious onset or in some cases paraplegia can develop with only a few prior symptoms.
>
> Spinal cord compression neurological findings include bilateral upper motor neuron lesions in the legs and a sensory level. Signs and symptoms in the arms should raise suspicion of involvement of the cervical cord. The cauda equina syndrome may cause signs of a lower limb lower motor neuron lesion, sensory loss and urinary dysfunction.
>
> It is imperative to act quickly in patients with suspected spinal cord compression. It is essential for clinicians to have a high index of suspicion and to initiate the diagnosis and treatment as quickly as possible. The main determinant of outcome has been shown to be the severity of neurological damage at the time of treatment initiation.
>
> If there is any suspicion of a patient having spinal cord compression, high dose steroids should be initiated immediately. Dexamethasone 8mg BD is usually prescribed. All patients require a whole spine MRI scan. A whole spine CT is an alternative for patients unable to have an MRI. The whole spine must be imaged as it is not uncommon for there to be multiple levels of spinal cord compression. It is essential that the initiation of steroids is not delayed whilst waiting for the outcome of the whole spine MRI scan.
>
> The definitive treatment options include surgical decompression (with post-operative radiotherapy) and radiotherapy alone. This decision should be made in conjunction with the neurosurgical team and the factors which need to be considered are the patient's performance status, neurology, site of the primary and the histology, other sites of disease, prognosis, further treatment options, and prior radiotherapy.
>
> (continued)

Indications for surgical intervention (which will involve an anterior decompression and spine stabilization) include an unknown primary tumour (this will also provide an opportunity to obtain a histological diagnosis), unstable spine, recurrence post-radiotherapy, worsening neurology during radiotherapy, and sudden onset paralysis. Evidence suggests that patients who receive emergency spinal decompression, followed by post-operative radiotherapy, have an improved functional outcome. In those patients who have very chemo-sensitive tumours, such as lymphoma or small cell lung cancer it may appropriate to initiate urgent chemotherapy prior to considering radiotherapy.

Barrett A, Dobbs J, Morris S and Roques T. Emergency and Palliative Radiotherapy. In: Barrett A, Dobbs J, Morris S and Roques T,editors. Practical Radiotherapy Planning. New York: CRC press; 2009.

Following treatment of his cord compression, the patient had further restaging scans which showed disease progression. He was initiated on abiraterone 1g od, with 10 mg of prednisolone. His PSA responded to the initiation of abiraterone and remained controlled for 3 months. Following this, his PSA rose, and he became increasingly symptomatic from worsening bone metastases, despite analgesia and palliative radiotherapy. His abiraterone was discontinued, as his PS declined. He received palliative care review and required hospice admission, following which he died.

🕐 **Evidence base** Abiraterone, compared with placebo, in castration-resistant prostate cancer [13]

- Patients with castration-resistant prostate cancer who had previously received docetaxel ($n = 1195$) were randomly assigned to receive 1000 mg of abiraterone acetate ($n = 797$ patients) or placebo ($n = 398$ patients) with prednisolone.
- OS was prolonged in the abiraterone group (14.8 months versus 10.9 months; HR 0.65, 95% CI 0.54–0.77; $p < 0.001$).
- Time to PSA progression (10.2 months versus 6.6 months; $p < 0.001$), PFS (5.6 months versus 3.6 months; $p < 0.001$), and PSA response rate (29% versus 6%; $p < 0.001$) favoured the abiraterone group.
- Abiraterone was associated with more frequent mineralocorticoid-related adverse events, including fluid retention, hypertension, and hypokalaemia.

Source: data from de Bono JS *et al*., Abiraterone and increased survival in metastatic prostate cancer, *New England Medical Journal*, Volume 364, Number 21, pp. 1995–2005, Copyright © 2011 Massachusetts Medical Society. All rights reserved.

Discussion

Prostate cancer comprises 12% of all cancers. In the UK there are approximately 32,000 new diagnoses and 10,000 prostate cancer related deaths each year. It tends to affect those aged 70 and above. An increase in PSA testing and surgery related to benign prostatic disease has led to the rising incidence of prostate cancer over the last 10-15 years. The exact aetiology is unknown. Suggested risk factors include a high-fat diet, anabolic steroids, oestrogen exposure, and family history [1].

This case illustrates the complexities in the management of early prostate cancer. The clinician and patient must undertake a joint decision-making process to balance the intended benefits, life expectancy, co-morbidities and treatment related toxicities [15]. Risk stratification tables place patients into low-,intermediate-, and high-risk groups, based on their PSA, Gleason grade, and MRI findings. This guides specific treatments according to risk and aids as a potential predictor of clinical outcome.

In recent years, a number of new treatments for prostate cancer have been approved, predominantly in the setting of hormone-refractory disease. Those patients who are not fit for systemic therapy may benefit from a low dose of steroids (0.5–1 mg of dexamethasone). Bisphosphonates can help with bone pain in those who can easily attend hospital on a monthly basis for monthly infusions. Zolendronic acid is effective in controlling metastatic bone pain and has also been shown to reduce the incidence of skeletal events. EBRT is also highly effective at controlling bone pain from bone metastases, as well as symptoms of prostatic tumour invasion such as haematuria or pain. Radiotherapy is also essential in the management of spinal cord compression.

> **⚠ Expert comment**
>
> NICE currently recommends bisphosphonates for the management of pain in men with prostate cancer and bone metastases [14]. Denosumab is an mAb that binds to RANKL and results in reduced osteoclast function. It has been demonstrated to be superior to zoledronic acid in reducing skeletal related events from bone metastases in most solid tumours. Denosumab has not yet been NICE-approved for use in prostate cancer.

A final word from the expert

Over recent years, the management of prostate cancer has undergone many changes, due to developments in our understanding of the natural history of prostate cancer and its response to treatment, the introduction of functional imaging, and technological advances in both radiotherapy and surgery.

This case nicely demonstrates the issues surrounding the diagnosis and risk stratification of prostate cancer, such that treatment options can be presented and an informed decision made.

The issue of PSA recurrence, subsequent metastatic disease, and its sequelae are discussed. The limitations of success from radical local treatment relate either to resistant disease, local disease, or the presence of early micrometastatic disease at diagnosis which is not treated with local therapies.

Management of metastatic disease requires a multimodality treatment approach, as demonstrated with the use of systemic therapies and palliative radiotherapy. Addressing the QoL and symptom control are important, in addition to therapies aimed at disease control.

References

1. Beresford M. Cancers of the prostate. In: Ajithkumar TV Hatcher HM, editors. *Specialist Training in Oncology.* China: Elsevier; 2011.
2. Edge SB, Byrd DR, Compton CC *et al.* eds. *AJCC cancer staging manual*, 7th edn. New York: Springer, 2010.
3. Resnick MJ, Koyama T, Fan KH *et al.* Long-term functional outcomes after treatment for localized prostate cancer. *The New England Journal of Medicine* 2013; **368**(5): 436–45.
4. Horwitz EM, Bae K, Hanks GE *et al.* Ten-year follow-up of radiation therapy oncology group protocol 92–02: a phase III trial of the duration of elective androgen deprivation in locally advanced prostate cancer. *J Clin Oncol.* 2008 **20**;26(15): 2497–504

5. Bolla M, de Reijke TM, Van Tienhoven G *et al.*; EORTC Radiation Oncology Group and Genito-Urinary Tract Cancer Group. Duration of androgen suppression in the treatment of prostate cancer. *The New England Journal of Medicine* 2009; **360**(24): 2516–27.

6. Dearnaley D, Syndikus I, Sumo G *et al.* Conventional versus hypofractionated high-dose intensity-modulated radiotherapy for prostate cancer: preliminary safety results from the CHHiP randomised controlled trial. *The Lancet Oncology* 2012; **13**(1): 43–54.

7. Sydes MR, Parmar MK, Mason MD *et al.* Flexible trial design in practice—stopping arms for lack-of-benefit and adding research arms mid-trial in STAMPEDE: a multi-arm multi-stage randomized controlled trial. *Trials* 2012; **13**: 168.

8. Ryan CJ, Smith MR, de Bone JS *et al.* Abiraterone in metastatic prostate cancer without previous chemotherapy. *The New England Journal of Medicine* 2013; **368**(2): 138–48.

9. Scher HI, Fizazi K, Saad F *et al.* Increased survival with enzalutamide in prostate cancer after chemotherapy. *The New England Journal of Medicine* 2012; **367**(13): 1187–97.

10. Berthold DR, Pond GR, Soban F, de Wit R, Eisenberger M, Tannock IF. Docetaxel plus prednisone or mitoxantrone plus prednisone for advanced prostate cancer: updated survival in the TAX 327 study. *Journal of Clinical Oncology* 2008; **26**(2): 242–5.

11. de Bono JS, Oudard S, Ozguroglu M *et al.* Prednisone plus cabazitaxel or mitoxantrone for metastatic castration-resistant prostate cancer progressing after docetaxel treatment: a randomised open-label trial (TROPIC). *The Lancet* 2010; **376**(9747): 1147–54.

12. Barrett A, Dobbs J, Morris S and Roques T. Emergency and Palliative Radiotherapy. In: Barrett A, Dobbs J, Morris S and Roques T, editors. *Practical Radiotherapy Planning.* New York: CRC press; 2009.

13. de Bono JS, Logothetis CJ, Molina A *et al.* Abiraterone and increased survival in metastatic prostate cancer. *The New England Journal of Medicine* 2011; 364(21): 1995–2005.

14. National Institute for Health and Care Excellence. *Prostate cancer: diagnosis and management.* 2008. Available at: <http://guidance.nice.org.uk/CG58>.

15. Shariat SF, Kattan MW, Vickers AJ, Karakiewicz PI, Scardino PT. Critical review of prostate cancer predictive tools. *Future Oncol.* 2009; **5**(10): 1555–84.

15 Transformed follicular lymphoma

Chern Siang Lee

✦ Expert commentary Andrew Davies

Case history

A 59-year-old man was originally diagnosed with follicular lymphoma in 2005, after investigations for cholecystitis led to the discovery of incidental lymphadenopathy. Diagnostic lymph node biopsy, at that time, confirmed grade 2 follicular lymphoma with a clinical stage of IIIA. The patient had a normal FBC and LDH, with a good prognosis based on the Follicular Lymphoma International Prognostic Index (FLIPI).

The patient's additional medical history included cholecystectomy, obesity, hypertension, depression, and type 2 diabetes. He was taking ramipril, citalopram, and gliclazide. He had no history of any cardiopulmonary disease. There was a family history of coronary heart disease and breast cancer in a first-degree relative. He was an ex-smoker of 15 pack years and drank 10 units of alcohol per week. He worked as a self-employed plumber.

> **✪ Learning point** Follicular lymphoma
>
> Follicular lymphoma is the commonest subtype of indolent NHL and the second commonest type of lymphoma in the Western world. It is thought to originate from germinal centre B cells and morphologically is composed of clonally related centrocytes (small cells) and centroblasts (large cells).
>
> Patients typically present in their sixties, at an advanced stage, with a history of asymptomatic lymphadenopathy. Half of patients are stage IV at presentation. The clinical course is usually long. The disease is chemosensitive and characterized by symptom-free intervals, followed by repeated relapses and diminishing sensitivity to each subsequent line of therapy. The median survival of patients presenting with advanced-stage disease is about 8–10 years.
>
> Patients with true stage I or II follicular lymphoma (15–20%) may be amenable to involved field radiotherapy treatment which may be curative; otherwise, follicular lymphoma is not usually considered curable.

> **✪ Learning point** Summary of investigations in suspected lymphoma
>
> Lymphoma may present as an incidental finding, during investigation of lymphadenopathy, or indeed as an oncological emergency. In the latter circumstance, discussion with a histopathologist, prior to obtaining an urgent diagnostic biopsy, is vital to ensure the tissue is handled, fixed, and stained appropriately.
>
> Tissue diagnosis
>
> - Whole lymph node excision biopsy preferable
> - Satisfactorily sized core biopsy is acceptable
> - Fine needle aspirate is insufficient for diagnosis
> - Specialist haematopathology review is required

(continued)

> **✦ Expert comment**
>
> Sufficient diagnostic material and review by an expert haematopathologist are essential. The use of needle biopsies should be limited to anatomically restricted sites, as contextualizing the malignant lymphocytes in their surrounding architecture is essential for accurate diagnosis.

> **✦ Expert comment**
>
> Rituximab with chemotherapy can cause reactivation of latent viral hepatitis. You must know the hepatitis status of your patients.

Staging and baseline information

- Standard bloods, including FBC (with immunophenotyping if lymphocytosis), T-cells, B-cells and natural killer cells (TBNK) subsets, blood film, group and save, direct antiglobulin test, ESR, U&Es, LFTs, LDH, urate, beta-2-microglobulin, immunoglobulin (and serum protein electrophoresis)
- Viral screen (including CMV, EBV, human T-cell leukaemia virus (HTLV), hepatitis, and human acquired immunodeficiency virus (HIV))
- CT of neck/chest/abdomen/pelvis with contrast
- Bone marrow aspirate and trephine

Optional investigations/comments

- Echocardiogram: elderly, diabetic, previous cardiac history, previous anthracycline exposure
- Consider PET/CT in certain circumstances (e.g. true early stage for curative radiotherapy).
- Other site-specific investigations such as endoscopy
- If CNS involvement suspected, then imaging with MRI and CSF analysis: cytospin, flow cytometry.
- Pregnancy testing in fertile women.
- Fertility preservation: consider sperm banking or embryonic cryopreservation. No routine place for ova/ovarian strip cryopreservation

---

✚ Clinical tip Grading of follicular lymphoma

The pathological grading of follicular lymphoma relies on the numbers of centroblasts in neoplastic follicles (Table 15.1). The 2008 WHO classification merges grades 1 and 2 into a single low-grade category [1]. Importantly, grade 3B lymphoma is regarded as akin to diffuse large B-cell lymphoma (DLBCL) and is treated with a similarly aggressive approach.

Table15.1 Follicular lymphoma grading system, based on centrocyte/centroblast count [2]

Grade	Criteria
1	0–5 centroblasts per high power field (HPF)
2	6–15 centroblasts per HPF
3	>15 centroblasts per HPF
3A	Centrocytes present
3B	Centrocytes absent

Adapted with permission from N. L. Harris *et al.*, The World Health Organization Classification of Neoplastic Diseases of the Hematopoietic and Lymphoid Tissues Report of the Clinical Advisory Committee Meeting, Airlie House, Virginia, November, 1997, *Annals of Oncology*, Volume 10, Issue 12, pp. 1419–1432, Copyright © 1999 Kluwer Academic Publishers, with permission of Oxford University Press.

✪ Learning point The classification of lymphomas

The current WHO (2008) classification of tumours of haematopoietic and lymphoid tissues [1] integrates morphological features, IHC, cytogenetics, molecular biology, and clinical behaviour as the basis for defining distinct clinicopathological diagnoses. It has been the globally adopted standard since 2001.

Although the name 'Non-Hodgkin's lymphoma (NHL)' no longer appears in the WHO classification, it remains widely used. Figure 15.1 shows a skeletal outline of the major disease categories.

(continued)

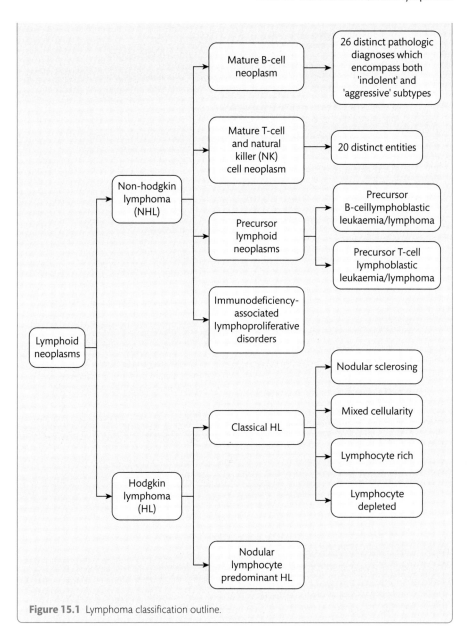

Figure 15.1 Lymphoma classification outline.

The Ann Arbor staging system (Table 15.2) was initially developed for use in Hodgkin's lymphoma. It provides the anatomical basis for staging in NHL, together with the Cotswold modifications, and is universally adopted in clinical practice. A shortcoming of this system is that it fails to account for the histological grade of the disease and the predilection for extranodal manifestation in certain NHL subtypes.

(continued)

❝ Expert comment

The WHO classification was a landmark event in the management of malignant lymphoma.

Table 15.2 Ann Arbor staging [3]

Stage	Features	Lymph node regions
I	Involvement of one lymph node region or lymphoid structure	Left and right sides are considered separate anatomical regions when displayed as italicized fonts:
II	Involvement of two or more lymph node regions on the same side of the diaphragm	• cervical (including cervical, supraclavicular, occipital, and preauricular lymph nodes)
III	Involvement of lymph nodes on both sides of the diaphragm	• axillary
IV	Involvement of extranodal sites other than one contiguous or proximal extranodal site	• infraclavicular • mediastinal
Suffix(es)		• hilar
A	No constitutional symptoms	• para-aortic • mesenteric
B	Any of:	• pelvic • inguinofemoral
	• unexplained fever >38°C • drenching night sweats • unexplained weight loss of >10% in preceding 6 months prior to diagnosis	Other sites or structures: these include Waldeyer's ring, epitrochlear, popliteal, occipital, and other small lymph node areas. Each of these is considered a separate lymph node site and is used in the distinction between stages I and II
E	Involvement of single extranodal site, contiguous or proximal to a known nodal site	
X	Bulky disease—any of:	Organ involvement of the bone marrow, liver, pleura, and CSF are always considered stage IV by convention
	• mediastinal mass of >33% of internal thoracic diameter at T5/6 on CXR • nodal mass >10 cm in diameter	
S	Splenic involvement	

Other symptoms, such as chills, pruritus, alcohol-induced pain, or fatigue, should be recorded but do not form part of the formal staging system.

Adapted from Armitage J. O., Staging Non-Hodgkin Lymphoma, *CA: A Cancer Journal for Clinicians* Volume 55, Issue 6, pp. 368–376, Copyright © American Cancer Society, Inc., 2005, with permission from John Wiley & Sons.

⊗ **Learning point FLIPI and FLIPI2**

The FLIPI is a prognostic score for newly diagnosed follicular lymphoma, which was originally developed in 2004 [4], prior to the advent of rituximab-containing treatment regimens. Its role in the stratification of prognosis has been confirmed in more recent prospective clinical trials involving the use of rituximab.

The adverse factors used in FLIPI are: age ≥60 years, stage III or IV disease, anaemia with Hb <120 g/L, elevated serum LDH, and five or more nodal sites involved. Patients are stratified, depending on the number of factors present, into three distinct risk groups: low (≤1 factor), intermediate (two factors), or high (≥3 factors). The corresponding 5-year OS rates are: 91%, 78%, and 53%, respectively.

FLIPI2 was developed in 2009 for the rituximab era in patients requiring chemoimmunotherapy treatment [5]. The scores for the three risk groups remain the same, but there are changes to the adverse factors used. These are: age ≥60 years, Hb <120 g/L, bone marrow involvement, elevated beta-2-microglobulin, and the longest diameter of the largest involved node (LoDLIN) >6 cm. The corresponding 5-year OS rates are: 98%, 88%, and 77%, respectively.

Both indices are used in clinical practice to guide prognostication. They do not predict when to initiate treatment or what treatment to use.

With asymptomatic low tumour burden, the patient was managed on a 'watch and wait' basis for 2 years, before he started experiencing progressive pressure symptoms in his abdomen and fatigue. Repeat CT staging and lymph node biopsy confirmed disease progression with follicular lymphoma histology. He proceeded to receive six cycles of immunochemotherapy with rituximab (375 mg/m^2), cyclophosphamide (750 mg/m^2), vincristine (1.4 mg/m^2), and prednisolone (100 mg, days 1–5) (R-CVP) to a complete remission (CR) in 2008.

> **❝ Expert comment**
>
> In patients with advanced-stage symptomatic follicular lymphoma, systemic immunochemotherapy is the standard of care. The choice of chemotherapy backbone is not firmly established, and options include R-CHOP, R-CVP, R-bendamustine, and R-fludarabine combinations. Treatment choices should be individualized, remembering that these therapies are not curative. R-CVP may have perhaps lower response rates and shorter PFS but is very well tolerated. R-bendamustine is non-inferior to R-CHOP, with less immediate toxicity, but long-term follow-up data are limited. Fludarabine may compromise the ability to collect stem cells in the future. R-CHOP as initial therapy may preclude anthracycline use in the future, should transformation occur. Each choice has its compromise, and future recurrence is inevitable.

> **✓ Evidence base** Watch and wait, compared to immediate systemic therapy [6]
>
> - Watch and wait until clinical progression ($n = 151$) versus immediate systemic therapy with chlorambucil ($n = 158$) in 309 asymptomatic, advanced-stage low-grade NHL.
> - RCT.
> - Daily oral chlorambucil 0.2 mg/kg of body weight (to maximum of 10 mg daily), continued for 3 months beyond CR in responding disease. Discontinued if no response at 3 or 6 months or if clinical progression.
> - Low-dose radiotherapy to localized symptomatic nodes allowed in both groups.
> - Median length of follow-up of 16 years.
> - No significant difference in OS or cause-specific survival between the two groups. Actuarial chance of not needing chemotherapy at 10 years was 19% (40% if older than 70 years old).
> - Conclusion: no advantage to immediate treatment in advanced asymptomatic cases.
>
> *Source:* data from *The Lancet*, Volume 362, Issue 9383, Ardeshna KM *et al.*, Long-term effect of a watch and wait policy versus immediate systemic treatment for asymptomatic advanced-stage non-Hodgkin lymphoma: a randomised controlled trial, pp. 516–22, Copyright © 2003 Elsevier Ltd All rights reserved.

> **✓ Evidence base** Rituximab plus chemotherapy, compared to chemotherapy only [7]
>
> - Meta-analysis examining the survival benefit of adding rituximab to chemotherapy as first-line treatment in indolent lymphoma or mantle cell lymphoma.
> - Combined survival data from seven RCTs, pooled survival analysis of patients with follicular lymphoma favoured chemotherapy plus rituximab versus chemotherapy only, with HR of 0.63 (95% CI 0.51–0.79).
>
> *Source:* data from Schulz H *et al.*, Chemotherapy plus Rituximab versus chemotherapy alone for B-cell non-Hodgkin's lymphoma, *Cochrane Database System Review*, Volume 17, Issue 4, 2007, CD003805, Copyright ©2009 The Cochrane Collaboration.

The patient's GP requested an urgent follow-up appointment in the lymphoma clinic, as the patient had been complaining of a 2-week history of progressive shortness of breath and a cough, which had not improved despite rest and a course of antibiotics. In addition, he had been feeling unwell for the previous 2 months, with increasing fatigue, loss of appetite, and intermittent drenching night sweats.

Clinical examination in outpatients revealed reduced air entry in the right lung base with a dull percussion note, a distended abdomen with a palpable liver edge, and lymphadenopathy in both groins. The PS score of the patient was 1.

Urgent blood tests were requested (Table 15.3) which notably showed a significantly elevated LDH.

Table 15.3 Blood test results

Haematology		Biochemistry	
Hb	10.8 g/dL	Na	138 mmol/L
MCV	88 fL	K	4.2 mmol/L
Plt	139 × 10⁹/L	Urea	7.6 mmol/L
WCC	5.8 × 10⁹/L	Creatinine	77 mmol/L
Neutrophils	3.1 × 10⁹/L	Bilirubin	13 umol/L
Lymphocytes	1.8 × 10⁹/L	Total protein	55 g/L
Monocytes	0.6 × 10⁹/L	Albumin	30 g/L
Eosinophils	0.2 × 10⁹/L	ALT	34 IU/L
Basophils	0.1 × 10⁹/L	ALP	150 IU/L
ESR	27 mm/hour	LDH	1034 IU/L
INR	1.1	Uric acid	0.49 mmol/L
Virology		Corrected calcium	2.44 mmol/L
CMV IgG	Positive	Phosphate	0.78 mmol/L
HIV Ab	Negative	Immunology	
Hep B surface antigen	Negative	Beta-2-microglobulin	3.0 mg/L
Hep B core Ab	Negative	IgA	2.3 g/L
Hep C IgG	Negative	IgG	12.3 g/L
HTLV 1 and 2 total Ab	Negative	IgM	1.0 g/L
EBV nuclear antigen	Detected		
EBV serology	Consistent with past infection		

It was felt that the current clinical presentation was consistent with rapid progression of the patient's disease, and there was suspicion of a histological transformation to a more aggressive type of lymphoma. An urgent outpatient CT staging scan of the neck, chest, abdomen, and pelvis demonstrated multiple enlarged lymph node stations above and below the diaphragm, with bulky intra-abdominal lymphadenopathy, right lower lobe pulmonary involvement associated with a pleural effusion, and hepatic involvement. A bone marrow aspirate and trephine biopsy and CT-guided core biopsies of the abdominal nodal mass were performed within the same week.

The case was reviewed in the regional lymphoma multidisciplinary meeting. The histopathology of the bone marrow trephine biopsy demonstrated features of follicular lymphoma, whereas the lymph node biopsy showed areas of high-grade diffuse large B-cell infiltration with a Ki-67 of >70% (Figure 15.2). Despite the discordant pathological findings between the two samples, the aggressive clinical picture of extranodal pulmonary and hepatic involvement identified on CT was consistent with the diagnosis of stage IVB histological transformation of follicular lymphoma to DLBCL.

The patient was seen in the lymphoma clinic to discuss the results of the investigations and recommended management plan. He appeared unwell in clinic and reported progressive night sweats, with abdominal distension. He was admitted to hospital and immediately commenced on allopurinol (300 mg bd), dexamethasone (4 mg bd),

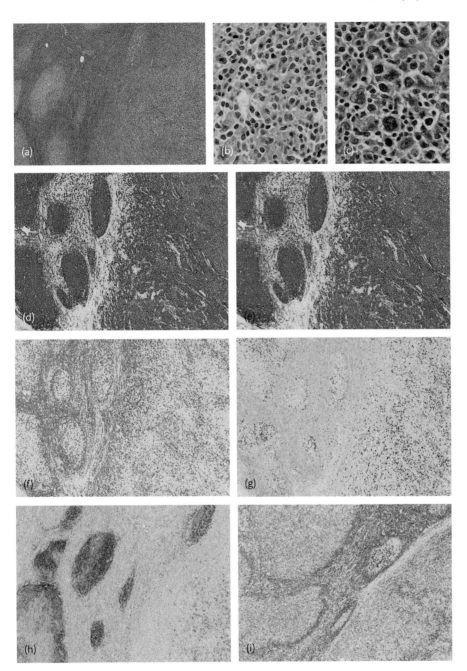

Figure 15.2 Photomicrographs of a transformed follicular lymphoma.
(A) Low power view demonstrating both follicular and diffuse large B-cell components. (B) High power view of the follicles showing mainly centrocytes. (C) High power view of the diffuse large B-cell component with many blasts. (D) CD10 highlighting both components and confirming the germinal centre phenotype. (E) There is strong uniform CD20 expression in both the follicles and diffuse areas. (F) CD3 highlights admixed small T-cells within the diffuse component and a perifollicular distribution in the follicular area. (G) Ki-67 shows a low proliferation fraction in the follicles and a high proliferation fraction in the diffuse large B-cell area. (H) The follicles have a CD23-positive follicular dendritic cell meshwork; this is lost in the transformed area. (I) Both components are expressing Bcl-2 protein. Images courtesy of Dr Margaret Ashton-Key.

> ⭐ **Learning point** DLBCL
>
> DLBCL is the most common aggressive NHL subtype, accounting for about 30% of all new lymphomas diagnosed worldwide. Patients typically present with symptomatic nodal or extranodal disease that exhibit rapid tumour growth. It has an aggressive natural history, with a median survival of <1 year, if left untreated. DLBCL is potentially curable with standard first-line combination chemoimmunotherapy, but patient-related factors can make treatment challenging, with the median age at diagnosis of around 64 years.

> ⭐ **Learning point** Transformation of follicular lymphoma (tFL)
>
> Histological transformation is a well-documented phenomenon in the natural history and clinical course of follicular lymphoma. tFL confers an adverse prognosis. The transformed subtype is usually DLBCL or, less commonly, Burkitt's lymphoma (BL). Histological transformation is also observed in other indolent B-cell NHL.
>
> There are no clinical characteristics at initial diagnosis that predict future high-grade transformation. The frequencies of histological transformation, based on retrospective series, vary considerably; overall, published studies suggest an estimated cumulative rate of transformation of about 3% per year [8]. In a retrospective series, no cases of histological transformation were observed after 16 years, at which time the cumulative probability of transformation was 39% [9]. The impact of 'watch and wait' at diagnosis on the risk of transformation is unclear; published retrospective series have been conflicting, and only one prospective study reported no differences between 'watch and wait' and early intervention [10]. There is no evidence to support the notion that early treatment reduces the risk of histological transformation.

omeprazole (20 mg od), and IV hydration. An urgent baseline transthoracic echocardiogram was performed after admission and showed an adequate LVEF of 56%.

He consented to receive combination chemoimmunotherapy with six cycles of rituximab (375 mg/m^2), cyclophosphamide (750 mg/m^2), doxorubicin (50 mg/m^2), vincristine (1.4 mg/m^2), and prednisolone (100 mg days 1–5) (R-CHOP 21) the next day.

> ⭐ **Learning point** Management of transformed follicular lymphoma (tFL)
>
> tFL is managed along similar lines to *de novo* DLBCL; patients are usually treated with anthracycline-containing regimes like CHOP, with a reported CR of about 40% and an ORR of about 60% [9]. The most important prognostic factor determining long-term outcome is the achievement of CR with treatment. This consideration explains the UK practice favouring R-CVP over R-CHOP, in order to avoid anthracycline exposure in the initial management of patients with symptomatic follicular lymphoma that has not transformed. CNS prophylaxis should be offered, according to the local policy. The prognosis of tFL has been historically poor in the pre-rituximab era, with a median survival of around 1 year from transformation [9]. Rituximab has improved outcome, with a retrospective analysis of 108 cases, comparing rituximab-naïve patients treated with R-CHOP (*n* = 23) or a CHOP-like regime without rituximab, showing a 5-year post-transformation OS of 61% versus 33% (*p* = 0.01) [11].

Twenty-four hours after receiving R-CHOP, his routine blood results became progressively deranged in association with oliguria (Table 15.4). A diagnosis of early tumour lysis syndrome (TLS) with urate nephropathy was made, and rasburicase was immediately administered. Aggressive IV hydration was instituted, a urinary catheter inserted, and careful fluid balance maintained.

Table 15.4 Blood test results 24 hours post-chemotherapy

Biochemistry		Reference ranges
Na	142 mmol/L	133–146 mmol/L
K	5.9 mmol/L	3.5–5.3 mmol/L
Urea	5.3 mmol/L	2.5–7.8 mmol/L
Creatinine	102 mmol/L	53–97 mmol/L
LDH	1201 IU/L	225–425 IU/L
Uric acid	1.6 mmol/L	0.16–0.48 mmol/L
Corrected calcium	2.19 mmol/L	2.15–2.60 mmol/L
Phosphate	1.2 mmol/L	0.78–1.53 mmol/L

❻ Expert comment

Before initiating any therapy for lymphoma, you should know the urate. Analyse the risk factors for TLS in each individual patient—histology, disease burden, renal dysfunction, etc. In those at risk, watch the renal function and electrolytes very closely.

The use of the recombinant urate oxidase rasburicase has, no doubt, resulted in a considerable reduction in the morbidity and mortality from acute TLS. It is important to risk-assess any patient prior to the initiation of therapy. Always be mindful of the risk of TLS in patients with aggressive lymphomas, and be proactive in its prevention and management.

➕ Clinical tip Tumour Lysis Syndrome (TLS)

TLS is caused by the rapid and massive release of intracellular metabolites, such as potassium, nucleic acids (catabolized t o uric acid), phosphorus, and proteins, into the blood. The risk varies, depending on the tumour type being treated [12]. The ensuing hyperkalaemia, hyperuricaemia, and hyperphosphataemia (with or without secondary hypocalcaemia) lead to renal failure, cardiac arrhythmias, seizures, and death. This oncological emergency can occur spontaneously or, more usually, 12–72 hours following the initiation of cytotoxic chemotherapy.

✪ Learning point (Acute Oncology) Management of Tumour Lysis Syndrome

Tumour lysis syndroe (TLS) is caused by the rapid and massive release of intracellular metabolites, such as potassium, nucleic acids (catabolized to uric acid), phosphorus, and proteins, into the blood. The risk varies, depending on the tumour type being treated [12]. The ensuing hyperkalaemia, hyperuricaemia, and hyperphosphataemia (with or without secondary hypocalcaemia) lead to renal failure, cardiac arrhythmias, seizures, and death. This oncological emergency can occur spontaneously or, more usually, 12–72 hours following the initiation of cytotoxic chemotherapy.

Management includes pre-chemotherapy risk evaluation to instigate appropriate prophylactic measures, close monitoring, and prompt recognition, with aggressive management in the event of its occurrence

Prevention

- Maintain hydration and urine output (low risk: increased oral fluids; intermediate/high risk: IV fluids without potassium supplementation)
- Commence allopurinol at least 24 hours prior to chemotherapy
- Consider rasburicase (recombinant uric oxidase) prophylaxis in high-risk category

Monitoring

- Monitor fluid balance and urine output
- Intermediate/high risk: serial biochemistry monitoring of uric acid, potassium, phosphate, and calcium every 6–12 hours post-chemotherapy initiation for up to 72 hours

Treatment

- Hyperuricaemia: stop allopurinol, and commence IV rasburicase (0.2 mg/kg/day) until normalization. * Rasburicase is contraindicated in glucose-6-phosphate dehydrogenase (G6PD) deficiency, in which case use allopurinol
- Hypocalcaemia: secondary to hyperphosphataemia. Do not replace if asymptomatic. Cardiac monitoring is required in case of arrhythmia which necessitates calcium replacement (this increases the risk of renal tubular failure from calcium phosphate deposition)
- Hyperphosphataemia: difficult to treat once established. Maintain high urine output
- Hyperkalaemia: standard medical treatment applies. Cardiac monitoring
- Uncontrolled biochemical TLS or TLS with clinical symptoms: refer for haemodialysis

The patient's biochemistry stabilized and improved after the administration of rasburicase. The patient was discharged from the ward 4 days later, with a supply of allopurinol for the duration of the first cycle of treatment.

The B symptoms experienced by the patient improved after the first cycle of R-CHOP. Subsequent cycles were supported through the use of G-CSF, and other side effects of the treatment were manageable with mainly grades 1–2 nausea, mucositis, anorexia, and fatigue. He also received CNS prophylaxis with intrathecal methotrexate with cycles 2–5 of R-CHOP.

Interim CT scan after four cycles of R-CHOP showed a very good partial response, and the outcome CT scan after six cycles of induction chemotherapy showed a complete response. The patient is currently under close follow-up in the lymphoma clinic.

Discussion

This case illustrates the fairly standardized diagnostic pathway for all suspected lymphomas. 'Watch and wait' is an appropriate strategy for patients with follicular lymphoma, who are asymptomatic at diagnosis. The advent of rituximab, however, has prompted a re-examination of this policy [13].

For patients with symptomatic advanced-stage disease, the goal of therapy is to decrease the disease burden and alleviate symptoms, with the expectation that the disease will pursue a relapsing and remitting course, requiring several lines of therapy. No universal agreement exists on the optimal initial management of advanced-stage disease, so patients should be encouraged to enrol into a clinical trial, if possible. Rituximab is the backbone of treatment, and evidence now exists to recommend rituximab maintenance after completion of first-line therapy.

⊘ **Evidence base** PRIMA (Primary RItuximab and MAintenance) study [14]

- A total of 1217 treatment-naïve follicular lymphoma patients needing induction chemoimmunotherapy with one of three commonly used regimes (R-CHOP, R-CVP, or R-FCM).
- A total of 1019 responding patients were randomized to 2 years of maintenance rituximab (375 mg/m^2) every 8 weeks for 2 years ($n = 505$) or observation ($n = 513$).
- Median follow-up of 36 months.
- PFS: rituximab maintenance 74.9% (95% CI 70.9–78.9) versus observation 57.6% (95% CI 53.2–62.0) (HR 0.55, 95% CI 0.44–0.68; $p < 0.0001$).
- No difference in OS, and no difference in the QoL between the two groups.

Source: data from *The Lancet*, Volume 377, Issue 9759, Salles G *et al.*, Rituximab maintenance for 2 years in patients with high tumour burden follicular lymphoma responding to rituximab plus chemotherapy (PRIMA): a phase 3, randomised controlled trial, pp. 42–51, Copyright © 2003 Elsevier Ltd All rights reserved.

The clinical picture at transformation is typically characterized by an increase in the pace of the disease, declining PS, rapidly growing lymphadenopathy, the development of B symptoms, the involvement of extranodal sites, raised LDH, and hypercalcaemia. The presence of raised LDH, elevated beta-2-microglobulin, abnormal FBC, and LFT from involvement of extranodal sites is evident in this case study (Table 15.3). This patient had discordant (bone marrow shows follicular lymphoma) and composite histologies (lymph node shows both follicular lymphoma and DLBCL), which illustrates the inherent heterogeneity of this phenomenon.

> **❻ Expert comment**
>
> Rituximab maintenance therapy for 2 years after completion of immunochemotherapy is associated with a significant improvement in PFS, but no OS benefit has been reported. There is a higher rate of infection, due to chronic B-cell depletion, in those receiving maintenance, compared to those observed after, immunochemotherapy, which needs to be remembered in making therapeutic choices.

A final word from the expert

This case illustrates many aspects of the challenges that are faced in the management of B-cell lymphomas.

In patients with asymptomatic, low-tumour-burden follicular lymphoma, with no evidence of organ compromise, the dogma has been to manage these patients expectantly, as there is no survival advantage to immediate initiation of chemotherapy. This is because the chemotherapy is not curative, and relapse is inevitable. We call it 'watch and wait', but sometimes the patients 'watch and worry'. The median time from diagnosis to initiation of therapy is 2.5–3 years, although 20% of patients may still not have an indication for therapy 10 years after diagnosis. Although the early data that have examined the use of single-agent rituximab in asymptomatic patients are provocative, full study reporting is required, before there is a change in practice.

Transformation of follicular lymphoma to DLBCL, or other aggressive histologies, is a relatively common event and associated with a poor outcome. It can occur anytime in the disease course, and the risk is not modified by treatment. The molecular aberrations that underlie this phenotypic switch are not well understood (but include the acquisition of *TP53* mutations and c-*MYC* rearrangements/mutation). The optimal therapy is not clear either but should be treated as would the *de novo* histology. We should strive to perform a repeat biopsy at every episode of progression of follicular lymphoma to diagnose or exclude transformation.

The treatment approach should be tailored to the individual, with a clear strategy focussed on the long clinical course of follicular lymphoma, whilst recognizing that it will be punctuated by episodes of disease. When talking to patients with follicular lymphoma, we need to communicate clearly the rationale for the various options that we present.

Acknowledgement

The author would like to thank Dr Margaret Ashton-Key for kindly providing the pathology images.

References

1. Swerdlow SH, Campo E, Harris NL *et al. WHO classification of tumours of haematopoietic and lymphoid tissues*, 4th edn. Lyon: IARC, 2008.
2. Harris NL, Jaffe ES, Diebold J *et al.*, World Health Organization classification of neoplastic diseases of the hematopoietic and lymphoid tissues: report of the Clinical Advisory Committee meeting-Airlie House, Virginia, November 1997. *Journal of Clinical Oncology* 1999; **17**(12): 3835–49.

3. Armitage JO. Staging non-Hodgkin lymphoma. *Cancer* 2005; **55**(6): 368–76.

4. Solal-Celigny P, Roy P, Colombat P *et al.* Follicular lymphoma international prognostic index. *Blood* 2004; **104**(5): 1258–65.

5. Federico M, Bellei M, Marcheselli L *et al.* Follicular lymphoma international prognostic index 2: a new prognostic index for follicular lymphoma developed by the international follicular lymphoma prognostic factor project. *Journal of Clinical Oncology* 2009; **27**(27): 4555–62.

6. Ardeshna KM, Smith P, Norton A *et al.* Long-term effect of a watch and wait policy versus immediate systemic treatment for asymptomatic advanced-stage non-Hodgkin lymphoma: a randomised controlled trial. *The Lancet* 2003; **362**(9383): 516–22.

7. Schulz H, Bohlius J, Skoetz N *et al.* Chemotherapy plus rituximab versus chemotherapy alone for B-cell non-Hodgkin's lymphoma. *Cochrane Database of Systematic Reviews* 2007; **4**: CD003805.

8. Lossos IS, Gascoyne RD. Transformation of follicular lymphoma. *Best Practice & Research Clinical Haematology* 2011; **24**(2): 147–63.

9. Montoto S, Davies AJ, Matthews J *et al.* Risk and clinical implications of transformation of follicular lymphoma to diffuse large B-cell lymphoma. *Journal of Clinical Oncology* 2007; **25**(17): 2426–33.

10. Brice P, Bastion Y, Lepage E *et al.* Comparison in low-tumor-burden follicular lymphomas between an initial no-treatment policy, prednimustine, or interferon alfa: a randomized study from the Groupe d'Etude des Lymphomes Folliculaires. Groupe d'Etude des Lymphomes de l'Adulte. *Journal of Clinical Oncology* 1997; **15**(3): 1110–17.

11. Al-Tourah AJ, Savage KJ, Gill KK *et al.* Addition of rituximab to CHOP chemotherapy significantly improves survival of patients with transformed lymphoma. *Blood* 2007; **110**(11): 790.

12. Cairo MS, Coiffier B, Reiter A, Younes A. Recommendations for the evaluation of risk and prophylaxis of tumour lysis syndrome (TLS) in adults and children with malignant diseases: an expert TLS panel consensus. *British Journal of Haematology* 2010; **149**(4): 578–86.

13. Ardeshna KM, Qian W, Smith P *et al.* An intergroup randomised trial of rituximab versus a watch and wait strategy in patients with Stage II, III, IV, asymptomatic, non-bulky follicular lymphoma (Grades 1, 2 and 3a). A preliminary analysis. *Blood* 2010; **116**(21): 6.

14. Salles G, Seymour JF, Offner F *et al.* Rituximab maintenance for 2 years in patients with high tumour burden follicular lymphoma responding to rituximab plus chemotherapy (PRIMA): a phase 3, randomised controlled trial. *The Lancet* 2011; **377**(9759): 42–51.

16 Metastatic germ cell cancer

Jennifer Bradbury

ⓘ **Expert commentary** Jonathan Shamash

Case history

A 20-year-old male presented with right testicular swelling and a 2-week history of cough with haemoptysis. In the preceding few days, he had experienced several episodes of numbness in the right hand and around the right side of his mouth, suggestive of partial seizures. He had no significant past medical history and was a non-smoker. On examination, he had gynaecomastia, a palpable abdominal mass, and a right-sided testicular mass.

Investigations showed AFP 1.01 ng/mL, HCG 507 000 IU/mL, and LDH 1684 IU/L. Testicular ultrasound showed a 2.5 cm × 2 cm right testicular mass with calcification, suggestive of a teratoma. CXR showed multiple lung metastases (Figure 16.1). CT CAP imaging demonstrated gross bilateral lung metastases (largest 32 mm diameter), moderate-volume liver metastases, and retroperitoneal lymphadenopathy (78 mm transverse diameter), with a right-sided hydronephrosis. He also had a single lesion in the left frontal lobe on an MRI of the brain, consistent with a metastasis.

The patient was given a diagnosis of International Germ Cell Consensus Classification (IGCCC) poor prognosis metastatic non-seminoma, specifically choriocarcinoma [2]. This diagnosis was made on the basis of the presentation and tumour markers alone, without pathological confirmation, due to a serum HCG >50 000 IU/L and the presence of non-pulmonary visceral metastases. In view of the extent of his disease, he went on to receive urgent chemotherapy with the 5-day BEP (bleomycin, etoposide, cisplatin) regimen, after undergoing sperm storage. He also had a right ureteric stent inserted, in order to decompress the right kidney.

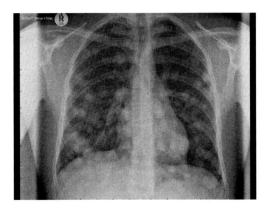

Figure 16.1 CXR at diagnosis.

ⓒ Expert commênt

Avoidance of cranial irradiation would be an advantage, as it is clear that the long-term side effects of cranial irradiation are significant. Chemotherapy regimens, including high-dose methotrexate, have been proposed as an alternative.

✪ Learning point Classification and prognosis

Germ cell tumours are classified histologically as either seminomas or non-seminomas. The non-seminomas are a heterogeneous group and include the combination of seminoma and non-seminoma (mixed tumours).

Patients are staged according to the TNM classification [1], with the use of the histopathological report of the testicular tumour, tumour markers, CXR, and CT CAP imaging. Patients with stage I non-seminoma are managed, according to their level of risk of recurrence.

All other patients are considered to have metastatic germ cell tumours and are classified, according to the International Germ Cell Consensus Classification (IGCCC), with three identified prognostic groups (good risk, intermediate risk, or poor risk), defined on the basis of serum tumour markers before chemotherapy, the primary tumour site, and the presence or absence of extra-pulmonary visceral metastases [2].

✪ Learning point Brain metastases

In the context of a patient presenting with brain metastases and widespread systemic metastatic disease, the need to proceed with systemic chemotherapy is apparent. What is less clear is the role and sequencing of other treatment modalities for cerebral metastatic disease in combination with chemotherapy. A multivariate analysis suggested that cranial irradiation, in addition to systemic chemotherapy, led to an improvement in the overall prognosis of patients presented with brain metastases [3], although earlier reports had not demonstrated a benefit from this approach [4].

✪ Learning point Post-orchidectomy risk stratification of stage I non-seminoma and management

Clinical stage I disease in both seminoma and non-seminoma is defined as disease limited to the testes, with no radiological evidence of metastatic disease and normal serum tumour markers after orchidectomy [5]. Patients presenting post-orchidectomy with stage I non-seminoma are assessed for their level of risk of recurrence and managed accordingly.

Low risk of relapse

- No vascular invasion.
- Management: active surveillance (preferred, although some may wish for adjuvant therapy).

High risk of relapse

- Vascular invasion.
- Management options include [5,6]:
  1. active surveillance, or
  2. adjuvant chemotherapy with one cycle of BEP (etoposide 500mg/m^2) or two cycles of BEP (etoposide 360mg/m^2), or
  3. retroperitoneal LND, with or without adjuvant chemotherapy, e.g. if retroperitoneal lymph nodes of equivocal size.

The patient received four cycles of BEP chemotherapy which he tolerated well. He had no further seizures. He developed a DVT and PEs during his fourth cycle of chemotherapy and required anticoagulation with LMWH.

⭐ **Learning point** Curative treatments for metastatic disease

BEP chemotherapy remains the standard of care for the treatment of metastatic seminoma and non-seminoma. The recommended first-line treatment for good-prognosis disease is three cycles of BEP chemotherapy (or four cycles of EP chemotherapy if there are contraindications to bleomycin) [5]. Radiotherapy may be considered as a treatment option for early-stage IIA seminoma with retroperitoneal lymph node metastases of <2 cm, but chemotherapy may be preferred [7]. Four cycles of BEP is the standard treatment for intermediate-prognosis and poor-prognosis disease [5].

The efficacy of 5-day BEP chemotherapy has been shown to be equivalent to 3-day BEP in patients with good-prognosis advanced disease [8]. Increased long-term ototoxicity is seen with 3-day BEP, compared with 5-day treatment, particularly if four cycles are administered [9]. Therefore, four cycles of 5-day BEP are recommended for patients with poor- and intermediate-prognosis disease.

🔟 **Expert comment**

An alternative to the use of bleomycin in situations where lung function is compromised at the start of the therapy is to use etoposide, ifosfamide, and cisplatin (VIP).

➕ **Clinical tip** BEP chemotherapy

BEP is the 3-weekly chemotherapy regimen, combining bleomycin 30 mg on days 1, 8, and 15 with cisplatin 100 mg/m^2 and etoposide 500 mg/m^2 in week 1.

- *3-day* BEP: cisplatin 50 mg/m^2 days 1 and 2; etoposide 165 mg/m^2 days 1, 2, and 3. *5-day BEP*: cisplatin 20 mg/m^2 days 1–5; etoposide 100 mg/m^2 days 1–5.

The 3-day BEP is highly emetogenic, and patients receiving this require an anti-emetic regimen, comprising a neurokinin 1 (NK1) antagonist, e.g. aprepitant, a 5-hydroxytryptamine-3 (5HT3) antagonist, e.g. ondansetron, plus dexamethasone [13,14]. It would be common practice to also offer a dopamine antagonist (metoclopramide or domperidone). The 5-day BEP contains a lower daily dosage of cisplatin and may therefore be considered moderately emetogenic, but current guidance recommends using the same anti-emetic regimen [13,14].

✅ **Evidence base** Three versus four cycles of BEP, and 5-day versus 3-day BEP, in good-prognosis germ cell cancer [8]

- A 2 × 2 factorial study testing the equivalence of three versus four cycles of BEP and a 5-day versus 3-day schedule in good-prognosis germ cell cancer.
- Aiming to rule out a 5% decrease in the 2-year PFS rate.
- A total of 812 patients randomly assigned to receive three or four cycles of BEP; 681 of these were also randomly assigned to the 5-day or 3-day schedule.
- At the time of analysis, the median follow-up was 25 months, with a minimum follow-up of 2 years available for 93% of the patients.
- The 2-year PFS rate was 90.4% on three cycles, and 89.4% on four cycles; a difference of –1.0% (80% confidence limit –3.8% to +1.8%).
- The 2-year PFS rate was 89.7% on the 3-day schedule, and 88.8% on the 5-day schedule; a difference of –0.9% (80% confidence limit –4.1% to +2.2%).

Source: data from de Wit R *et al.*, Equivalence of three or four cycles of bleomycin, etoposide and cisplatin chemotherapy and of a 3- or 5-day schedule in good-prognosis germ cell cancer: a randomized study of the European Organization for Research and Treatment of Cancer Genitourinary Tract Cancer Cooperative Group and the Medical Research Council, *Journal of Clinical Oncology*, Volume 19, Number 6, pp. 1629–40, Copyright © 2001 by American Society of Clinical Oncology.

⭐ **Learning point (Acute Oncology)** Bleomycin-induced lung disease

Bleomycin-induced lung disease may take a number of forms, but the commonest pattern is interstitial pneumonitis which can progress to pulmonary fibrosis [10]. The pathophysiology appears to be immune-mediated with the induction of cytokines and free radicals, leading to endothelial damage and the activation of fibroblasts with subsequent collagen deposition [10–12].

(continued)

Factors predicting for an increased risk of bleomycin-induced pulmonary toxicity are [11]:

- GFR <80 mL/min before chemotherapy
- stage IV disease
- age >40 years
- cumulative dose of bleomycin >300 000 IU.

Cigarette smoking is less well defined as a risk factor, but smoking history should be considered when planning treatment [12].

There is no specific test for bleomycin-induced pneumonitis, and it should be suspected on the basis of a combination of clinical features, radiographic abnormalities, and pulmonary function test results [10]. The most usual treatment is steroids (prednisolone 1 mg/kg/day), but there has been recent interest in the use of novel therapies, such as imatinib and nilotinib [12], which are thought to have an anti-inflammatory effect due to their inhibitory activity at the PDGFR.

⊕ **Learning point** Induction chemotherapy

The 'choriocarcinoma syndrome' was identified in the early 1980s as respiratory failure due to adult respiratory distress syndrome (ARDS) occurring early during the course of treatment, typically in patients with extensive lung metastases and very high HCG levels at presentation [15,16].

This led to a study looking at an initial reduction in chemotherapy doses during the first cycle of treatment in patients with poor-prognosis non-seminoma with extensive lung metastases plus dyspnoea and/or hypoxia (pO_2 <80 mmHg) at presentation [16]. The median HCG was 200 000 IU/L (range 11–8 920 000). The induction regime consisted of reduced doses of EP, with bleomycin delayed or omitted for the first cycle, followed by classic BEP. This small, non-randomized study demonstrated a significant reduction in the incidence of ARDS in patients treated with the modified regime, compared with a full-dose regimen, from 13/15 (87%) to 3/10 (30%) ($p = 0.01$).

The principle of using a short course of reduced-dose induction chemotherapy, prior to full-dose treatment, is recognized as a possible management option for patients with extensive metastatic disease or poor PS at presentation, although data on how to optimally administer a pre-phase induction chemotherapy are limited [5].

After completion of BEP chemotherapy, the patient's HCG had fallen to 61 IU/mL but had failed to normalize. His imaging showed an improvement in his retroperitoneal tumour mass (62 mm transverse diameter), liver and lung metastases, but still over 40 residual lung metastases. His MRI of the brain showed resolution of the left frontal lesion. Approximately a month from completion of chemotherapy, his HCG had risen to 131 IU/mL. This was felt to represent a relapse of his metastatic choriocarcinoma, and salvage chemotherapy was planned. The option of a standard second-line chemotherapy with TIP (paclitaxel, ifosfamide, cisplatin) was offered to the patient, or the alternative of involvement in a phase II clinical trial of TIP chemotherapy in combination with gemcitabine.

He opted to participate in the trial, receiving four cycles of gemcitabine plus TIP chemotherapy. Again, this was well tolerated, except for myelosuppression requiring blood and platelet transfusions. There was a fall in his HCG to near normal levels at 9.5 IU/mL. Repeat imaging showed a dramatic improvement in the lung and liver metastases. There had been a marginal reduction in the 5 cm retroperitoneal mass which appeared more cystic. There was no visible disease in the brain on MRI imaging. PET-CT imaging showed no tracer uptake in the majority of pulmonary lesions, no abnormal uptake in the liver, and subtle FDG uptake at the margin of the cystic retroperitoneal mass.

> ✪ **Learning point** Options in relapsed disease
>
> Patients who relapse after surveillance for stage I non-seminoma should be managed as patients with *de novo* metastatic disease with three or four cycles of BEP chemotherapy, according to their IGCCC score [2,5].
>
> Patients who relapse after first-line chemotherapy may be managed with either conventional-dose chemotherapy 'salvage' regimens or high-dose chemotherapy. There is not currently a consensus of opinion as to the recommended approach [5]. Options for conventional-dose regimens include VIP, TIP, or VeIP (cisplatin, ifosfamide, and vinblastine) [17,18]. High-dose regimens are usually combinations of carboplatin and etoposide and require stem cell support [19–21].

> ❻ **Expert comment**
>
> Recent data from a multicentre consortium have meant that the prognosis for patients at relapse can be more acutely predicted [22], based on the time to first-line treatment failure, sites of disease at relapse, height of markers at relapse, and primary site of disease and histology. No particular second-line treatment could be preferred over another. Retrospective matched-control series have suggested that high-dose chemotherapy provides a greater overall cure rate, and this should certainly be considered if first-line relapse therapy fails.
>
> Enrolment in a clinical trial is also an appropriate option for salvage treatment, given the lack of an established second-line management option. This patient was treated in a phases I/II study with the combination of gemcitabine and TIP chemotherapy [23]. Gemcitabine has previously shown promising activity as a single agent in intensively pretreated patients with metastatic germ cell cancers [24]. The initial phase I component of the study demonstrated that gemcitabine could be combined with standard TIP chemotherapy, with tolerable toxicity [23].

Two months after completion of chemotherapy, the patient underwent retroperitoneal LND and right orchidectomy. Pathology showed necrotic tissue only, with no evidence of viable germ cell tumour or teratoma differentiated. Post-operatively, his HCG level normalized for the first time since diagnosis.

> ✪ **Learning point** Resection of residual disease
>
> The role for resection of residual disease post-chemotherapy in the event of normalization of tumour markers is firmly established, and current recommendations are that residual tumours of 1 cm or more in diameter should be resected within 4–8 weeks of chemotherapy [5]. However, if residual disease persists in multiple sites, the sequence and exact nature of such surgery may need to be determined on an individual patient basis. This particular patient was left with numerous small pulmonary metastases post-chemotherapy and a retroperitoneal mass. As the resected residual mass from the retroperitoneum showed necrosis only, no resection of pulmonary metastases was undertaken, and an observational strategy was followed.

A year after completion of his second-line chemotherapy, his tumour markers remained within normal limits. A repeat CT scan confirmed ongoing improvement in the pulmonary metastases, with a suggestion that some of the residual abnormalities were areas of scar tissue only. No residual hepatic lesions were seen.

One year after completion of chemotherapy, he was found to have a normal testosterone level, but low free testosterone at 0.198 nmol/L (normal range >0.245) and high luteinizing hormone (LH) at 14.4 IU/L (normal range 1.2–8.6). He was therefore commenced on testosterone replacement in the form of intramuscular (IM) injections.

> ⊕ **Clinical tip** Management of testosterone deficiency
>
> Gonadal dysfunction can occur after orchidectomy alone and is more likely when chemotherapy is also given. Follicle-stimulating hormone (FSH) and LH levels rise, and testosterone levels fall. In one series of 272 patients, it was found that 13% had hypogonadism, which may require testosterone supplementation [25]. This has been identified to have an impact on the QoL as well as other consequences, in terms of bone health and cardiac risk factors.
>
> Therefore, the determination of testosterone is recommended during follow-up, with replacement offered to all patients with low testosterone levels and/or symptoms of hypogonadism [5]. Testosterone is most commonly replaced through the use of IM injections (most often every 3 months), but other routes of administration are available such as patches, gels, and implanted pellets [25].

During his follow-up, the patient has continued to complain of residual peripheral neuropathy which has slowly improved but not resolved completely. Continuing out-patient review focussed on the assessment for relapse, as well as on the development of potential long-term treatment-related sequelae.

> ✪ **Learning point** Long-term effects of treatment
>
> As testicular germ cell tumours are potentially curable malignancies, it has become increasingly important over recent years to consider survivorship issues and the long-term complications of treatment. Testicular cancer patients are at risk of fertility problems and hypogonadism. Sperm storage is typically offered to patients prior to treatment, if their clinical condition allows this.
>
> Population studies have demonstrated an increased risk of cardiovascular events, following chemotherapy for testicular cancer. One of the largest studies included over 30 000 testicular cancer survivors drawn from North American and European cancer registries, with a median follow-up of 10 years [26]. Amongst patients who received chemotherapy, with or without radiotherapy, they found a standardized mortality ratio of 1.58 for all circulatory diseases. A Norwegian study, with a median follow-up of 19 years, included 364 patients who received chemotherapy and observed an increased risk for atherosclerotic disease in age-adjusted Cox regression analyses for chemotherapy versus surgery alone (HR 2.6, 95% CI 1.1–5.9) [27]. In this study, the risk of myocardial infarction was significantly increased after treatment with BEP chemotherapy (HR 3.1, 95% CI 1.4–11.7), compared with normal controls.
>
> One potential mechanism for the increased risk of cardiovascular complications, following chemotherapy for testicular cancer, may be a higher incidence of the metabolic syndrome, which includes hypertension, dyslipidaemia, obesity, and insulin resistance. There appears to be an association between this syndrome and hypogonadism, and it has been suggested that adequate testosterone replacement may help to prevent the metabolic syndrome [28]. Another possible mechanism may be direct endothelial damage, demonstrated by microalbuminuria [29], which has been shown to be an independent risk factor for coronary artery disease in large trials.
>
> Survivors of testicular cancer are also at an increased risk of developing secondary malignancies. A large population-based study in 40 576 testicular cancer survivors showed that, for patients diagnosed with seminomas or non-seminomatous tumours at age 35 years, cumulative risks of solid cancer by the age of 75 years were 36% and 31%, respectively, compared with 23% for the general population [30]. The greatest site-specific relative risks were observed for cancers of the stomach, pancreas, and connective tissue, followed by cancers of the pleura and bladder, with increased risks persisting for at least 30 years for most sites. Combination chemotherapy has also been shown to be associated with an increased risk of myelodysplastic syndrome and secondary leukaemias [31].

Twenty-four months following the completion of second-line chemotherapy, the patient remains well, with normal tumour markers, a normal CXR appearance (Figure 16.2), and no clinical evidence of recurrence of his metastatic disease.

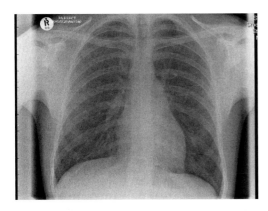

Figure 16.2 Post-treatment CXR.

Discussion

This is an example of a patient presenting with a testicular mass and widespread metastatic disease, including brain metastases. The recommended therapy for intermediate- and poor-prognosis disease, according to the European Germ Cell Cancer Consensus Group (EGCCCG) guidelines, is four cycles of BEP chemotherapy [5]. Using this approach, the 5-year survival for patients with poor-prognosis disease was reported in the IGCCC series to be 48% [2]. More recent data suggest that the outcome for this patient group may be somewhat better, particularly for those who fall into the poor-prognosis group as a result of marker elevation alone (i.e. no non-pulmonary visceral metastases and gonadal/retroperitoneal primary site) [32,33].

In this patient, the decision was made to proceed with systemic chemotherapy, leading to a complete radiological remission of the cerebral disease. In the event of a complete response within the brain, there is currently no consensus of opinion as to the role of cranial radiotherapy [5]. In the case of a residual cerebral mass post-chemotherapy, the role of surgical resection is also unclear.

His tumour markers did not normalize, and his disease progressed fairly soon after first-line treatment. There is no standard second-line regimen, and he therefore enrolled on a clinical trial, using an established combination of drugs with gemcitabine. His disease responded well to this, and, following the subsequent resection of key sites of residual disease, he remains well, with no evidence of metastatic disease 2 years later.

A final word from the expert

Patients with metastatic germ cell tumours with poor-prognosis disease continue to recur—the use of more intensive initial therapies seems to yield better PFS and, in one study, an improvement in OS. Increasingly, prognostic factors will be used at relapse to guide further therapy, in the absence of any definitive randomized trial. To date, the use of newer targeted agents has been associated with disappointing results.

References

1. Edge S, Byrd D, Compton C, Fritz AG, Greene FL, Trotti A, eds. *AJCC cancer staging manual*, 7th edn. New York: Springer, 2010; pp 469–78.
2. [No authors listed]. International Germ Cell Consensus Classification: a prognostic factor-based staging system for metastatic germ cell cancers. International Germ Cell Cancer Collaborative Group. *Journal of Clinical Oncology* 1997; **15**(2): 594–603.
3. Hartmann JT, Bamberg M, Albers P *et al.* Multidisciplinary treatment and prognosis of patients with central nervous system metastases (CNS) from testicular germ cell tumour (GCT) origin. *Proceedings of the American Society of Clinical Oncology* 2003; **22**: 1607.
4. Fossa SD, Bokemeyer C, Gerl A *et al.* Treatment outcome of patients with brain metastases from malignant germ cell tumours. *Cancer* 1999; **85**(4): 988–97.
5. Beyer J, Albers P, Altena R *et al.* Maintaining success, reducing treatment burden, focusing on survivorship: highlights from the third European consensus conference on diagnosis and treatment of germ-cell cancer. *Annals of Oncology* 2013; **24**(4): 878–88.
6. Maroto P, Garcia del Muro X *et al.* Multicentre risk-adapted management for stage I non-seminomatous germ cell tumours. *Annals of Oncology* 2005; **16**(12): 1915–20.
7. Tandstad T, Smaaland R, Solberg A *et al.* Management of seminomatous testicular cancer: a binational prospective population-based study from the Swedish Norwegian testicular cancer study group. *Journal of Clinical Oncology* 2011; **29**(6): 719–25.
8. de Wit R, Roberts JT, Wilkinson PM *et al.* Equivalence of three or four cycles of bleomycin, etoposide and cisplatin chemotherapy and of a 3- or 5-day schedule in good-prognosis germ cell cancer: a randomized study of the European Organization for Research and Treatment of Cancer Genitourinary Tract Cancer Cooperative Group and the Medical Research Council. *Journal of Clinical Oncology* 2001; **19**(6): 1629–40.
9. Fossa SD, de Wit R, Roberts JT *et al.* Quality of life in good prognosis patients with metastatic germ cell cancer: a prospective study of the European Organization for Research and Treatment of Cancer Genitourinary Group/Medical Research Council Testicular Cancer Study Group (30941/TE20). *Journal of Clinical Oncology* 2003; **21**(6): 1107–18.
10. Sleijfer S. Bleomycin-induced pneumonitis. *Chest* 2001; **120**(2): 617–24.
11. O'Sullivan JM, Huddart RA, Norman AR, Nicholls J, Dearnaley DP, Horwich A. Predicting the risk of bleomycin lung toxicity in patients with germ-cell tumours. *Annals of Oncology* 2003; **14**(1): 91–6.
12. Froudarakis M, Hatzimichael E, Kyriazopoulou L *et al.* Revisiting bleomycin from pathophysiology to safe clinical use. *Critical Reviews in Oncology/Haematology* 2013; **87**(1): 90–100.
13. Roila F, Herrstedt J, Aapro M *et al.*; ESMO/MASCC Guidelines Working Group. Guideline update for MASCC and ESMO in the prevention of chemotherapy- and radiotherapy-induced nausea and vomiting: results of the Perugia consensus conference. *Annals of Oncology* 2010; **21**(Suppl 5): v232–43.
14. Basch E, Prestud AA, Hesketh PJ *et al.* Antiemetics: American Society of Clinical Oncology Clinical Practice Guideline Update. *Journal of Clinical Oncology* 2011; **29**(31): 4189–98.
15. Logothesis CJ. Choriocarcinoma syndrome. *Cancer Bulletin* 1984; **36**: 118–20.
16. Massard C, Plantade A, Gross-Goupil M *et al.* Poor prognosis nonseminomatous germ-cell tumours (NSGCTs): should chemotherapy doses be reduced at first cycle to prevent acute respiratory distress syndrome in patients with multiple lung metastases? *Annals of Oncology* 2010; **21**(8): 1585–8.
17. Loehrer PJ, Lauer R, Roth BJ, Williams SD, Kalasinski LA, Einhorn LH. Salvage therapy in recurrent germ cell cancer: ifosfamide and cisplatin plus either vinblastine or etoposide. *Annals of Internal Medicine* 1988; **109**(7): 540–6.

18. Kondagunta GV, Bacik J, Donnadio A *et al.* Combination of paclitaxel, ifosfamide, and cisplatin is an effective second-line therapy for patients with relapsed testicular germ cell tumours. *Journal of Clinical Oncology* 2005; **23**(27): 6549–55.

19. Einhorn LH, Williams SD, Chamness A, Brames MJ, Perkins SM, Abonour R. High-dose chemotherapy and stem-cell rescue for metastatic germ-cell tumors. *The New England Journal of Medicine* 2007; **357**(4): 340–8.

20. Kondagunta GV, Bacik J, Sheinfeld J *et al.* Paclitaxel plus ifosfamide followed by high-dose carboplatin plus etoposide in previously treated germ cell tumours. *Journal of Clinical Oncology* 2007; **25**(1): 85–90.

21. Lorch A, Kleinhans A, Kramar A *et al.* Sequential versus single high-dose chemotherapy in patients with relapsed or refractory germ cell tumours: long-term results of a prospective randomized trial. *Journal of Clinical Oncology* 2012; **30**(8): 800–5.

22. Lorch A, Bascoul-Mollevi C, Kramar A *et al.* Conventional-dose versus high-dose chemotherapy as first salvage treatment in male patients with metastatic germ cell tumors: evidence from a large international database. *Journal of Clinical Oncology* 2011; **29**(16): 2178–84.

23. ClinicalTrials.gov. *Gemcitabine, paclitaxel, ifosfamide, and cisplatin in treating patients with progressive or relapsed metastatic germ cell tumors (GemTIP).* Available at: <http://clinicaltrials.gov/show/NCT00551122>. Accessed 6 June 2013.

24. Bokemeyer C, Gerl P, Schöffski A *et al.* Gemcitabine in patients with relapsed or cisplatin-refractory testicular cancer. *Journal of Clinical Oncology* 1999; **17**(2): 512–16.

25. Huddart R, Norman A, Moyniham C *et al.* Fertility, gonadal and sexual function in survivors of testicular cancer. *British Journal of Cancer* 2005; **93**(2): 200–7.

26. Fossa SD, Gilbert E, Dores GM *et al.* Noncancer causes of death in survivors of testicular cancer. *Journal of the National Cancer Institute* 2007; **99**(7): 533–44.

27. Haugnes HS, Wethal T, Aass N *et al.* Cardiovascular risk factors and morbidity in long-term survivors of testicular cancer: a 20-year follow-up study. *Journal of Clinical Oncology* 2010; **28**(30): 4649–57.

28. Haugnes HS, Aass N, Fossa SD *et al.* Components of the metabolic syndrome in long-term survivors of testicular cancer. *Annals of Oncology* 2007; **18**(2): 241–8.

29. Meinardi MT, Gietama JA, van der Graaf WTA *et al.* Cardiovascular morbidity in long-term survivors of metastatic testicular cancer. *Journal of Clinical Oncology* 2000; **18**(8): 1725–32.

30. Travis LB, Fossa SD, Schonfeld SJ *et al.* Second cancers among 40 576 testicular cancer patients: focus on long-term survivors. *Journal of the National Cancer Institute* 2005; **97**(18): 1354–65.

31. Kollmansberger C, Hartmann JT, Kanz L, Bokemeyer C. Risk of secondary myeloid leukaemia and myelodysplastic syndrome following standard-dose chemotherapy or high dose-chemotherapy with stem cell support in patients with potentially curable malignancies. *Journal of Cancer Research and Clinical Oncology* 1998; **124**(3–4): 207–14.

32. Kollmannsberger C, Nichols C, Meisner C, Mayer F, Kanz L, Bokemeyer C. Identification of prognostic subgroups among patients with metastatic 'IGCCCG poor-prognosis' germ-cell cancer: an explorative analysis using cart modelling. *Annals of Oncology* 2000; **11**(9): 1115–20.

33. Van Dijk MR, Steyerberg EW, Stenning SP, Habbema JD. Identifying subgroups among poor prognosis patients with nonseminomatous germ cell cancer by tree modelling: a validation study. *Annals of Oncology* 2004; **15**(9): 1400–5.

34. Fizazi K, Pagliaro LC, Flechon A *et al.* A phase III trial of personalized chemotherapy based on serum tumor marker decline in poor-prognosis germ-cell tumors: Results of GETUG 13. Proceedings of the American Society of Clinical Oncology 2013. *Journal of Clinical Oncology* 2013; **31**(18 Suppl): abstr LBA4500.

17 Osteosarcoma and the use of high-dose chemotherapy

Kai-Keen Shiu

Expert commentary Sandra Strauss

Case history

A 17-year-old boy presented to his GP with a 3-month history of intermittent pain in his right thigh and knee that was partially relieved with paracetamol and ibuprofen. He was a fit and very active student, and his main concerns were not being able to play football to his best ability and being distracted from his A-level revision. The patient was referred for physiotherapy, but, over the following 4 weeks, the pain progressed and woke him up at night. There was no associated history of weight loss, fevers, or other malaise. After two further visits to the GP, a plain X-ray of his right femur was performed which demonstrated an organized periosteal reaction with mixed dense and lytic areas of bone from the upper mid third to the middle of the shaft of the right femur, covering approximately 9 cm in length. The concern was to exclude a primary bone tumour, and the patient was urgently referred to a specialist diagnostic sarcoma referral centre for further investigation.

Clinically, his gait was normal, and there was no neurovascular deficit. Hip and knee joint examination was normal. He went on to have an MRI of his right leg that demonstrated a distal right femoral intramedullary lesion, measuring 8.6 cm in length and extending to 8 cm from the distal femoral articular surface. No joint involvement was seen. A CT-guided diagnostic needle core biopsy of the lesion was performed under general anaesthetic. This confirmed a diagnosis of high-grade osteoblastic osteosarcoma. The patient completed staging investigations, including a fine-cut CT scan of the chest and a bone scan which showed no evidence of metastatic disease. His preoperative stage was T2bN0M0.

> **⭐ Learning point** Epidemiology of sarcoma
>
> Primary malignant tumours of the bone are rare. Their annual incidence accounts for <0.2% of all malignancies, and, on average, 379 patients are diagnosed per year in the UK [1]. The peak incidence occurs during puberty, although a second peak occurs in adults (>50 years old).
>
> The three commonest histological types are osteosarcoma, chondrosarcoma, and Ewing sarcoma. Osteosarcoma can occur as part of familial cancer predisposition syndromes, such as Li–Fraumeni and retinoblastoma gene mutations, and therefore a family history is important.
>
> Osteosarcoma is the commonest primary bone tumour in the adolescent population. Differential diagnoses include primary bone lymphomas and myelomas. The commonest primary site of disease is the distal femur, and over 80% of tumours occur in the long bones of the leg. With increasing age, the incidence of pelvic and other axial tumours increases [1].

> **➕ Clinical tip** Signs and symptoms of osteosarcoma
>
> *Pain:*
>
> - often thought to relate to a sporting injury or 'growing pains'
> - not relieved by rest
> - progressive despite change in activity and physiotherapy
> - requiring increasing analgesia
> - night pain.
>
> *Swelling:*
>
> - may relate to oedema associated with the tumour or increased soft tissue extension of the disease.
>
> *Systemic symptoms, such as weight loss, are rare and usually relate to advanced disease.*

✪ Learning point Prognostic factors in osteosarcoma

The primary site of tumour is important in determining the outcome; patients with axial tumours have a worse outcome than those with extremity tumours. Recent analyses demonstrate that children have a better prognosis than adolescent and adult patients, and that females too have a better prognosis [2,3].

The histological subtype and tumour size have prognostic significance in some analyses, but studies are hampered by a lack of consistent data collection, methodological differences, and contradictory results.

The strongest prognostic factor in patients with resectable disease is histological response to preoperative chemotherapy. Prior surgery with fixation of a pathological fracture and contamination of the surgical field confers a poor outcome.

✪ Learning point Staging investigations for sarcoma

A plain X-ray of the symptomatic bone is usually the first and most important modality of imaging, followed by an MRI scan of the suspicious bone lesion and adjacent joints, using T1, T2, and STIR sequences. This is particularly helpful to diagnose skip bony metastases which have prognostic value (Figure 17.1 and Figure 17.2). Skip lesions are classified as T3, whatever the size. Lesions involving joints may preclude limb-sparing surgery.

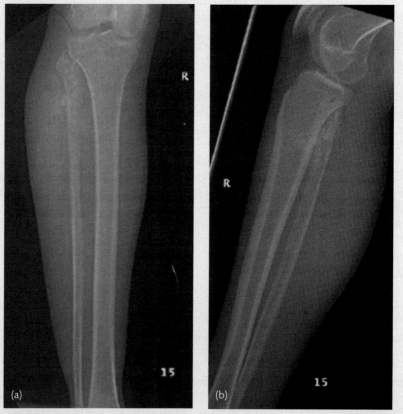

(a) (b)

Figure 17.1 Plain X-ray—lesion in the head of the left fibula.

(continued)

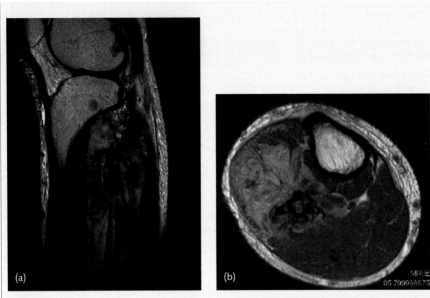

(a)

(b)

Figure 17.2 MRI scan showing a primary in the head of the fibula and a skip lesion in the head of the tibia.

Accurate histology and staging at diagnosis are fundamental and allow the MDT to determine if all sites of disease are potentially resectable. Bone tumours spread haematogenously, and the commonest site of metastases is the lungs; bone metastases are less frequent. The protocol for staging of an osteosarcoma includes a fine-cut (1 mm slices) CT chest scan and a bone scan. In patients with Ewing's sarcoma, bone marrow aspirate and trephines are performed, as bone marrow involvement and bone metastases are more common [4]. Imaging of other sites can be directed to clinical symptoms. Whole-body MRI scans and PET-CT scans are not standard imaging techniques but may detect metastatic disease, if other imaging is inconclusive and it will alter prognosis and therapeutic modalities offered.

The patient was informed of the diagnosis with his family present. His case had been discussed at the MDT, and it was determined that limb-sparing surgical excision would be possible with an endoprosthetic reconstruction. Neoadjuvant chemotherapy was recommended, and he was referred to a sarcoma oncologist for pretreatment investigations and commencement of treatment. He was provided with crutches to allow for partial weight-bearing, avoiding the complications of a pathological fracture.

The patient attended a teenage young adult (TYA) unit at a regional sarcoma centre to discuss the diagnosis and planned treatment with the oncology team. He was provided with written information about osteosarcoma and its treatment and information about support groups, including the Bone Cancer Research Trust (<http://www.bcrt.org.uk/>) and Teenage Cancer Trust (<http://www.teenagecancertrust.org/>). The patient was also discussed at the TYA MDT and allocated a clinical nurse specialist and a social worker to ensure his educational, social, financial, and psychological needs could be met. He had an EDTA GFR that showed a corrected GFR of 110 mL/min. An echocardiogram showed normal fractional shortening of 43% and LVEF of 76%. Bilateral audiometry was normal. He also was consented for, and underwent, fertility testing and semen storage. Blood tests, including FBC, renal, liver, and bone profiles, were normal. Virology testing, including HIV, CMV, and hepatitis A, B, and C, was also normal.

⊗ **Learning point** Specialist sarcoma MDT

Management of high-grade sarcomas requires an expert, multidisciplinary, and multimodality therapeutic approach [5]. This should be within a sarcoma specialist centre where the delivery and management of side effects from treatment are established, as well as provide patients access to trials that require multicentre collaboration in these rare cancers.

Even in the presence of metastatic disease, MDT discussion should include a decision about local therapy to manage the primary site and determine whether the tumour is resectable, potentially resectable after chemotherapy, or inoperable due to its site and proximity to vital structures. The aim of surgery is to achieve a complete resection of the tumour with as wide a margin and as little loss of function as possible. It is one of the reasons why osteosarcomas of the extremities/long bones have a better prognosis than those affecting axial bones such as the spine or pelvis.

Radiotherapy is not an alternative to surgery as local management of the primary, as these tumours are radioresistant, and, in general, if a tumour is unable to be completely resected, the patient is not thought to be 'curable'. Radiotherapy should be reserved for palliative treatment in unresectable disease or as adjuvant therapy in highly selected cases. The evidence for the value of adjuvant radiotherapy in this setting is limited. In line with improving outcome guidance, all teenagers and young adults with cancer should be discussed at an age-appropriate MDT to enable the provision of support and services tailored to their needs [6].

⊕ **Clinical tip** Biopsies should be performed in a specialist centre

If the suspicion of a primary bone tumour is raised on imaging, a biopsy should *not* be attempted, unless performed at a specialist bone sarcoma unit after all local imaging, including MRI, is performed. This is to maintain staging accuracy and to avoid tumour contamination and compromising potential curative surgery, as there is a risk of seeding of the tumour, either down the bone shaft (e.g. with an intramedullary nail for a pathological fracture) or along the needle tract. It should be planned, so that the biopsy site, biopsy tract, and entire tumour can be resected en bloc.

⊗ **Learning point** Chemotherapy in osteosarcoma

Nine historical surgery-only studies have shown 5-year DFS of only 16% [8]. The OS has increased significantly since the introduction of chemotherapy, but outcomes are similar, whether chemotherapy is given before or after surgery [2,8–10]. If a patient is fit, the preferred regimen includes methotrexate, cisplatin, and Adriamycin® (doxorubicin) (MAP), which reduces relapse rates at 5 years for localized disease to approximately 30%. Many studies have explored the effect of the addition of ifosfamide to this regimen, but its contribution remains undefined, and, in the UK, MAP would be considered the standard induction therapy in patients <40 years who are able to tolerate methotrexate. Preoperative intensification of treatment, although showing increased rates of good pathological response, to date, have not led to significant changes in post-treatment OS.

The oncology team recommended neoadjuvant MAP chemotherapy on the EURAMOS-1 trial. The patient consented to treatment on this trial and was admitted 2 days later for insertion of a peripherally inserted central catheter (PICC) line and for his first cycle of chemotherapy. This was uneventful, apart from mild nausea, despite prophylactic anti-emetics, including aprepitant. He was discharged 3 days later, with prophylactic G-CSF injections from days 5 to 15. Shared care arrangements were made with his local oncology team, if he became unwell with neutropenic sepsis or other complications of chemotherapy, as he lived over 60 miles away.

➕ **Clinical tip** MAP chemotherapy

The MAP regimen includes doxorubicin 75 mg/m^2 and cisplatin 120 mg/m^2 (AP) given on days 1–3, followed by methotrexate (M) 12 g/m^2 given on days 22 and 29 of a 5-week cycle. Close monitoring of renal and cardiac function is important. Patients on the EURAMOS-1 trial have mandatory EDTA creatinine clearance after cycles 2 and 4 of doxorubin, and LVEF testing at 300 mg/m^2 (prior to cycle 5) and 375 mg/m^2 (prior to cycle 6), due to the increased incidence of cardiac toxicity after cumulative exposure of 300 mg/m^2 which is increased in teenagers and young adults. Furthermore, nephrotoxic antibiotics, such as amikacin and gentamicin, which are usually recommended as part of first-line broad-spectrum antibiotics in neutropenic sepsis, should be avoided in the management of patients who are already receiving high doses of cisplatin, methotrexate, and ifosfamide, all of which already can cause significant renal impairment.

✪ **Learning point** Induction chemotherapy

Induction chemotherapy is generally recommended prior to surgical resection, even in resectable disease.

Pathological response to neoadjuvant therapy is one of the strongest prognostic factors of outcome in patients with localized osteosarcoma.

- 5-year survivals of approximately 70% are seen with >90% of tumour necrosis after two cycles of induction therapy.
- The 5-year survival falls to around 50% when there is >10% of residual viable tumour.

The potential for limb salvage and joint-preserving surgery, with better functional outcome for the patient, increases with prior chemotherapy. Amputation can be reserved, if resection margins are positive or in cases of local recurrence. The rate of local recurrence is significantly higher in patients who have had previous limb-sparing surgery (8% versus 2%) [11] and in patients who decline amputation when limb salvage surgery is thought likely to be marginal; patients are counselled on this carefully preoperatively.

Patients with metastatic disease also receive intensive chemotherapy to prolong the time to disease progression and maintain the QoL.

✔ **Evidence base** EURAMOS-1: addition of ifosfamide and etoposide to MAP chemotherapy

- The EURAMOS study group was set up in 2001 (<http://www.euramos.org>) to improve survival from osteosarcoma by conducting large collaborative randomized studies with parallel biological studies.
- EURAMOS-1 aimed to investigate the impact on outcome of the addition of ifosfamide and etoposide to MAP in patients with a poor response to neoadjuvant chemotherapy, and the role of immunomodulation with IFN given as maintenance therapy in those with a good response to neoadjuvant MAP.
- Largest randomized phase III study conducted in osteosarcoma.
- A total of 2260 patients registered and 1332 randomized from April 2005 to December 2011 across 17 countries.
- The study demonstrated an estimated event-free survival at 5 years of 77% in patients randomized to IFN, compared to 74% on the standard arm. This difference was not significant.[13]
- The results of the poor responder group were presented recently at the Connective Tissue Oncology society meeting 2014 and showed no benefit for the addition of ifosfamide and etoposide with increased toxicity, so the standard of care remains MAP

Source: data from *European and American Osteosarcoma Study Group* (EURAMOS), available from <http://www.euramos. org>, Copyright © 2006 Medical Research Council, Clinical Trials Unit.

The patient was admitted for day 22 high-dose methotrexate. Apart from grade 2 fatigue from days 3–10, and grade 2 mucositis from days 7–14, he had tolerated his doxorubicin and cisplatin chemotherapy well. He commenced methotrexate after adequate pre-hydration and alkalinization of his urine (pH >7) using IV fluids and sodium bicarbonate. At 24 hours after the commencement of his methotrexate infusion, simultaneous U & Es and methotrexate levels were done. His 24-hour methotrexate level was 12 µmol/L. Folinic acid at 15 mg/m^2 orally every 6 hours was given, and daily methotrexate levels and renal function were continued, until the methotrexate level was <0.2 µmol/L.

⊕ Clinical tip High-dose methotrexate and folinic acid rescue

Methotrexate is an anti-metabolite/folic acid analogue that competitively inhibits dihydrofolate reductase. It is given at the highest IV dose in osteosarcoma—usually 12 g/m^2 (compared to 3–6 g/m^2 in primary CNS lymphomas, and 40 mg/m^2 boluses for CMF chemotherapy in breast cancer).

The efficacy of the treatment is believed to be due to the peak dose achieved at 24 hours, but thereafter clearance of methotrexate is vital, in order to avoid significant toxicities, particularly renal failure and mucositis/stomatitis. Folinic acid facilitates clearance and is administered in the washout period, until the level of methotrexate is below a threshold of 0.2 µmol/L. Close clinical monitoring of methotrexate levels, in addition to urine output, urine pH, and renal function, is mandatory.

Algorithms are available at treating hospitals, based on local practice and/or trial protocols, to calculate the level of methotrexate and the dose of folinic acid required to protect end-organs—in particular, the kidney—and when it is safe to stop folinic acid rescue.

If worsening renal function or poor methotrexate clearance occurs, consultant advice should be sought immediately for further management. Drugs, such as glucarpidase, may be used to reduce ongoing complications. Glucarpidase, a recombinant form of the bacterial enzyme carboxypeptidase G2, converts methotrexate into glutamate and 2,4-diamino-N(10)-methylpteroic acid but is expensive. Current studies are ongoing, examining the role of glucarpidase in reducing complications from methotrexate treatment in osteosarcoma (GLU1; EudraCT 2006-003203-40) and primary CNS lymphoma (NCT00727831Clinicaltrials.gov).

⊕ Clinical tip Drugs to avoid with concomitant administration of high-dose methotrexate

A number of common drugs can increase methotrexate toxicities, by altering the pharmacokinetic profile, and should not be used within 24 hours prior to methotrexate infusion, nor used until at least 24 hours after clearance of methotrexate.

The following drugs should be used with caution or are contraindicated in patients receiving methotrexate (recommendations adapted from the GLU1 trial protocol):

- salicylates, sulfonamides, probenecid, cephalothin, penicillins (carbenicillin, ticarcillin) in high concentrations, omeprazole: known to compete with methotrexate for membrane transport and thus may reduce renal tubular secretion
- salicylates, sulfonamides, phenylbutazone, hypoglycaemics, diphenylhydantoins, tetracyclines, chloramphenicol, p-aminobenzoic acid, and acidic anti-inflammatory drugs: known to displace methotrexate from its binding sites on plasma proteins and thus may increase free methotrexate levels in plasma
- theophylline or methionine could enhance methotrexate cytotoxicity
- NSAIDs reduce the tubular secretion of methotrexate
- co-trimoxazole and trimethoprim are folate antagonists and may increase methotrexate cytotoxicity
- chloramphenicol and tetracycline could interfere with the enterohepatic circulation.

The patient was readmitted on day 28 for his next high-dose methotrexate. On examination, he had two ulcers, measuring over 1 cm, over the hard palate with overlying *Candida*, grade 3, all of which were causing odynophagia and reduction in oral intake, but he was maintaining adequate fluid intake. His FBC was normal. Supportive care, including antibacterial and anaesthetic mouthwashes, analgesia, and oral fluconazole, were given for 3 days, and treatment delayed until toxicity had resolved to grade 1.

> ⏱ **Expert comment**
>
> Dose reductions of methotrexate are not utilized in the management of patients with osteosarcoma, as it is believed the peak methotrexate concentration is important in determining efficacy. Patients with mucositis are managed supportively, and treatment is delayed until toxicity recovers. A recent meta-analysis of 24 prospectively conducted studies and registries of patients with osteosarcoma demonstrated that patients who experience grades 3/4 mucositis have a better outcome than those who do not (HR 0.77, 95% CI 0.59–0.98; $p = 0.03$), and that females experience this toxicity more frequently than males, contributing to their better outcome in this analysis ($p = 0.002$) [3]. Patients over 40 years generally will not tolerate methotrexate, due to delayed excretion and subsequent renal impairment, so standard chemotherapy is with AP alone. The Italian Sarcoma Group has trialled a regimen that incorporates 8 g/m^2 of methotrexate in this population, and the results are encouraging but have not been compared with AP [14].

The delivery of the second cycle of MAP chemotherapy was uncomplicated, apart from an infected PICC line that grew Gram-negative cocci. This was removed, prior to the subsequent cycle of methotrexate, and replaced with a left suprabrachial PICC line. At this point, the patient underwent restaging MRI scan of his right leg and CT scan of the chest, and repeat EDTA GFR, echocardiogram, and audiometry after two cycles of MAP chemotherapy. Tests showed neither progression of disease nor significant impairment of renal or cardiac function.

> ➕ **Clinical tip** PICC/Hickman lines
>
> Long lines are inserted under ultrasound or X-ray screening guidance and allow for ease of administration of fluids and chemotherapy and taking blood samples. The chance of vesicant drugs causing significant complications is also reduced. Correct placement and ongoing care of the line is essential, including the use of aseptic techniques when assessing the line and weekly flushing to maintain patency.
>
> One of the main complications of indwelling lines is sepsis, particularly in the context of neutropenia.
>
> Management should include swabbing the line insertion site, taking blood cultures from all line ports, and at least one peripheral blood culture (not from the line). Lines can be 'salvaged' with high-dose antibiotics, preferably treating known sensitive organisms. Teicoplanin may be used as 'blind' treatment for suspected line infections, until sensitivities are known. Removal of the line and culture of the tip may, however, still be required.
>
> Other complications of long lines include increased risk of thrombosis, which requires anticoagulation and line removal, and palpitations if the line tip is near the right atrium. Recently, the use of ECGs during line placement has been introduced to improve line placement and may reduce the need for a CXR. If palpitations occur, line placement must be checked and the line pulled back, if appropriate.

The patient had resection of his tumour, with a distal femoral endoprosthesis, and his resection histology was discussed at the sarcoma MDT meeting. This confirmed an osteoblastic sarcoma, with a good response to therapy with >90% tumour necrosis and clear margins.

> ➕ **Clinical tip** Management of chemotherapy-induced mucositis
>
> Mucositis is commonly associated with doxorubicin and usually occurs 5–7 days after chemotherapy. To date, there are no RCTs that have demonstrated effectiveness of any treatment directed against mucositis. Unlike radiation-induced mucositis, the mucositis usually resolves with conservative management that includes good oral hygiene with supportive care and prophylactic or treatment doses of anti-fungal antibiotics. Although parental nutrition can be used in severe cases, the requirement for this is unusual.

He was randomized to standard consolidation MAP chemotherapy, as per the EURAMOS-1 protocol, and completed a further four cycles of MAP. Close monitoring of cardiac and renal function continued, with a repeat GFR performed after cycle 4 and repeat echocardiography prior to cycle 5 (after a cumulative dose of 300 mg/m^2 of doxorubicin) and prior to cycle 6 (cumulative dose of 375 mg/m^2) due to increasing incidence of cardiac toxicity. These were satisfactory, and his end of treatment investigations, including a CT of the chest, showed no evidence of lung metastases, normal renal and cardiac function, and unimpaired hearing.

The patient was followed up with 2-monthly CXRs and 4-monthly X-rays of his right leg. Eight months later, he developed pleuritic chest pain. A plain CXR showed a rounded lesion in the right upper lobe. A CT of the chest showed a 3 cm pulmonary metastasis, abutting the right pleura, and two satellite nodules in the right upper lobe, suspicious of metastases. No disease was noted in the left lung. MDT discussion with specialist sarcoma thoracic surgeons determined the disease to be resectable, but, in view of the short disease-free interval, preoperative chemotherapy was recommended. He was treated with high-dose ifosfamide and etoposide chemotherapy, incorporating 14 g/m^2 of ifosfamide given over 5 days and 500 mg/m^2 of etoposide.

The night after the third dose of ifosfamide during the first cycle, he became agitated and confused and was attempting to leave the ward. It was felt that he had developed ifosfamide-induced encephalopathy (IIE). The ifosfamide infusion was stopped, and methylene blue, 50 mg given IV every 4 hours, was commenced, and he was closely monitored with neurological observations and urine output. Twelve hours later, the patient was improving and not confused. He was given prophylactic IV methylene blue (50 mg IV 6-hourly) for subsequent treatment with ifosfamide.

Clinical tip Ifosfamide-induced encephalopathy

Ifosfamide can cause some degree of CNS toxicity in 10–30% of patients, if given IV. The exact mechanism is unknown.

Confusion is the commonest symptom, ranging from lethargy to delirium. Hallucination or psychosis can occur in up to 30% of patients, and incontinence of muscles twitching in 9% of patients [17].

Variables that predict the likelihood of IIE include [18]:

- low serum albumin (<30 g/L)
- high creatinine (>150 µmol/L)
- pelvic disease
- hypokalaemia
- hyponatraemia.

However, a retrospective study of 82 patients failed to support using these variables [19]. There are no conclusive randomized controlled prospective trials of treatment of IIE. Management is based on retrospective studies of the use of methylene blue, albumin, or thiamine [17,20,21]. This strategy is based on a widely accepted hypothesis that the encephalopathy is caused by one or more of the metabolites of ifosfamide, especially chloroacetaldehyde, which may cause a form of Wernicke's encephalopathy. In the absence of proven treatments, a pragmatic strategy is to stop ifosfamide, monitor any deterioration in neurology, treat signs or symptoms as they occur, e.g. IV replacement of fluids and electrolytes, and consider haemodialysis and sedation, if the patient is critically unwell with seizures. Ventilatory support may be needed in severe cases.

> ⊕ **Clinical tip** Late effects of treatment
>
> Long-term follow-up of patients to monitor for late effects of chemotherapy (and/or radiotherapy) is essential. Late effects can include (sub) fertility, chronic renal impairment, cardiomyopathy, early coronary heart disease, and second malignancies [22]. Psychosocial, educational, employment, and insurance support after treatment should be optimized for the individual. It therefore requires a multidisciplinary approach to the long-term care and management of patients with osteosarcoma.

> ⊕ **Expert comment**
>
> To date, there are no randomized studies comparing the treatment of patients at first recurrence. Treatment is given according to whether patients are being treated with curative intent and treatment received at diagnosis. In the curative setting, high doses of ifosfamide and etoposide are recommended. If a patient has unresectable lung metastases, then palliative doses of these agents can be employed.

After four cycles of ifosfamide and etoposide, reassessment CT scans showed a partial response, and the patient underwent pulmonary metastasectomy. An additional two ipsilateral pulmonary nodules were palpated at the time of surgery and were also resected. He had an uneventful intra- and post-operative course. Histology revealed no residual metastatic tumour in the pulmonary resections. He remained on surveillance under the sarcoma team, with 2-monthly CXRs and 6-monthly CT chest scans, as well as long-term monitoring of cardiac and renal function and other late effects of chemotherapy.

Discussion

This case illustrates the management of a patient with osteosarcoma from the initial diagnostic work-up, primary therapy, management at first relapse, and long-term follow-up. It emphasizes the importance of full diagnostic work-up and careful MDT discussion to define the extent of disease and aims of treatment which are not without morbidity (and rarely mortality).

In the UK, there are specialist sarcoma centres linked in with TYA services to provide a comprehensive multidisciplinary approach in the management of this challenging disease in children and young adults. Experienced oncologists should manage these patients, and, if involved in their care, early advice should be sought to ensure appropriate management of complications of therapy.

Careful follow-up after curative therapy is vital, in order to detect relapse, the risk of which is highest within the first 2–3 years. Early recurrence within 2 years predicts worse OS, although late recurrences after 5 years do occur [23]. In a meta-analysis of three European RCTs, the median recurrence-free survival was 31 months, and median survival after first relapse was only 14 months [11]. Metastatic recurrence is most likely to occur in the lungs (90%). Routine CXRs are used to identify asymptomatic lung metastases. There is no evidence to suggest that more invasive surveillance, using CT chest scans or bone scans, will alter outcome, but prompt clinical assessment and investigation of new symptoms are essential.

Any patient who relapses should be considered for surgical resection, if possible. Patients who relapse with resectable disease may still survive long-term, even with >1 episode of relapse if surgically resectable [2,11]. Perioperative chemotherapy can be used, but no prospective randomized trial has been conducted to demonstrate its benefit. CT chest scans may under-report pulmonary metastases, so careful intraoperative lung palpation to examine for other metastases should be performed. Patients with recurrent metastases may still achieve long-term disease control, so MDT discussion that includes consideration of surgery at subsequent relapses should also occur.

A final word from the expert

This case illustrates the complexities in the management of a rare tumour in a challenging age group and the importance of MDT involvement and specialist care. Aggressive management and meticulous attention to assessing toxicity from chemotherapy is paramount to avoid acute and long-term sequelae of treatment and ensure successful outcome. The importance of collaboration in trials is also discussed, as, in a rare disease such as osteosarcoma, these studies are essential. Few improvements have been made in outcome over the last decade, and there is an urgent need to develop novel therapies. It is hoped that further understanding of the biology of osteosarcoma, including current genetic sequencing studies, will identify novel therapeutic targets, which should be investigated collaboratively to ensure any evidence of efficacy can be translated swiftly to the first-line setting to improve outcome in this group of patients (<http://icgc.org/icgc/cgp/60/508/70116>). Unfortunately, the fragmented use of MTP across Europe, its unavailability in the US, and the reluctance of pharmaceutical partners to conduct further randomized studies using this agent will hamper the ability of the osteosarcoma community to conduct such trials.

References

1. Whelan J, McTiernan A, Cooper N *et al.* Incidence and survival of malignant bone sarcomas in England 1979-2007. *International Journal of Cancer* 2012; **131**(4): E508–17.
2. Whelan JS, Jinks RC, McTiernan A *et al.* Survival from high-grade localised extremity osteosarcoma: combined results and prognostic factors from three European Osteosarcoma Intergroup randomised controlled trials. *Annals of Oncology* 2012; **23**(6): 1607–16.
3. Collins M, Wilhelm M, Conyers R *et al.* Benefits and adverse events in younger versus older patients receiving neoadjuvant chemotherapy for osteosarcoma: findings from a meta-analysis. *Journal of Clinical Oncology* 2013; **31**(18): 2303–12.
4. Seddon BM, Whelan JS. Emerging chemotherapeutic strategies and the role of treatment stratification in Ewing sarcoma. *Paediatric drugs* 2008; **10**(2): 93–105.
5. Bielack S, Carrle D, Casali PG. Osteosarcoma: ESMO clinical recommendations for diagnosis, treatment and follow-up. *Annals of Oncology* 2009; **20**(Suppl 4): 137–9.
6. Taylor RM, Pearce S, Gibson F, Fern L, Whelan J. Developing a conceptual model of teenage and young adult experiences of cancer through meta-synthesis. *International Journal of Nursing Studies* 2013; **50**(6): 832–46.
7. Edge S, Byrd DR, Compton CC, Fritz AG, Greene FL, Trotti A, eds. *AJCC cancer staging handbook*, 7th edn. New York: Springer, 2010.
8. Anninga JK, Gelderblom H, Fiocco M *et al.* Chemotherapeutic adjuvant treatment for osteosarcoma: where do we stand? *European Journal of Cancer* 2011; **47**(16): 2431–45.
9. Whelan JS. Osteosarcoma. *European Journal of Cancer* 1997; **33**(10): 1611–18; discussion 8–9.
10. Meyers PA, Heller G, Healey J *et al.* Chemotherapy for nonmetastatic osteogenic sarcoma: the Memorial Sloan-Kettering experience. *Journal of Clinical Oncology* 1992; **10**(1): 5–15.
11. Gelderblom H, Jinks RC, Sydes M *et al.* Survival after recurrent osteosarcoma: data from 3 European Osteosarcoma Intergroup (EOI) randomized controlled trials. *European Journal of Cancer* 2011; **47**(6): 895–902.
12 Marina, N; Smeland S; Bielack, SS *et al.* MAPIE VS MAP as Post-operative chemotherappthy in patients with a poor response to pre-operative chemotherapy for newly

diagnosed osteosarcoma: results from EURAMOS-1. Proceedings Connective Tissue Oncology society Meeting, Berlin, 2014, abstract 032

13. Bielack S, Smeland S, Whelan J *et al.* MAP plus maintenance pegylated interferon α-2b (MAPIfn) versus MAP alone in patients with resectable high-grade osteosarcoma and good histologic response to preoperative MAP: First results of the EURAMOS-1 'good response' randomization. *Journal of Clinical Oncology* 2013; **31**(Suppl): abstr LBA10504.

14. Ferrari SS. Smeland S. Bielack A *et al.* A European treatment protocol for bone sarcoma in patients older than 40 years. *Journal of Clinical Oncology* 2009; **15**(Suppl): abstr 10516.

15. National Institute for Health and Care Excellence. *Mifamurtide for the treatment of osteosarcoma.* 2011. Available from: <http://guidance.nice.org.uk/TA235>.

16. Meyers PA, Schwartz CL, Krailo MD *et al.* Osteosarcoma: the addition of muramyl tripeptide to chemotherapy improves overall survival—a report from the Children's Oncology Group. *Journal of Clinical Oncology* 2008; **26**(4): 633–8.

17. Ajithkumar T, Parkinson C, Shamshad F, Murray P. Ifosfamide encephalopathy. *Clinical Oncology* 2007; **19**(2): 108–14.

18. Meanwell CA, Blake AE, Kelly KA, Honigsberger L, Blackledge G. Prediction of ifosfamide/mesna associated encephalopathy. *European Journal of Cancer & Clinical Oncology* 1986; **22**(7): 815–19.

19. Watkin SW, Husband DJ, Green JA, Warenius HM. Ifosfamide encephalopathy: a reappraisal. *European Journal of Cancer & Clinical Oncology* 1989; **25**(9): 1303–10.

20. Pelgrims J, De Vos F, Van den Brande J, Schrijvers D, Prove A, Vermorken JB. Methylene blue in the treatment and prevention of ifosfamide-induced encephalopathy: report of 12 cases and a review of the literature. *British Journal of Cancer* 2000; **82**(2): 291–4.

21. Richards A, Marshall H, McQuary A. Evaluation of methylene blue, thiamine, and/or albumin in the prevention of ifosfamide-related neurotoxicity. *Journal of Oncology Pharmacy Practice* 2011; **17**(4): 372–80.

22. Janeway KA, Grier HE. Sequelae of osteosarcoma medical therapy: a review of rare acute toxicities and late effects. *The Lancet Oncology* 2010; **11**(7): 670–8.

23. Strauss SJ, McTiernan A, Whelan JS. Late relapse of osteosarcoma: implications for follow-up and screening. *Pediatric Blood & Cancer* 2004; **43**(6): 692–7.

18 Melanoma and immunotherapy

Sarah Ellis

ⓘ **Expert commentary** **Mark Harries**

Case history

A 54-year-old woman presented to her GP with a 3-month history of worsening right upper quadrant pain and malaise. She had also noted several new dark-coloured cutaneous lesions on her left arm.

Six years previously, she had a wide local excision for an ulcerated, 2 mm thickness, malignant melanoma on her left forearm (stage IIA). She had discussed the option of sentinel node biopsy, but, due to concerns regarding lymphoedema and in the absence of clinical or radiological evidence of lymph node metastases, she opted to have clinical observation, rather than surgery. She had completed follow-up with the dermatological team, with no evidence of recurrence after surgery. Other past medical history included depression, for which she was on citalopram, and mild asthma. She had spent the first 15 years of her life in Australia and had used sunbeds in her twenties occasionally.

➕ **Clinical tip** Surgical excision of melanoma [1]

The biopsy should aim to result in the complete removal of the whole lesion and a 2 mm margin of normal skin and include the whole depth of the skin, including a cuff of subcutaneous fat. In cosmetically sensitive areas or for very large lesions, the urgent advice of plastic surgery should be sought before biopsy. When a histological diagnosis of melanoma has been made, the patient should undergo a wide local excision. The margin of this excision required is judged, according to the Breslow depth. All melanocytic lesions should be examined by a pathologist involved in a local or specialist skin cancer MDT.

Breslow thickneSS	Excision margin
In situ	5 mm
<1 mm	1 cm
1.01–2 mm	1–2 cm
2.1–4 mm	2–3 cm
>4 mm	3 cm

✖ **Learning point** Genetic and environmental risk factors

Multiple risk factors for the development of melanoma have been identified. Only 5% of cases are thought to be familial; a third of familial cases are seen to have a variety of germline mutations in the *CDKN2A* gene, which is involved in entry into the cell cycle. Most melanoma cases are not related to high penetrance genes but likely a combination of low penetrance genes and environmental exposures [2].

(continued)

ⓘ **Expert comment**

The margins of excision for intermediate-thickness melanoma remain controversial, but all international guidelines recommend at least 2 cm.

Risk factors

- Caucasian skin/type 1 or 2.
- Red or blond hair.
- Melanoma in ≥1 first-degree relative.
- >100 benign melanocytic naevi.
- ≥3 dysplastic naevi.
- High sun exposure in childhood.
- Past history of blistering sunburn.
- Sunbed use.

✪ Learning point Prognostic factors in melanoma

The AJCC released new melanoma staging guidelines in 2009 [3]. Using a database of over 38 000 patients with melanoma, and multivariate analysis, the factors most significantly affecting prognosis were identified:

- Increased thickness:
  - <1.0 mm, 10-year survival of 92%
  - >4.0 mm, 10-year survival of 50%.
- Presence of ulceration indicates a higher rate of relapse, independent of the tumour depth.
- Mitotic rate.
- T1 lesions are subdivided to T1a and T1b, according to a mitotic rate of ≥1 mm/m^2, with a reduction in survival from 95% to 88% at 10 years [3].
- Lymph node burden.

For patients with distant metastatic disease, the presence of extra-pulmonary visceral disease is a poor prognostic factor.

- 62% survival at 1 year in the absence of visceral disease.
- 33% survival at 1 year with extra-pulmonary visceral disease or raised serum LDH [3].

Serum LDH is an independent prognostic indicator and should be measured in stage IV disease.

✪ Learning point Assessment of nodal disease

In the UK, patients with tumours of greater than stage IA should have the option of sentinel node biopsy at the same time as their wide local excision [1]. Around 20% of patients will have occult nodal disease at presentation. Sentinel lymph node biopsy offers prognostic information and potential stratification for clinical trial entry, but it has no therapeutic value [4].

Routine cross-sectional imaging is not recommended for patients with low-risk early-stage disease. The role of imaging for patients at high risk of relapse is controversial, as there are no randomized trials to support a proactive imaging approach. However, with the advent of new therapies for melanoma, it is possible that the detection of small-volume or oligometastatic disease will become important.

❝ Expert comment

Sentinel node biopsy for melanoma remains controversial, as, in itself, it has no impact on OS for the patient. It should be considered for three reasons: first, as a staging procedure to help guide prognosis and follow-up; second, to minimize the risk of nodal recurrence and to gain locoregional control of the disease in the 20% of patients with nodal metastases; and third, as an important stratification procedure that is often required prior to entry into adjuvant clinical trials.

❝ Expert comment

Recent UK recommendations advocate the testing of all high-risk melanomas for the *BRAF* mutation, so that appropriate therapies can be initiated without delay on relapse.

✔ Evidence base Sentinel node biopsy or nodal observation in melanoma (MSLT-1) [4]

- Large international prospective RCT.
- A total of 1269 patients recruited between 1994 and 2002.
- Melanoma thickness of 1.2–3.5 mm.
- Randomly assigned 60:40 to biopsy or observation.
- At 5 years:
  - no difference in melanoma-specific survival: 86% versus 87.1% (HR 0.92, 95% CI 0.67–1.25; p = 0.58).
  - relapse at any site: 26.8% in the observation group and 20.7% in the biopsy group
  - statistically significant DFS benefit: 78.3% versus 73.1% (HR 0.74, 95% CI 0.59–0.93; p = 0.009)

(continued)

○ subgroup analysis of OS in those who underwent sentinel node biopsy and immediate nodal dissection and those who later relapsed and underwent delayed LND were 72.3% versus 52.4% (HR for death 0.51, 95% CI 0.32–0.81; p = 0.004).

> ⊗ **Learning point** Adjuvant treatment for melanoma
>
> In the UK, there is no standard systemic adjuvant treatment offered to those at high risk of relapse following resection of their primary tumour, outside clinical trials.
>
> Adjuvant therapy with IFN-alpha is licensed in the US. Many phase III trials have been carried out, with varying results, and initial meta-analyses failed to show a definitive improvement in OS [5,6]. An individual patient data meta-analysis (ASCO 2007) showed an absolute OS benefit of 3% (CI 1–5%) at 5 years [6]. A more recent systematic review and meta-analysis, with the addition of two more RCTs, found an 18% risk reduction in DFS and 11% risk reduction in OS; however, it was unable to identify the duration or optimal dosing strategy [5]. Treatment courses can have a duration of 1–2 years. Side effects of IFN-alpha include profound flu-like symptoms, fatigue, and severe depression, leading to some patients stopping treatment early.
>
> Adjuvant radiotherapy to the nodal basin, following LND, for those at high risk of regional recurrence can be considered. There are few prospective randomized trials. A recent international randomized trial included 217 patients. Radiotherapy significantly reduced recurrence in the lymph node field (HR 0.56, 95% CI 0.32–0.98; p = 0.041). There was no benefit in relapse-free survival [7].
>
> Eligibility criteria to receive radiotherapy included ≥1 parotid nodes, ≥2 cervical or axillary nodes, ≥3 inguinal nodes, or extranodal spread. Patients received 48 Gy to the involved nodal field. At 3 years, 19% of those in the radiotherapy group had relapsed in the treated nodal basin, compared with 31% of those in the observation arm [7].

The GP noted a palpable liver edge and several black nodular lesions on her forearm and chest. He requested LFTs and referred her urgently to her dermatology team. A CT scan demonstrated enlarged lymph nodes in the left axilla, multiple liver metastases, and several suspicious lung nodules (Figure 18.1).

Following discussion in the skin MDT meeting, she underwent liver biopsy, which confirmed malignant melanoma. Samples were analysed for the *BRAF* mutation; the presence of a *V600E* mutation was found.

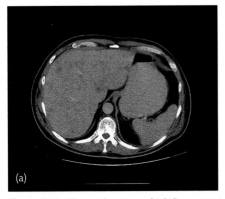
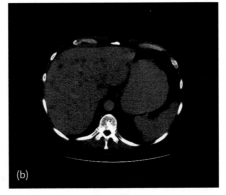

Figure 18.1 CT scan showing multiple liver metastases. (A) Standard setting and (B) liver window.

She was referred to an oncologist. It was explained that cure of her disease was unlikely, and treatments would be aimed at prolonging the quality and length of her life. Due to the presence of the *BRAF* mutation in her tumour and large volume of disease, treatment with Vemurafenib, the oral inhibitor of the mutated *BRAF*, was recommended as first-line treatment at a dose of 960 mg bd. This was felt to be more likely to offer rapid control of her symptoms, compared with conventional chemotherapy options.

✪ Learning point Chemotherapy options in metastatic melanoma

Dacarbazine

- Given IV every 3 weeks.
- Side effects include nausea and vomiting, constipation, and bone marrow suppression.
- Standard melanoma treatment used for head-to-head comparisons. There have been no placebo-controlled phase III trials of its efficacy.
- Response rates of around 10–15% are seen, and complete responses are rare, with PFS in the order of 3–6 months [8].
- No survival benefit has been seen for combination therapy when compared with single-agent chemotherapy, although response rates are higher.

    Combination chemotherapy regimens, such as the Dartmouth regimen (DTIC/cisplatin/carmustine/tamoxifen), have shown increased response rates in phase III trials versus single-agent dacarbazine but have failed to show an OS benefit [9]. Toxicity is significantly increased, so these regimens are not commonly used.
    The addition of IFN and IL-2 to chemotherapy regimens has also shown an increase in response rate, but again toxicity is increased, without significant prolongation of survival [8].

Temozolomide

- Oral alkylating agent given at 150–200 mg/m^2 orally for 5 days every 4 weeks.
- Side effects include nausea and vomiting and bone marrow suppression.
- Similar efficacy to dacarbazine:
    o Median PFS in the largest trial, including 305 patients, was 7.7 months in the temozolamide arm versus 6.4 months in the DTIC arm ($p = 0.2$). Overall response rates were similar at 14% and 12%, respectively [10].
- CNS penetration: evidence from a number of small trials has demonstrated increased responses in the brain and reduced occurrences of brain metastases, following treatment [10]. It is used by some physicians to treat patients with CNS disease or those who prefer to use an oral regimen.

❝ Expert comment

Combination chemotherapy (e.g. CVD or carboplatin–paclitaxel) is still sometimes used in patients with significant symptoms from their disease and with melanoma that does not harbour a BRAF mutation. In these circumstances, the extra toxicity of therapy may be justified to increase the likelihood of palliation.

✪ Learning point Small molecule inhibitors in melanoma

Around 50% of melanomas have an activating mutation in BRAF. This is a serine–threonine protein kinase, downstream from RAS and upstream from the MAP kinase/ERK signalling pathway. Constitutive activation of mutant BRAF leads to increased cell proliferation and survival. Ninety per cent of the mutations are due to a single nucleotide substitution of glutamic acid for valine at codon 600 (V600E) [11].

✔ Evidence base BRIM-3 [12]: vemurafenib, compared to DTIC, in BRAF-mutant advanced melanoma

- Phase III open-label trial.
- Stages IIIc/IV melanoma with V600 mutation.
- A total of 675 patients.
- Vemurafenib 960 mg bd PO or DTIC 1000 mg/m^2 3-weekly IV.
- Primary endpoints were OS and PFS.
- Median OS: 13.2 months vemurafenib versus 9.6 months DTIC.
- Median PFS: 6.9 months vemurafenib versus 1.6 months DTIC.
- Overall response rates: 57% PR, 5.6% CR vemurafenib versus 8.6% PR, 1.2% CR DTIC.
- Patients in the DTIC arm were allowed to cross-over after initial interim analysis.

Source: data from PB Chapman et al., Improved survival with Vemurafenib in melanoma with V600E mutation, New England Journal of Medicine, Volume 364, Number 26, pp. 2507–16, Copyright © 2011 Massachusetts Medical Society. All rights reserved.

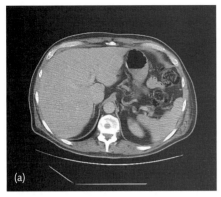 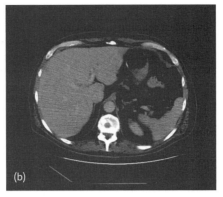

Figure 18.2 CT scan showing response of liver metastases to vemurafenib after 10 weeks of treatment. (A) Standard setting and (B) liver window.

Within the first 2 weeks of treatment, the patient noted her right upper quadrant pain had gone and several of the cutaneous nodules had regressed on the arm. She was seen by the acute oncology service, with widespread painful erythema over her face, forearms, and feet, following a day out. There was evidence of blistering on her lips and nose. She was given emollient creams and reminded to avoid sun exposure, wear strong sun protection factors (SPFs) when outside, due to photosensitivity. After 10 weeks on treatment, a nodular lesion with a necrotic centre developed on her right arm. She was referred to dermatology who removed the lesion which was found to be an SCC. A CT scan at 12 weeks confirmed a good partial response to treatment at all disease sites (Figure 18.2).

✛ Clinical tip Side effects of vemurafenib and dose modification for toxicity

These include arthralgia, rash, fatigue, alopecia, nausea, and diarrhoea. The drug can also cause significant photosensitivity and keratoacanthomas and SCCs of the skin.

Intolerable grade 2 or 3 toxicities require dose interruption until grades 0–1, and dose reduction from 960 mg bd to 720 mg bd. If they then recur, the dose can be further reduced to 480 mg bd. If grade 4 toxicity occurs, a dose reduction to 480 mg bd is recommended when toxicity has resolved to grades 0–1. The occurrence of an SCC does not necessitate discontinuation of treatment or dose reduction but requires referral to dermatology for removal.

Giving vemurafenib treatment breaks to help improve tolerability in those who find side effects debilitating is an option, although there is no trial evidence to support this.

✪ Learning point Skin cancers with BRAF inhibition [13]

Eighteen per cent of those treated with vemurafenib in BRIM-3, and 10% of those treated with dabrafenib in BREAK-3, developed keratoacanthomas and SCCs of the skin. The median time to presentation was 8 weeks from starting the drug. This recognized complication requires referral to dermatology for examination and removal of the lesions. Importantly, the drugs do not need to be stopped because of this. The exact mechanism for the development of the keratoacanthomas and SCCs is unknown but is thought to be due to the paradoxical activation of the MAP kinase/ERK pathway in cells with wild-type BRAF. The SCCs have shown high rates of mutant RAS activity which is not typically seen in sporadic SCCs. The promotion of CRAF dimerization leads to downstream signal activation and cell proliferation.

✓ **Evidence base** BREAK-3 Trial [14]: Dabrafenib, compared to DTIC, for BRAF-mutant advanced melanoma

- Dabrafenib is another oral BRAF inhibitor.
- BREAK-3 was a phase III trial which randomized patients to dabrafenib 150 mg bd or DTIC chemotherapy (n = 250).
- Median PFS was 5.1 months and 2.7 months, respectively (HR 0.3, 95% CI 0.18–0.51; p <0.0001) [14].
- Median OS reported at ASCO 2013 was 18.2 months in the dabrafenib group and 15.6 months in the DTIC group.
- Cross-over was allowed.
- Side effects were arthralgia, fatigue, headache, and fever; again, a proportion of patients developed keratoacanthomas and SCCs.

Source: data from *The Lancet*, Volume 380, Issue 9839, A Hauschild *et al.*, Dabrafenib in BRAF-mutated metastatic melanoma: a multicenter, open-label, phase 3 randomised controlled trial, pp. 358–65, Copyright © 2012 Elsevier Ltd All rights reserved.

After 8 months, the cutaneous metastases on her left arm began to increase in number, and she noted mild abdominal discomfort. A CT scan was requested which confirmed progression of the disease in the liver, retroperitoneal nodes, and lungs (Figure 18.3).

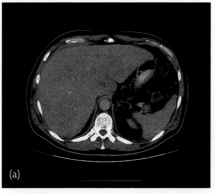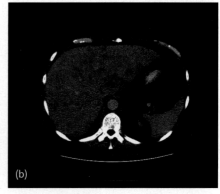

(a)   (b)

Figure 18.3 CT scan showing disease progression in the liver on (A) standard setting and (B) liver window.

✪ **Learning point** Resistance to BRAF inhibition

Although response rates are high with BRAF inhibitors, there are few complete responses, and those who initially respond eventually develop progressive disease at around 6–7 months.

A number of putative mechanisms of resistance have been put forward. These include upstream NRAS mutations or upregulation of cell surface receptor tyrosine kinases, leading to increased RAS activity, subsequent CRAF dimerization, and reactivation of the MAP kinase pathway. Mutations in MEK, downstream of BRAF, or increased activity of COT kinase, an activator of MEK1/2, have been suggested. Another potential factor is the activation of parallel pathways, independent of MAP kinase, such as the PI3K pathway, possibly due to an increased expression of PDGF and insulin-like growth factor (IGF) receptors on the cell surface [11].

✪ **Learning point** MEK inhibition

MEK inhibition in V600-mutant patients has also proved beneficial in phase III trials.

In METRIC, patients were randomized to trametinib 2 mg orally or chemotherapy with DTIC or paclitaxel. Median PFS was 4.8 months with trametinib versus 1.5 months with chemotherapy. The HR for disease progression or death was 0.45 (95% CI 0.33–0.63; p <0.001). At publication, median OS had not been reached, and response rates were 22% (95% CI 17–28) and 8% (95% CI 4–15) (p = 0.01). Side effects were rash, diarrhoea, and peripheral oedema; there were no secondary skin neoplasms [16].

✪ **Learning point** Combined MEK and BRAF inhibition

Combining inhibitors of the MAP kinase pathway may delay the onset of resistance and prevent secondary skin neoplasms.

A phase I/II trial of dabrafenib and trametinib [17] has been published:

- patients received dabrafenib (150 mg) and trametinib (1 or 2 mg), or dabrafenib alone
- response rates were high in the combination arm 76% versus 54% in the monotherapy arm (p = 0.03)
- median PFS was 9.4 months and 5.8 months, with HR for progressive disease or death 0.39 (95% CI 0.25–0.62; p <0.001)
- at 12 months, 41% of the combination arm, and 9% of the monotherapy arm, were alive without progression
- main side effects from the combination were fever (71%), fatigue, nausea and vomiting, and diarrhoea; grade 3 or 4 events were rare
- low-dose oral glucocorticoids were required for recurrent fever.

The COMBI-V study has been reported [18]:

- patients received dabrafenib (150 mg) and trametinib (2 mg) daily, or vemurafenib (960 mg bd) daily
- median PFS of 11.4 months versus 7.3 months, in favour of combination (HR 0.56; p <0.01)
- overall response rate of 64% versus 51% (p <0.01)
- fewer cutaneous malignancies were reported in the combination arm.

The COBRIM study [19]:

- a total of 495 BRAF-positive patients randomly assigned to receive vemurafenib/cobimetinib or vemurafenib/placebo
- the combination arm showed median PFS of 9.9 months, compared with 6.2 months (HR 0.51)
- non-significantly higher risk of adverse events in the combination arm, but fewer cutaneous malignancies.

⭐ **Learning point** Ipilimumab

- Monoclonal, fully human IgG targeted at the T-lymphocyte-associated antigen 4 (CTLA-4) receptor on T-cells.
- It is thought to work by blocking CTLA-4 binding and prevent the functional inactivation of the T-cell, hence upregulating the immune response against the tumour cells.

As she remained PS 1, she was offered treatment with Ipilimumab, an immunotherapeutic agent. Although response rates were not as good as with Vemurafenib, this was recommended, as durable disease control can be achieved for a proportion of patients. Treatment was administered every 3 weeks IV 3 mg/kg and was planned for four cycles.

⭐ **Learning point** IL-2 in melanoma

In 1998, the FDA approved IL-2 for the treatment of stages III/IV melanoma. This is a cytokine which regulates T-cell growth and proliferation and has anti-tumour activity in melanoma and renal cell cancer.

High-dose recombinant IL-2 is given by IV infusion 8-hourly over 5 days and repeated after 7 days. Repeated courses can be given. It must be given in hospital with intensive care support, as complications, such as capillary leak syndrome, sepsis, and hepatorenal toxicity, can necessitate vasopressor support.

A review of eight trials between 1985 and 1993, including 270 patients, demonstrated an overall response rate of 16% (95% CI 12–21%); 6% of these were complete responses. Median survival was 11.4 months, and six patients died due to sepsis on treatment [20].

The selection of fit patients is imperative. The continued use in the face of the risks of treatment is due to the potential for prolonged remissions and cures in a small percentage of patients. Ten of the 17 patients with complete response, and two of the 26 with partial responses, remained progression-free for over 2 years, and, after surgical removal of isolated sites of progression, 6% of the cohort remained alive at over 5 years post-treatment [20].

✅ **Evidence base** Ipilimumab in melanoma

Ipilimumab, with or without gp100 cancer vaccine, compared to vaccine alone [21]

- 676 HLA-A*0201-positive patients with unresectable stages III/IV melanoma.
- ≥1 previous treatment regime.
- Ipilimumab 3 mg/kg every 3 weeks for four cycles.
- Assigned 3:1:1 to (a) ipilimumab plus gp100 cancer vaccine, (b) ipilimumab alone, (c) gp100 alone.
- Median survival: (a) 10 months, (b) 10.1 months, (c) 6.4 months (HR for death 0.68; p <0.001); statistically significant survival benefit of 3.6 months.
- Disease control rate (SD + PR + CR) of 28% of patients.
- Overall response rates (CR and PR) on completion of therapy were in the region of 10%.
- 60% of patients suffered an immune-related adverse event (irAE); 10–15% of these were grades 3 and 4 [13]. The skin and GI tract were most frequently involved, with 30% of patients developing diarrhoea or colitis. Five of the seven deaths attributed to an irAE were due to colitis and bowel perforation.
- Like IL-2, a subset of patients obtained durable response after ipilimumab, and, at the time of publication, 2% of the ipilimumab-treated cohorts had ongoing objective responses at 2 years [21].

DTIC plus ipilimumab versus DTIC in previously untreated metastatic melanoma [22]

- Placebo-controlled RCT (n = 502).
- Ipilimumab plus dacarbazine, compared to dacarbazine plus placebo.
- If stable disease or objective response, without significant toxicity, patients randomized to ipilimumab or placebo maintenance every 12 weeks.
- OS benefit of 2.1 months for the chemoimmunotherapy combination.
- Grade 3 or 4 adverse events in 56.3% with chemoimmunotherapy, compared to 27.5% in the chemotherapy and placebo arm. These were most commonly deranged LFTs.

Source: data from FS Hodi *et al.*, Improved survival with Ipilimumab in Patients with Metastatic Melanoma, *New England Journal of Medicine*, Volume 363, Number 8, pp. 711–23; Copyright © 2010 Massachusetts Medical Society; and C Robert et al., Ipilimumab plus dacarbazine for previously untreated metastatic melanoma, *New England Journal of Medicine*, Volume 364, Number 26, pp. 2517–26, Copyright © 2011 Massachusetts Medical Society.

After the second cycle, she presented with diarrhoea, with bowels opening 4–6 times per day, despite anti-diarrhoeal medications. She was commenced on prednisolone 40 mg od, with an improvement in her symptoms over the next 48 hours. Over the next month, the steroid dose was successfully tapered off.

✪ Learning point (Acute Oncology) Management of immune-related adverse events (irAEs) [23]

Initial trials had several toxic deaths, and it became apparent that the removal of T-cell checkpoint blockade resulted in a variety of irAEs. These included autoimmune dermatitis, enterocolitis, hypophysitis, and hepatitis.

Recognition and early treatment of these phenomena has meant that treatment-related deaths are now rare. Patients may need multidisciplinary input from dermatology, gastroenterology, surgery, and endocrinology teams.

Skin

- 47–68% of patients develop rash on treatment.
- Typically seen within 2–3 weeks of starting ipilimumab.
- Diffuse maculopapular and often pruritic.
- Histology—perivascular lymphocytic infiltrate, extending from the dermis to the epidermis.
- Grade 1 or 2—topical steroids and oral antihistamines for the relief of itch.
- Grade 3—withhold ipilimumab, and start 1 mg/kg of oral prednisone, tapering off over 30 days.
- Discontinue if grade 4 toxicity; rarely, toxic epidermal necrolysis and Stevens–Johnson syndrome have been seen to occur which can be life-threatening.

GI tract

- Diarrhoea and colitis were seen in 30% of patients treated at 3 mg/kg in initial phase III trial.
- Typically 6–7 weeks into the treatment regime.
- Histology—neutrophilic, mixed neutrophilic/lymphocytic, or lymphocytic infiltrates in the bowel wall.
- Those with persistent diarrhoea or rectal bleeding should have sigmoidoscopy or colonoscopy.

NCI grade	Definition	Management
1	<4 stools/day above baseline	Loperamide, oral hydration
2	4–6 stools/day above baseline	Send stool for M, C & S, Clostridium difficile toxin. Start oral prednisone 40 mg, and taper over 30 days
3	≥7 stools/day above baseline, incontinence	Stop ipilimumab. Give IV methylprednisolone 125 mg, followed by oral prednisone 1–2 mg/kg daily, and taper according to symptoms. If no improvement in 48–72 hours, give infliximab 5 mg/kg IV. Low threshold for imaging to rule out perforation.
4	Life-threatening consequences	

Source: data from JS Weber *et al.*, Management of Immune-Related Adverse Events and Kinetics of Response with Ipilimumab, *Journal of Clinical Oncology*, Volume 30, Number 21, pp. 2691–97, Copyright © 2012 by the American Society of Clinical Oncology.

Hepatic

- Seen in 3–9% of patients who may have an asymptomatic rise in bilirubin and transaminases; it can be accompanied with fever and malaise in some cases.
- Typically seen 6–7 weeks into treatment.
- Histology—diffuse T-cell infiltrate.
- Grade 1—monitor.
- Grade 2—oral prednisone 40 mg daily, and wean over 30 days.

(continued)

- Grade 3 or 4—discontinue ipilimumab. High-dose IV glucocorticoids for 24–48 hours, then prednisolone 1–2 mg/kg; taper over 30 days.
- If no reduction in serum transaminases within 48 hours, then mycophenolate mofetil can be considered at 500 mg bd.

Endocrinopathy

- 1–6% of patients seen to develop hypophysitis.
- Other endocrine organs can be affected such as the thyroid, adrenals.
- Typically seen around 9 weeks into treatment.
- Symptoms include headache, weakness, and dizziness.
- Before starting ipilimumab, patients should have baseline morning cortisol, ACTH, free tri-iodothyronine (T3), free T4, TSH, testosterone in males, and FSH, LH, and prolactin in females.
- Symptomatic panhypopituitarism should be treated with 1–2 mg/kg of IV methylprednisolone, then prednisolone 1–2 mg/kg, tapering over 30 days. Endocrine referral will be required, as patients are likely to need lifelong hormone replacement.

A CT scan at the end of treatment showed minor progression in the liver lesions and stable disease elsewhere. This was repeated 6 weeks later and showed stable disease at all sites.

⊗ **Learning point** Response criteria

Immune-related response criteria (irRC) have been proposed as an alternative to the traditional imaging criteria used to delineate response (WHO/RECIST). Tumour burden is estimated from a combination of measurements taken from original index lesions pre-treatment and any new lesions which appear through the course of treatment. Unlike the WHO and RECIST criteria, the appearance of new lesions does not automatically mean progression. Disease progression is only assumed, if the total tumour burden is increased by 25%, and confirmed on the next assessment at least 1 month later [22]. The criteria therefore take into account the cohort of patients who can be seen to progress, then stabilize or regress several months post-treatment.

irRC [24]

SPD is the sum of the products of the two largest perpendicular diameters of the index lesions.

$$\text{Tumour burden} = \text{SPD}_{\text{index lesions}} + \text{SPD}_{\text{new, measurable disease}}$$

Immune-related complete response	irCR	Disappearance of all measurable and non-measurable lesions, confirmed by interim imaging >4 weeks later
Immune-related partial response	irPR	≥50% reduction in tumour burden from baseline assessment, confirmed on interim imaging >4 weeks later
Immune-related stable disease	irSD	<50% reduction, but <25% increase, in tumour burden from baseline
Immune-related progressive disease	irPD	≥25% increase in tumour burden from baseline measurement, confirmed on interim imaging >4 weeks later

Source: data from JD Wolchok *et al.* Guidelines for the Evaluation of Immune Therapy Activity in Solid Tumours: Immune-related Response Criteria, *Clinical Cancer Research*, Volume 15, Issue, pp. 7412–7420, Copyright © 2009 American Association for Cancer Research.

She remained on follow-up with her oncologist, 4 months after completion of ipilimumab.

Discussion

Until very recently, treatment options for metastatic melanoma were limited. Locoregional relapse, in the first few years after surgery (60% within 3 years), is the commonest presentation; however, patients can present later, and the time course is not always predictable.

Incidence increases with age, although a substantial proportion (27%) are now diagnosed in those under 50 years of age, as in this case. Higher sun exposure during her childhood in Australia, where rates are as high as 37 per 100 000 people, increased her risk. Prior sunbed use is also thought to be a causative factor. In the UK, malignant melanoma is the fifth commonest malignancy, with approximately 20 cases per 100 000 people [25].

Key questions in melanoma, particularly in patients with V600 mutations, relate to the sequencing of treatments. Small molecule inhibitors have much higher response rates, but most patients will ultimately develop resistance. Ipilimumab does not offer such rapid responses, and, in some cases, patients can progress and later respond many months later, and, for some, it can offer prolonged disease stabilization. Early-phase trials of combined vemurafenib and ipilimumab had to be abandoned, due to grade 3 liver toxicity in seven of the first 12 patients administered the drugs concomitantly [26]. Trials are now looking at sequential treatment strategies.

In the field of immunotherapy, anti-PD-1 antibodies are showing promising results in early-phase trials, and phase III trials are recruiting. The PD-1 receptor is present on T-cells. Its ligand PD-L1 is expressed both on cancer cells and tumour-infiltrating macrophages; another ligand PD-L2 is expressed on antigen-presenting cells. Binding of the PD-1 receptor to its ligand is seen to downregulate tumour-specific T-cells and contribute to immune evasion by tumour cells [27]. Anti-PD1 is thought to exert its effect by blocking the receptor and preventing ligand binding, allowing the activation of the immune response.

> ✪ **Learning point** PD-1 inhibition
>
> A number of mAbs targeting PD-1 are currently in trial. Safety and efficacy data for Nivolumab (BMS-936558) from the initial phase I trial and its expansion cohorts demonstrated impressive response rates (31%) and OS (16.8 months; 95% CI 12.5–NR) in the 107 patients with advanced melanoma [27]. Patients received 0.1–10 mg/kg 2-weekly for up to 12 cycles/48 infusions. Side effects included fatigue, rash, diarrhoea, pruritus, and nausea. Grade 3 or 4 toxicities were rare, although three patients (none in the melanoma group) died from pneumonitis, leading to increased monitoring and new management guidelines. Like Ipilimumab, a spectrum of irAEs are seen. Nivolumab is currently featured in a number of ongoing phase III trials, including a phase III trial of combination checkpoint blockade with Ipilimumab after evidence of high ORR and tolerability in early phase trials [28]. Nivolumab has demonstrated superiority over chemotherapy in patients pre-treated with Ipilimumab in a phase III trial, with overall response rates of 32%, compared with 11% with chemotherapy alone [29]. Recently published results from trials featuring another anti-PD1 antibody Lambrolizumab (MK-3475) have shown median PFS of over 7 months in a study population of 135 patients. Prior therapy with Ipilimumab was allowed and has not been seen to affect response in this cohort. Patients were dosed at 2 mg/kg or 10 mg/kg, with RECIST response rates of 38% (95% CI 25–44) and 52% (95% CI 38–66), respectively, at 12 weeks [30].

Advances in immune therapy and small molecule inhibitors have changed the disease course of advanced melanoma, and several other new agents are demonstrating promise. The best adjuvant therapy for those at high risk of relapse remains in question, but trials using the array of new therapeutic options will hopefully give answers over the next few years. Public health campaigns and raised awareness of the risk factors for melanoma remain important, as prevention and early pick-up of melanomatous skin lesions are key to reducing the rising incidence of what still remains for many a life-shortening disease.

A final word from the expert

The initial surgical management of melanoma has been established over many years, although controversy remains over margins of excision, sentinel lymph node biopsy, and follow-up protocols. However, there have been seismic changes in the systemic therapy for advanced melanoma, with the recent licensing of Vemurafenib and Ipilimumab. These drugs are now being tested in adjuvant trials. For patients with advanced disease, even newer therapies and combinations designed to modulate resistance are showing early promise. Entry into clinical trials continues to remain the gold standard for patients with advanced melanoma.

References

1. Marsden JR, Newton-Bishop JA, Burrows L et al. Revised U.K. guidelines for the management of cutaneous melanoma 2010. *British Journal of Dermatology* 2010; **163**(2): 238–56.
2. MacKie RM, Hauschild A, Eggermont AM. Epidemiology of invasive cutaneous melanoma. *Annals of Oncology* 2009; **20**(Suppl 6): vi1–7.
3. Balch CM, Gershenwald JE, Soong SJ et al. Final version of 2009 AJCC melanoma staging and classification. *Journal of Clinical Oncology* 2009; **27**(36): 6199–206.
4. Morton DL, Thompson JF, Cochran AJ et al. Sentinel-node biopsy or nodal observation in melanoma. *The New England Journal of Medicine* 2006; **335**(13): 1307–17.
5. Mocellin S, Pasquali S, Rossi CR, Nitti D. Interferon alpha adjuvant therapy in patients with high-risk melanoma: a systematic review and meta-analysis. *Journal of National of Cancer Institute* 2010; **102**(7): 493–501.
6. Wheatley K, Ives N, Eggermont A et al. on behalf of the International Malignant Melanoma Collaborative Group. Interferon-α as adjuvant therapy for melanoma: an individual patient data meta-analysis of randomised trials. *Journal of Clinical Oncology* 2007; **25**(18 Suppl): 8526.
7. Burmeister BH, Henderson MA, Ainslie J et al. Adjuvant radiotherapy versus observation alone for patients at risk of lymph-node field relapse after therapeutic lymphadenectomy for melanoma: a randomized trial. *The Lancet Oncology* 2012; **13**(6): 589–97.
8. LJ Jason, GK Schwartz. Chemotherapy in the management of advanced cutaneous malignant melanoma. *Clinics in Dermatology* 2013; **31**: 290–7.
9. Lui P, Cashin R, Machado M, Hemels M, Corey-Lisle PK, Einarson TR. Treatments for metastatic melanoma: synthesis of evidence from randomized trials. *Cancer Treatment Reviews* 2007: **33**(8): 665–80.
10. Quirt I, Verma S, Petrella T, Bak K, Charette M. Temozolamide for the treatment of metastatic melanoma: a systematic review. *The Oncologist* 2007; **12**(9): 1114–23.
11. Ascierto PA, Kirkwood JM, Grob JJ et al. The role of BRAF V600 mutation in melanoma. *Journal of Translational Medicine* 2012; **10**: 85.
12. Chapman PB, Hauschild A, Robert C et al. Improved survival with Vemurafenib in melanoma with V600E mutation. *The New England Journal of Medicine* 2011; **364**(26): 2507–16.
13. Anforth R, Fernandez-Penas P, Long GV. Cutaneous toxicities of RAF inhibitors. *The Lancet Oncology* 2013; **14**(1): e11–18.

14. Hauschild A, Grob JJ, Demidov LV *et al.* Dabrafenib in BRAF-mutated metastatic melanoma: a multicenter, open-label, phase 3 randomised controlled trial. *The Lancet* 2012; **380**(9839): 358–65.

15. Aplin AE, Kaplan FM, Shao Y. Mechanisms of resistance to RAF inhibitors in melanoma. *Journal of Investigative Dermatology* 2011; **131**(9): 1817–20.

16. Flaherty KT, Robert C, Hersey P *et al.* Improved survival with MEK inhibition in BRAF-mutated melanoma. *The New England Journal of Medicine* 2012; **367**(2): 107–14.

17. Flaherty KT, Infante JR, Daud A *et al.* Combined BRAF and MEK inhibition in melanoma with BRAF V600 mutations. *The New England Journal of Medicine* 2012; **367**(18): 1694–703.

18. Robert C, Karaszewska B, Schachter J *et al.* COMBI-V: A randomised, open-label, phase III study comparing the combination of dabrafenib (D) and trametinib (T) with vemurafenib (V) as first-line therapy in patients with unresectable or metastatic BRAF V600E/K mutation-positive cutaneous melanoma. *Annals of Oncology* 2014; **25**(5): 1–41.

19. Larkin J, Ascierto PA, Dréno B *et al.* Combined vemurafenib and cobimetanib in BRAF-mutated melanoma. *The New England Journal of Medicine* 2014; Sep 29. Epub ahead of print.

20. Atkins MB, Lotze MT, Dutcher JP *et al.* High-dose recombinant interleukin 2 therapy for patients with metastatic melanoma: analysis of 270 patients treated between 1985 and 1993. *Journal of Clinical Oncology* 1999; **17**(7): 2105–16.

21. Hodi FS, O'Day SJ, McDermott DF *et al.* Improved survival with ipilimumab in patients with metastatic melanoma. *The New England Journal of Medicine* 2010; **363**(8): 711–23.

22. Robert C, Thomas L, Bondarenko I *et al.* Ipilimumab plus dacarbazine for previously untreated metastatic melanoma. *The New England Journal of Medicine* 2011; **364**(26): 2517–26.

23. Weber JS, Kahler KC, Hauschild A. Management of immune-related adverse events and kinetics of response with ipilimumab. *Journal of Clinical Oncology* 2012; **30**(21): 2691–7.

24. Wolchok JD, Hoos A, O'Day S, Weber JS *et al.* Guidelines for the evaluation of immune therapy activity in solid tumours: immune-related response criteria. *Clinical Cancer Research* 2009; **15**(23): 7412–20.

25. Cancer Research UK. *Skin cancer incidence statistics.* Available at: < http:// www.cancerresearchuk.org/cancer-info/cancerstats/types/skin/incidence/ uk-skin-cancer-incidence-statistics#source12 >.

26. Ribas A, Hodi FS, Callahan M, Konto C, Wolchok J. Hepatotoxicity with combination of vemurafenib and ipilimumab. *The New England Journal of Medicine* 2013; **368**(14): 1365–6.

27. Topalian SL, Sznol M, Brahmer JR *et al.* Nivolumab (anti-PD-1; BMS-936558; ONO-4538) in patients with advanced solid tumors: Survival and long-term safety in a phase I trial. *Journal of Clinical Oncology* 2013; **31**(Suppl); abstr 3002^.

28. Wolchok JD, Kluger H, Callahan MK *et al.* Nivolumab plus ipilimumab in advanced melanoma. *The New England Journal of Medicine* 2013; **369**(2): 122–33.

29. Weber JS, Minor DR, D'Angelo SP *et al.* A phase 3 randomised open-label study of nivolumab (anti-PD1, BMS-936558, ONO-4538) versus investigator's choice chemotherapy in patients with advanced melanoma after prior anti-CTLA-4 therapy. *Annals of Oncology* 2014; **25**(Suppl 4): doi: 10.1093/annonc/mdu438.34.

30. Hamid O, Robert C, Daud A *et al.* Safety and tumor responses with lambrolizumab (anti-PD-1) in melanoma. *The New England Journal of Medicine* 2013; **369**(2): 134–44.

19 Laryngeal cancer and oral mucositis

Gemma Eminowicz

Expert commentary Amen Sibtain

Case history

A 58-year-old man presented to his GP with a 3-week history of cough and hoarseness. His past medical history included reflux, for which he took lansoprazole and Gaviscon®. He was a divorced architect and a smoker with a 38-pack-year history. He had a moderate alcohol intake of 10 units per week. His PS was 1. On examination, he had hoarseness and no evidence of cervical lymphadenopathy or distant metastases. His symptoms were attributed to an infection, and the patient was asked to return in 2 weeks, if there had not been any improvement.

Five weeks later, the patient re-presented with persistent hoarseness and was urgently referred to the ear, nose, and throat (ENT) surgeons.

✪ Learning point Presentation of head and neck cancers

Head and neck cancers comprise a range of neoplasms arising from any of the lining membranes of the upper aerodigestive tract. The head and neck region is divided into six major sites:

- nasal cavity and paranasal sinuses
- oral cavity
- nasopharynx
- oropharynx
- hypopharynx
- larynx.

Each major site can be further subdivided, and the presentation differs widely, according to the site and subsite involved and the size of the primary tumour. Head and neck tumours can be difficult to diagnose, as the initial presenting symptoms are often non-specific and insidious. It is not uncommon for patients to present late.

The head and neck cancer urgent referral guidelines for England are:

- hoarseness persisting for >6 weeks
- ulceration of the oral mucosa persisting for >3 weeks
- oral swellings persisting for >3 weeks
- all red or red and white patches of the oral mucosa
- dysphagia persisting for >3 weeks
- unilateral nasal obstruction, particularly when associated with purulent discharge
- unexplained tooth mobility not associated with periodontal disease
- unresolving neck masses for >3 weeks
- cranial neuropathies
- orbital masses
- the level of suspicion is increased if the patient is a heavy smoker or an alcohol drinker and is aged >45 and male. Other forms of tobacco use and/or betel use should raise suspicion.

(Continued)

Another risk factor is hardwood dust which increases the risk of adenocarcinoma of the nose and paranasal sinuses.

EBV causes some types of nasopharyngeal carcinoma.

Human papillomavirus (HPV) 16 is a causative agent in oropharyngeal and oral SCC, but doubt remains regarding other sites and HPV subtypes.

Rarely, patients present with symptoms of metastatic disease, including shortness of breath, haemoptysis, and bone pain.

✚ Clinical tip Subsites of the larynx and differing presenting symptoms

Subsite	Contents	Presentation
Supraglottis	Suprahyoid epiglottis, subhyoid epiglottis, false cords, aryepiglottic folds, arytenoids	Dysphonia 'Hot potato' voice Sore throat Referred ear pain Neck nodes
Glottis	True vocal cords, anterior and posterior commissures	Hoarse voice Sore throat—late sign Neck nodes—late sign
Subglottis	10 mm below the free edge of vocal cords to the inferior edge of the cricoid cartilage	Hoarse voice Dyspnoea Stridor

---

Nasendoscopy revealed an ulcerating lesion of the left vocal cord with impaired vocal cord mobility. All blood tests were normal. Staging CT scan of the head, neck, and chest confirmed a primary lesion on the left vocal cord with invasion of the paraglottic space, without involvement of the thyroid cartilage (Figure 19.1). No lymph nodes or distant metastases were seen. Subsequent panendoscopy did not reveal any additional abnormalities, and the biopsy confirmed squamous cell carcinoma (SCC).

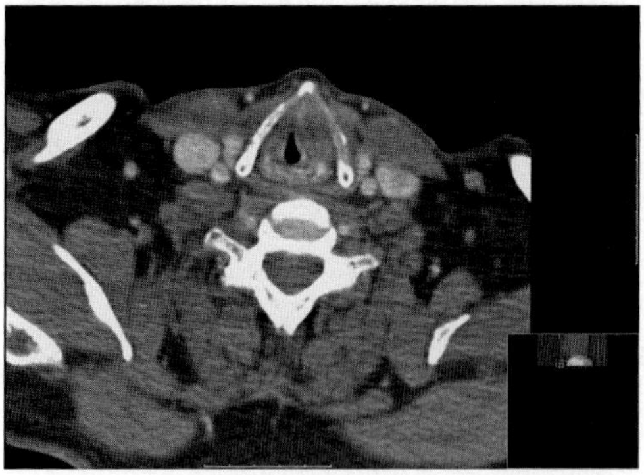

Figure 19.1 An axial contrast-enhanced CT slice through the level of the thyroid cartilage, demonstrating asymmetry and enlargement of the left vocal cord. The cartilage is intact, and nasendoscopy confirmed the cord was immobile.

> **⭐ Learning point**
> **Epidemiology of laryngeal cancer**
>
> Laryngeal cancer is the commonest of the head and neck tumours, although its incidence is only 4 per 100 000 in the UK. It typically occurs in the fifth and sixth decades and has a male:female ratio of 5:1.
>
> Ninety-five per cent of malignant laryngeal tumours are SCCs. The other 5% comprise spindle cell tumours, neuroendocrine tumours, minor salivary gland tumours, lymphoma, plasmacytoma, mucosal melanoma, and metastases.

After discussion at the head and neck MDT meeting, his final stage was confirmed as a glottic T3N0M0 due to paraglottic invasion (AJCC TNM, 7th edition 2010). Radical chemoradiotherapy (CRT) was the most suitable treatment option, due to functional preservation, but total laryngectomy was discussed as a potential alternative.

> ✪ **Learning point** Surgical options for laryngeal cancer
>
> | Procedure | Indications | Removes | Contraindications/notes |
> |-----------|-------------|---------|--------------------------|
> | Stripping/CO_2 laser | Tis | Mucosa of cord | No definitive pathology. Affects voice quality |
> | Cordectomy | T1a of middle third of one cord | Transoral excision of part of cord | Effect on voice quality |
> | Vertical partial (hemi-) aryngectomy | Voice preservation for T1 and T2 glottic lesions | Bisects larynx, removes half of thyroid cartilage, up to one vocal cord, and up to 5 mm of contralateral vocal cord | Contraindicated if vocal cord fixation |
> | Supraglottic partial laryngectomy | Voice preservation for T1/T2 supraglottic lesions | Removes epiglottis, false cords, aryepiglottic folds, upper portion of thyroid cartilage, ± hyoid bone | Contraindicated if exolaryngeal spread, vocal cord fixation, involvement of arytenoids |
> | Total laryngectomy | Extensive disease, transglottic or extensive subglottic extension, cartilage erosion, extralaryngeal extension | Removes hyoid bone, thyroid and cricoid cartilage, epiglottis, strap muscles. Patient left with permanent tracheostoma and pharynx reconstruction | Speech rehabilitation options include oesophageal speech, tracheoesophageal speech, and electrolarynges |
>
> Perioperative complications of surgery include bleeding, airway obstruction, infection, and wound complications. Post-operative complications include webs, stenosis, fistulae, aspiration, and chondritis.
> Reproduced from Hansen E, Roach M (Ed), *Handbook of Evidence-Based Radiation Oncology*, Second Edition, Springer Science+Business Media, New York, Copyright © 2010, with permission from Springer Science+Business Media.

The patient was consented for radical CRT, having been counselled to the practicalities, and short- and long-term side effects. An EDTA renal clearance test confirmed adequate glomerular filtration for high-dose cisplatin chemotherapy. His swallow was safe and his nutritional status adequate. He did not require elective placement of a feeding tube. Elective extraction of several teeth was arranged before radiotherapy, and he was referred to the dental hygienist.

> ✪ **Learning point** Chemoradiotherapy (CRT) preparation
>
> **Pre-CRT assessment**
>
> - Dental assessment with orthopantomogram (OPG).
> - Nutritional assessment by dietician.
> - Speech and language therapy (SALT) assessment of speech and swallow (insertion of NG tube/PEG or RIG if extensive weight loss before diagnosis).
> - Advise patient to stop smoking and to reduce alcohol intake.
> - Assessment of kidney function and hearing function.
>
> **Consent/side effects**
>
> - Acute: increasing hoarseness, odynophagia, dysphagia, skin erythema and localized hair loss, pain, fatigue, weight loss, thickened secretions, xerostomia, neutropenia, renal toxicity, ototoxicity.
> - Chronic: skin changes, dysphagia, hypothyroidism, second malignancy, xerostomia (reversible with IMRT), dental caries.
>
> (Continued)

⊕ **Clinical tip** Stop smoking

Smoking is an independent risk factor for head and neck SCC (HNSCC). For smokers, the risk of developing laryngeal cancer decreases after the cessation of smoking but remains elevated 11 years later, compared to that of non-smokers [1].

Smoking during radiotherapy appears to have an adverse effect on local control (HR 1.5) and survival (HR 1.7) [2]. Patients should therefore be counselled to stop smoking, prior to commencing radiotherapy.

Set-up/immobilization

- Supine.
- Straight spine, unless IMRT.
- Nine-point thermoplastic shell fixed, leg rest.
- Bolus considered for anterior commissure tumours or over a tracheostoma.

Localization

- CT planning scan from vertex to carina.

❝ **Expert comment**

There is no doubt that smoking during radiotherapy exacerbates the severity and chronicity of both acute and late side effects. This includes late soft tissue fibrosis and osteoradionecrosis, the treatment of the latter made, in turn, more challenging if smoking continues. Smokers also have a lower physiological reserve, and a direct discussion of the clear benefits of smoking cessation with the patient should improve compliance, especially when it leads to the patient starting a formal cessation programme.

Smoking reduces the oxygen-carrying capacity of blood via the generation of carboxyhaemoglobin, potentially exacerbating tumour hypoxia and thus radioresistance.

The radiotherapy was planned, using an IMRT technique. He received a total dose of 70 Gy in 35 fractions to planning target volume (PTV) 1 comprising the whole larynx. A dose of 56 Gy in 35 fractions was delivered to PTV2 comprising bilateral elective neck nodes, levels II, III, IV, and V. The radiotherapy was delivered with concurrent cisplatin 100 mg/m^2 on days 1, 22, and 43 of radiotherapy.

❝ **Expert comment**

Dose levels can be defined for treating gross disease, the surgical tissue bed, and the microscopic disease; 70 Gy is a standard dose that has become established worldwide, although there is no randomized evidence supporting it. It seems to be a dose level that produces manageable toxicity, although newer technologies have improved the therapeutic ratio and may allow dose escalation. 44 to 50 Gy in 2 Gy fractions to microscopic disease is a standard dose, and the 56 Gy in 35 fractions used here is the biologically equivalent dose for 1.6 Gy per fraction, based on the linear quadratic formula. Fowler has published an excellent analysis and discussion of the doses and overall time used in head and neck cancer [3,4].

The treatment volumes and dose levels are becoming more harmonized, due to protocol development in national and international studies. Dose levels can be manipulated with IMRT more easily. In this case, many would deliver a higher dose to the levels IIb and III nodes, given the perceived higher risk of microscopic disease at these sites for a T3N0M0 laryngeal tumour.

During the course of treatment, the patient was reviewed weekly by the clinical oncologists, SALT, dietician, specialist nurse, and dental hygienist. In the third week of CRT, he developed odynophagia and was started on regular soluble paracetamol, with codeine as breakthrough, to good effect.

In week 5, he was unable to swallow solids and had moderate to severe pain swallowing liquids. He had lost 5 kg in 2 weeks, was tachycardic, with a postural BP drop of 20 mmHg. There was grade 2 radiation dermatitis , grade 1 mucositis of the oropharynx, and thrush. On swallow assessment, he coughed on sipping water. Blood tests revealed urea of 40 and creatinine of 250, Hb of 9, and normal WCC. The patient was admitted and made 'nil by mouth', pending SALT review. He was treated with IV rehydration, fluconazole 100 mg IV od, paracetamol 1 g IV four times daily (qds), and 5 mg of morphine s/c every 4 hours and as required (PRN). Two units of blood were transfused. Diprobase® was applied to his skin tds, and saline mouthwash PRN. After 24 hours, his creatinine had reduced to 150, and his pain was better controlled.

✪ Learning point Blood transfusion during radiotherapy

A proportion of head and neck cancers have areas of hypoxia which predict for adverse prognosis. Low Hb concentration can be used as a surrogate marker of low tumour oxygenation, and further studies have supported this hypothesis by demonstrating reduced OS for HNSCC patients with Hb concentrations of <12.5 g/dL during treatment. A number of studies have shown lower locoregional control rates associated with low pretreatment Hb concentrations in patients with HNSCC. A number of centres therefore maintain Hb above 11.5 g/dL during head and neck chemoradiation, using blood transfusions. However, blood transfusion may be detrimental in patients receiving radical radiotherapy, and hypotheses for this are:

1. Blood products contain growth factors, e.g. VEGF, that influence the biology of HNSCC.
2. Blood products contain an excess of IL-10 and apoptotic cells, causing the activation of the inflammatory cascade, resulting in immune suppression.

🛈 Expert comment

This learning point discusses the association between a low initial Hb and compromised outcome. A literature review by Hoff concluded correction of anaemia does not improve outcome. This was true whether the Hb level was increased by transfusion or erythropoietin stimulation [5]. Practically, it is probably correct to transfuse anaemic patients pretreatment, if they are symptomatic, but not with the aim of improving therapeutic outcome.

✪ Learning point (Acute Oncology) Managing oral mucositis

Oral mucositis is defined as an inflammation of the mucosal membrane. In a systematic review [6], 80% of patients treated for head and neck cancer experienced some degree of mucositis. Grades 3 and 4 mucositis (assessed by the common toxicity criteria, version 4) was observed in 57% of patients receiving altered fractionation radiotherapy, 43% of patients receiving CRT, and 34% of those treated with radiotherapy alone.

The sequence of biological events is initiated by the production of reactive oxygen species, causing DNA strand breaks. These cause clonogenic death of basal stem cells and also trigger transduction pathways, resulting in the activation of several transcription factors and pro-inflammatory cytokines (Table 19.1) [7].

Table 19.1 Management of oral mucositis [8]

WHO grade	Description	Treatment
1	Erythema, unpleasant sensation (pain)	Ensure good oral hygiene and increase the frequency of saline rinses Monitor nutritional status
2	Erythema, ulcers, pain, can eat solids	Consider paracetamol mouthwash (2 × 500 mg tablets dissolved in water) qds Consider benzydamine 0.15% mouthwash (Difflam®) Monitor for oral infection; swab and treat, as required Consider Caphosol® Consider saliva replacement Consider mucosal protectants, e.g. Episil®, Gelclair®, or MuGard®
3	Ulcers, significant pain, only liquid diet possible	Consider opioid analgesics (severe oral mucositis may require a syringe driver)
4	Ulcers, intolerable pain, enteral or parenteral feeding necessary, cannot talk	Consider IV and/or enteral hydration and feeding Consider Caphosol® Consider mucosal protectants, e.g. Episil®, Gelclair®, or MuGard® Consider tranexamic acid to treat localized bleeding Take swabs to identify the nature of bacterial, fungal, and/or viral infections, and treat appropriately

Reproduced from *Oral Oncology*, Volume 45, Issue 12, Sonis ST, Mucositis; The impact, biology and therapeutic opportunities of oral mucositis, pp. 1015–20, Copyright © 2009 Elsevier Ltd, with permission from Elsevier, <http://www.sciencedirect.com/science/journal/13688375>.

SALT assessment revealed a safe swallow to thickened consistencies only. As he was unable to meet his nutritional requirements, a NG tube was inserted and NG feeding commenced. A further 2 units of blood transfusion was arranged to raise his Hb above 12. His renal function normalized, his NG feed increased, and analgesia converted to NG preparations and titrated. The patient was trained to use his NG tube and to administer his feeds and was discharged during his sixth week of radiotherapy. He completed the full course of treatment.

⊗ **Learning point** Principles of nutrition: management and supportive care

Patients with head and neck cancer are at risk of malnutrition as a result of the site of their cancer, the disease process, and the treatment. At diagnosis, 50–75% of patients already have malnutrition, and 80% will lose a significant amount of weight during treatment. Malnutrition itself can lead to problems such as increased risk of infection, delayed wound healing, increased mortality, and depression.

Oral supplementation ranges from food fortification to nutritionally complete liquid supplements. NICE guidelines on enteral feeding recommend gastrostomy placement, if enteral feeding is expected to last >4 weeks [9]. Whilst there are no UK selection criteria for gastrostomy placement in head and neck patients, the NCCN head and neck guidelines [10] recommend prophylactic feeding tubes in:

- patients with severe weight loss prior to treatment, 5% over prior 1 month, or 10% over 6 months
- patients with ongoing dehydration or dysphagia, anorexia, or pain interfering with the ability to eat or drink
- patients with significant co-morbidities that could be aggravated by poor tolerance of dehydration, lack of calorific intake, missing medication
- patients with severe aspiration or mild aspiration in those with compromised cardiopulmonary function
- patients for whom long-term swallowing disorders are likely, e.g. large fields of high-dose radiotherapy to the mucosa and adjacent connective tissue.

After his radiotherapy, his swallow recovered over the following 4 weeks, and the NG tube was removed when he was able to meet his nutritional requirements orally.

He was regularly reviewed in the joint head and neck clinic by the clinical oncologists and ENT surgeons. He was seen monthly for the first year, 2-monthly for the second year, and 3- to 6-monthly thereafter to 5 years. At each visit, he was assessed by clinical examination and flexible nasendoscopy.

Discussion

The outcomes of laryngeal cancer have improved over the last two decades. Developments in radiotherapy technique, transoral surgery, and multimodality treatment approaches offer improved clinical, functional, and QoL outcomes. The aim of treatment is to cure the disease, whilst retaining function, but how this is best achieved for an individual patient can often pose a challenge.

> ✪ **Learning point** Early (T1–T2aN0) glottic cancer
>
> Treatment options for early glottic cancer are endolaryngeal surgery (transorally, with or without laser), definitive radiotherapy, or open partial laryngectomy. For T1a glottic tumours, the 5-year local control (LC) is similar for radiotherapy and transoral laser, ranging from 90% to 93%. For T1b tumours, the LC is 85–89%. LC and OS rates for T2a glottic cancers are comparable when treated with laser, radiotherapy, or partial laryngectomy [11]. There is continuing debate regarding which of these modalities is the superior treatment. A Cochrane review, published in 2002 and updated in 2010, found insufficient evidence to advocate a particular treatment modality, with only one large-scale RCT comparing open surgery and radiotherapy [12]. A meta-analysis by Higgins *et al.* found no statistically significant difference in LC between endolaryngeal surgery, compared with radiotherapy (OR 0.66; 95% CI 0.41–1.05), nor was there a statistically significant difference in laryngectomy-free survival between these two modalities (OR 0.73; 95% CI 0.39–1.35) [13].
>
> A number of centres have published case series of patients treated with endolaryngeal resection. Voice quality, following transoral laser, is affected by the degree of cord resected and by resection of the anterior commissure. Whilst voice outcomes are equally good, following either radiotherapy or laser, for smaller tumours, the long-term voice quality for T2 glottic tumours is accepted to be better after radiotherapy [11]. A further benefit of endolaryngeal surgery is that salvage options include further endoscopic resection, open surgery, or radiotherapy.
>
> In the UK, radiotherapy remains the standard of care for *de novo* early disease. Hypofractionated radiotherapy schedules, using a fraction size >2 Gy, result in equivalent outcomes without increased toxicity. Typical dose schedules vary with the field size and include 50–52 Gy in 16 fractions and 53–55 Gy in 20 fractions over 4 weeks.
>
> Open partial laryngectomy procedures are not commonly used in the UK for the treatment of early *de novo* glottic cancer. However, they are an option for disease inaccessible by endolaryngeal techniques or for radiorecurrent disease.
>
> Individual treatment choice is thus dependent on patient factors, tumour factors, and local expertise available. Other practical considerations include fitness to tolerate general anaesthetic and patient cooperation for daily treatments for radiotherapy.

> ✪ **Learning point** Early (T1–T2N0) supraglottic cancers
>
> The supraglottis has a dense lymphatic supply, and these tumours are associated with a high incidence of occult positive nodes in levels II and III. Elective treatment of bilateral nodal levels II and III, either by surgery or radiotherapy, is therefore recommended.
>
> The treatment options for the primary disease are radiotherapy, endolaryngeal surgery, or open partial laryngectomy. If complete resection can be achieved, the oncologic results of transoral laser surgery appear to be comparable to those of open supraglottic laryngectomy. Ambrosch *et al.* reported 5-year LC rates of 100% for pT1, and 89% for pT2, for patients treated with transoral laser [14]. In addition, the functional results of endolaryngeal surgery are superior to those of open surgery, in terms of feeding tube duration, tracheostomy duration, videofluoroscopy outcomes, and length of hospital stay [15].
>
> Mendenhall *et al.* reported LC in 100% of 13 patients with T1, and 81% of 42 patients with T2 supraglottic cancer, following treatment with radiotherapy alone [16]. Treatment is delivered, using either a 2-phase technique or IMRT, taking the primary disease to 66–70 Gy in 33–35 fractions and electively treating levels Ib, II, and III bilaterally to 44–50 Gy.

✪ **Learning point** T2b–T3 glottic tumours

The majority of patients with T2b–T3 glottic cancer are suitable for radiation-based larynx-preserving therapy. The optimal timing of chemotherapy, radiotherapy, and surgery remains an area of debate.

Elective treatment is recommended to lymph node levels II, III, and IV bilaterally, due to the risk of occult nodal disease. In node-positive disease, it is recommended that lymph node levels II–V are also treated on the involved side. The potential of radiotherapy and chemotherapy for larynx preservation was established by the 1991 VA larynx trial. Following publication, induction chemotherapy with cisplatin/5-FU, followed by radiotherapy, became the standard alternative to total laryngectomy for patients with locally advanced laryngeal cancer. The subsequent RTOG 91-11 study demonstrated that concurrent CRT (CCRT) was superior to induction chemotherapy and radiotherapy, and radiotherapy alone, in terms of larynx preservation rates, and has since become the standard of care for advanced laryngeal cancer. The results are supported by phase III randomized trials and a meta-analysis [17]. Standard concurrent chemotherapy regimes include cisplatin (100 mg/m^2) on days 1, 22, and 43 of radiotherapy, or lower-dose cisplatin (40 mg/m^2) weekly for 5 weeks. CRT is significantly more toxic than radiotherapy alone, and the additional benefit of chemotherapy must be balanced against risk. Of note, the benefit of chemotherapy decreases with age and is non-significant for those above 70.

✪ **Learning point** Induction chemotherapy in HNSCC

The role of induction chemotherapy remains uncertain. Whilst the MACH-NC meta-analysis did not find an OS benefit from induction chemotherapy, a significant improvement in the rate of distant metastases was seen. Several trials have reported improved outcomes with the more potent induction regime of a taxane, cisplatin, and 5-FU (TPF). A meta-analysis by Blanchard *et al.* [18] confirms that TPF is more efficacious than induction cisplatin/5-FU for OS, PFS, locoregional failure, and distant failure. Questions regarding the tolerability of the regimen remain, as only 50% of patients commencing the three-drug regime completed CRT as planned. The meta-analysis was not able to answer the question as to the benefit of sequential therapy over standard CCRT.

❝ **Expert comment**

Induction chemotherapy may have the advantages of starting treatment more quickly, a potential reduction in tumour bulk with consequent lower tumour hypoxia, and stabilization of the patient outline in large-volume disease. The potential disadvantages are the increased overall treatment toxicity and the potential limitation in chemotherapy that can be given concomitantly with radiotherapy, due to renal or haematological factors, and possible triggering of accelerated repopulation which may compromise radiotherapy. Good evidence of benefit is lacking, with the PARADIGM [19] and the DeCIDE [20] trials both showing no improvement in survival from induction chemotherapy before CRT. However, both studies were underpowered from poor accrual, so there remains no definitive answer regarding the value of induction chemotherapy. Whilst TPF should be the induction regimen of choice, many clinicians dose-reduce by 25%, due to concerns about toxicity, as in the TREMPLIN study where only 43% of patients were able to complete the planned treatment [21].

✔ **Evidence base** Department of Veterans Affairs Laryngeal Cancer Study Group (VA Larynx Trial) [22]

- A total of 332 patients with stages III/IV laryngeal cancer, randomized to surgery and post-operative radiotherapy (50–74 Gy) versus induction cisplatin/5-FU × two cycles (with a third cycle if PR/CR), followed by radiotherapy 66–77 Gy. No routine neck dissections for node-positive patients.
- This landmark study demonstrated the value of non-surgical therapy, finding a 64% larynx preservation rate at 2 years, with no difference in 2-year OS (68%).
- CRT decreased distant recurrences but carried a higher local failure rate (12% versus 2%).
- Organ preservation improved the QoL.
- Rates of salvage laryngectomy were significantly lower in T3 than T4 disease (29% versus 56%; $p = 0.01$).

Source: data from The Department of Veterans AVairs Laryngeal Cancer Study Group, Induction chemotherapy plus radiation compared with surgery plus radiation in patients with advanced laryngeal cancer, *New England Journal of Medicine*, Volume 324, Number 24, pp. 1685–90, Copyright © 1991 Massachusetts Medical Society. All rights reserved.

> ✅ **Evidence base** RTOG 91-11 [23]
>
> A total of 547 patients with stages III/IV larynx (T2–3 or low-volume T4 without gross cartilage destruction or >1 cm base of tongue invasion or LN+) were randomized to radiotherapy alone, induction chemotherapy and radiotherapy, or CCRT.
>
> - Radiotherapy was to a total dose of 70 Gy in 2 Gy per fraction in all arms.
> - Induction chemotherapy comprised two cycles of cisplatin/5-FU, followed by reassessment. If progression or less than a PR, patients were treated with laryngectomy and post-operative radiotherapy. Those patients with a PR/CR proceeded to a third cycle of cisplatin/5-FU, and then to radiotherapy.
> - The concurrent chemotherapy regime was three cycles of cisplatin. All patients with cN2 disease proceeded to neck dissection within 8 weeks of radiotherapy.
> - CCRT improved 5-year larynx preservation rates (84%), compared with induction chemotherapy (71%) and radiotherapy alone (66%).
> - CCRT improved locoregional control (69%) versus induction chemotherapy (55%) and radiotherapy alone (51%).
> - OS in each arm was similar.
> - Chemotherapy reduced the rate of distant metastases (13% CCRT, 14% induction, compared to 22% for radiotherapy alone).
>
> *Source*: data from Forastiere A *et al.*, Long term results of Intergroup RTOG 91-11: A phase III trial to presreve the larynx -Induction Cisplatin/5FU and radiation therapy versus concurrent cisplatin and radiation therapy versus radiation therapy, *Journal of Clinical Oncology*, Volume 31, Number 7, pp. 845–52, Copyright © 2013 by American Society of Clinical Oncology.

> ✅ **Evidence base** MACH-NC meta-analysis of CCRT compared with induction chemotherapy [24]
>
> - A total of 93 phase III trials, encompassing 17 346 patients.
> - A 5-year OS benefit (4.5%) when chemotherapy was added to radiotherapy, with a greater 5-year OS benefit for CCRT (6.5%) versus induction chemotherapy. Increased benefit with platinum-based regimes, but no difference between mono- and polychemotherapy regimes. No benefit was seen in those aged 71 or over. No OS benefit from induction chemotherapy.
>
> *Source*: data from *Radiotherapy and Oncology*, Volume 92, Issue 1, Pignon JP *et al.*, Meta-analysis of chemotherapy in head and neck cancer (MACH-NC): an update on 93 randomised trials and 17,346 patients, pp. 4–14, Copyright © 2009 Elsevier Inc. All rights reserved.

> ✪ **Learning point** EGFR inhibitors and radiotherapy
>
> Cetuximab is an mAb that targets the EGFR. Bonner *et al.* randomly assigned 424 patients with locally advanced head and neck cancer to cetuximab and radiotherapy versus radiotherapy alone. Cetuximab improved locoregional control and DFS and did not worsen the QoL [25]. Cetuximab is approved in radical patients with contraindications to platinum. The TREMPLIN study was a randomized trial, comparing induction chemotherapy, followed by CCRT, with either cetuximab or cisplatin in locally advanced SCC of the larynx or hypopharynx. There was a non-significant trend towards increased local recurrences in the cetuximab arm (*p* = 0.08) [26]. The RTOG 05-22 trial looked at the addition of cetuximab to CRT and found no improvement in any outcome, even if stratified by the HPV status [27].

A final word from the expert

The management of laryngeal SCC serves as a useful paradigm to illustrate the oncological principles of organ preservation using non-surgical methods, bimodality treatment, radiosensitization with chemotherapy, proactive toxicity management, and abrogation of late effects using intensity modulation. It is also an excellent example of the need for a strong MDT to help patients through a complex treatment process. The case also shows how specialist supportive care in the community is important in that the patient was discharged with an NG tube. The evidence base for chemoradiation in this setting is secure, with generally good results. Further improvements are focussing on radiotherapy dose escalation, and the true benefit of induction therapy should be resolved in the near future.

References

1. Bosetti C, Garavello W, Gallus S *et al.* Effects of smoking cessation on the risk of laryngeal cancer: an overview of published studies. *Oral Oncology* 2006; **42**(9): 866–72.
2. Fortin A, Wang CS, Vigneault E. Influence of smoking and alcohol drinking behaviours on treatment outcomes of patients with squamous cell carcinomas of the head and neck. *International Journal of Radiation Oncology*Biology*Physics* 2009; **74**(4): 1062–9.
3. Fowler JF. Is there an optimum overall time for head and neck radiotherapy? A review, with new modelling. *Clinical Oncology* 2007; **19**(1): 8–22.
4. Fowler JF. Optimum overall times II: Extended modelling for head and neck radiotherapy. *Clinical Oncology* 2007; **20**(2): 113–16.
5. Hoff CM. Importance of hemoglobin concentration and its modification for the outcome of head and neck cancer patients treated with radiotherapy. *Acta Oncologica* 2012; **51**(4): 419–32.
6. Trotti A, Bellm LA, Epstein JB *et al.* Mucositis incidence, severity and associated outcomes in patients with head and neck cancer receiving radiotherapy with or without chemotherapy: a systematic literature review. *Radiotherapy Oncology* 2003; **66**(3): 253–62.
7. Sonis ST. Mucositis: the impact, biology and therapeutic opportunities of oral mucositis. *Oral Oncology* 2009; **45**(12): 1015–20.
8. UK Oral Mucositis in Cancer Group. *Mouth care guidance and support in cancer and palliative care.* 2012. Available at: <http://www.ukomic.co.uk>.
9. National Institute for Health and Care Excellence. *Nutrition support in adults: oral nutrition support, enteral tube feeding and parenteral nutrition.* 2006. Available at: <http://www.nice.org.uk/guidance/cg032>.
10. National Comprehensive Cancer Network. *Head and neck cancers. NCCN clinical practice guidelines in oncology. Version 2.2013.* 2013. Available at: <http://oralcancerfoundation. org/treatment/pdf/head-and-neck.pdf>.
11. Roland NJ, Paleri V, eds. *Head and neck cancer: multidisciplinary management guidelines*, 4th edn. London: ENT UK, 2011.
12. Dey P, Arnold D, Wight R, MacKenzie K, Kelly C, Wilson J. Radiotherapy versus open surgery versus endolaryngeal surgery (with or without laser) for early laryngeal squamous cell cancer. *Cochrane Database of Systematic Reviews* 2002; **2**: CD002027.
13. Higgins KM, Shah MD, Ogaick MJ, Enepekides D. Treatment of early-stage glottic cancer: meta-analysis comparison of laser excision versus radiotherapy. *Journal of Otolaryngology – Head & Neck Surgery* 2009; **38**(6): 603–12.
14. Ambrosch P, Kron M, Steiner W. Carbon dioxide laser microsurgery for early supraglottic carcinoma. *Annals of Otology, Rhinology & Laryngology* 1998; **107**(8): 680–8.
15. Peretti G, Piazza C, Cattaneo A, De Benedetto L, Martin E, Nicolai P. Comparison of functional outcomes after endoscopic versus open-neck supraglottic laryngectomies. *Annals of Otology, Rhinology & Laryngology* 2006; **115**(11): 827–32.
16. Mendenhall WM, Parsons JT, Stringer SP, Cassisi NJ, Million RR. Carcinoma of the supraglottic larynx: a basis for comparing the results of radiotherapy and surgery. *Head & Neck* 1990; **12**(3): 204–9.
17. Adelstein DJ, Rodriguez CP. Current and emerging standards of concomitant chemoradiotherapy. *Seminars in Oncology* 2008; **35**(3): 211–20.
18. Blanchard P, Bourhis J, Lacas B *et al.* Taxane-cisplatin-fluorouracil as induction chemotherapy in locally advanced head and neck cancers: an individual patient data meta-analysis of the meta-analysis of chemotherapy in head and neck cancer group. *Journal of Clinical Oncology* 2013; **31**(23): 2854–60.
19. Haddad R, O'Neill A, Rabinowits G *et al.* Induction chemotherapy followed by concurrent chemoradiotherapy (sequential chemoradiotherapy) versus concurrent chemoradiotherapy alone in locally advanced head and neck cancer (PARADIGM): a randomised phase 3 trial. *The Lancet Oncology* 2013; **14**(3): 257–64.

20. Cohen EEW, Karrison T, Kocherginsky M *et al.* DeCIDE: a phase III randomized trial of docetaxel (D), cisplatin , 5-fluorouracil (F) (TPF) induction chemotherapy (IC) in patients with N2/N3 locally advanced squamous cell carcinoma of the head and neck (SCCHN). *Journal of Clinical Oncology* 2012; **30**(Suppl): abstr 5500.

21. Lefebvre JL, Pointreau Y, Rolland F *et al.* Induction chemotherapy followed by either chemoradiotherapy or bioradiotherapy for larynx preservation: the TREMPLIN randomized phase II study. *Journal of Clinical Oncology* 2013; **31**(7): 853–9.

22. [No authors listed]. Induction chemotherapy plus radiation compared with surgery plus radiation in patients with advanced laryngeal cancer. The Department of Veterans AVairs Laryngeal Cancer Study Group. *The New England Journal of Medicine* 1991; **324**(24): 1685–90.

23. Forastiere AA, Zhang Q, Weber RS *et al.* Long-term results of RTOG 91-11: a comparison of three nonsurgical treatment strategies to preserve the larynx in patients with locally advanced larynx cancer. *Journal of Clinical Oncology* 2013; **31**(7): 845–52.

24. Pignon JP, le Maitre A, Maillard E, Bourhis J. Meta-analysis of chemotherapy in head and neck cancer (MACH-NC): an update on 93 randomised trials and 17,346 patients. *Radiotherapy and Oncology* 2009; **92**(1): 4–14.

25. Bonner JA, Harari PM, Giralt J *et al.* Radiotherapy plus cetuximab for locoregionally advanced head and neck cancer: 5-year survival data from a phase 3 randomised trial, and relation between cetuximab-induced rash and survival. *The Lancet Oncology* 2010; **11**(1): 21–8.

26. Lefebvre J, Pointreau Y, Rolland F *et al.* Sequential chemoradiotherapy (SCRT) for larynx preservation (LP): Results of the randomized phase II TREMPLIN study. *Journal of Clinical Oncology* 2012; **30**(360s, Suppl 15): abstr 5501.

27. Ang KK, Zhang QE, Rosenthal DI *et al.* A randomized phase III trial (RTOG 0522) of concurrent accelerated radiation plus cisplatin with or without cetuximab for stage III-IV head and neck squamous cell carcinomas (HNC). *Journal of Clinical Oncology* 2011; **29**(Suppl): abstr 5500.

20 Glioblastoma multiforme (GBM)

Kathryn Tarver

⏱ **Expert commentary** Eliot Sims

Case history

A 55-year-old man presented to his GP with a 3-week history of headaches, which responded only partially to analgesia. They tended to be worse in the mornings and were associated with nausea. He denied visual disturbance or neurological symptoms. Neurological examination was unremarkable. In view of symptoms suggestive of raised intracranial pressure (ICP), the GP referred him directly to Accident and Emergency where an urgent non-contrast CT of the brain was performed. This revealed a right-sided parietal mass lesion, with significant surrounding oedema causing midline shift and compression of the anterior horn of the right lateral ventricle. Neurosurgical advice was sought, and he was admitted for further investigations.

✪ **Learning point (Acute Oncology)** Management of raised ICP

Most patients with symptoms of raised ICP due to peri-tumoural oedema can be adequately managed with glucocorticoids. High-dose dexamethasone should be administered, and care should be taken to address subclinical seizure activity as a possible cause of reduced Glasgow coma score (GCS).

In patients with symptoms of severe raised ICP, such as reduced GCS, urgent cranial imaging and neurosurgical review should be sought. Imaging may reveal a reversible cause such as hydrocephalus or a large cystic component arising within the tumour, which may be amenable to neurosurgical drainage.

In the setting of glioblastoma multiforme (GBM), mannitol is used as a holding measure, whilst awaiting a definitive surgical solution such as an intracranial shunt or cyst drainage. If no such procedure is possible and the patient is not responding to high-dose dexamethasone, the outlook is extremely poor, and the role of mannitol is limited.

Dexamethasone

- May be associated with a lower risk of infection and cognitive impairment than other glucocorticoids [1].
- Given as a 16 mg loading dose, followed by 8 mg bd if symptoms severe.
- Given as a daily dose of 4–8 mg of dexamethasone if symptoms mild.
- Not recommended for asymptomatic patients.
- Fully absorbed within 30 min of oral administration.
- Avoid evening/night-time doses, as this often causes insomnia.
- Symptomatic improvement within hours.

(continued)

⊕ **Clinical tip** Common presenting symptoms of brain tumours

- Headache.
- Seizures (less common in glioblastoma multiforme (GBM) versus lower-grade gliomas).
- Memory loss.
- Motor weakness.
- Visual symptoms.
- Language deficit.
- Cognitive/personality changes.

- Maximum benefit within 24–72 hours; standard imaging may not reveal decreased oedema for at least a week.
- Once response has been achieved, subsequent dosing should be adjusted to use the lowest dose necessary to control symptoms, tapering slowly over a 2-week period or longer in very symptomatic patients [2].
- Common side effects include insomnia, gastritis, altered appetite, and mood changes, and more serious complications of peptic ulceration, myopathy, and opportunistic infections.

Mannitol

- Osmotic diuretics reduce brain volume by drawing free water out of the tissue and into the circulation, dehydrating the brain parenchyma and reducing the ICP.
- Mannitol is prepared as a 20% solution and given by IV infusion over 30–60 min at a dose of 0.25–2 g/kg.
- Effects usually peak at about 1 hour and can last for up to 24 hours.
- Monitor serum sodium, serum osmolality, and renal function.

Dexamethasone 8 mg twice daily was commenced, in view of his symptoms and the degree of midline shift and oedema seen. A CT CAP showed no evidence of malignancy outside the brain. An MRI was performed.

MRI of the brain with gadolinium showed a solitary irregularly ring-enhancing lesion in the right frontal lobe, which was hypointense on T1-weighted images, with a central area of low signal, consistent with necrosis (Figure 20.1). It appeared hyperintense on T2-weighted images, with marked surrounding vasogenic oedema. The patient's case was discussed in the neuro-oncology MDT meeting. Radiological appearances were highly suggestive of a high-grade glioma, and the decision was made to proceed to surgical debulking. Pathology from the debulking surgery confirmed GBM.

✚ Clinical tip Diagnosis of GBM

The gold standard imaging modality of choice in primary brain tumours is MRI with gadolinium contrast. GBM displays a characteristic appearance. In many cases, CT and MRI appearances are so typical of GBM that patients proceed to surgery on this basis alone. On CT, GBM often appears as a ring-enhancing lesion with irregular thick margins and a central area of hypodense necrosis. Marked mass effect due to surrounding vasogenic oedema is common.

✚ Clinical tip Differential diagnosis

An important differential of such a lesion on CT is a solitary metastasis or an abscess.

If there is doubt, based on radiological appearances, or elements in the presenting history suggest the possibility of disseminated malignancy, a staging CT CAP should be performed to rule out the presence of a primary cancer having metastasized to the brain.

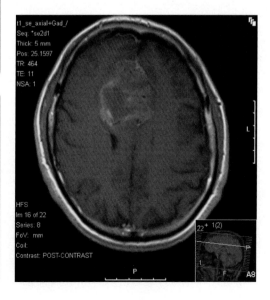

Figure 20.1 T1-weighted MRI with gadolinium showing an irregularly enhancing lesion in the right frontal lobe.

✪ **Learning point** Surgical management of GBM

Surgery is the initial therapeutic approach in patients with GBM, with the dual aims of obtaining tissue for diagnosis and tumour debulking. Where possible, patients should undergo maximal debulking, with removal of the visibly abnormal tissue seen intraoperatively or abnormally enhancing on preoperative MRI. When this is not feasible, due to the location of the tumour or the condition of the patient, stereotactic biopsy should be undertaken.

Advantages of maximal debulking surgery

- Rapid improvement of symptoms, including seizure control and recovery of neurological or cognitive deficits.
- More representative tissue sample for detailed histopathological analysis.
- Possible impact on survival: there is evidence for a survival benefit in patients achieving complete macroscopic resection within a study looking at the use of fluorescence-guided resection using 5-aminolevulinic acid (ALA) [3]. Whether this benefit is also seen in patients undergoing 'standard' surgical debulking is unknown.

GBMs are widely infiltrative tumours, with microscopic disease extending into the adjacent brain parenchyma, often far beyond the apparent macroscopic tumour margin. Therefore, the addition of adjuvant chemoradiation results in an improvement in local control and survival.

✪ **Learning point** Classification of primary brain tumours

The majority of primary brain tumours arising from the brain parenchyma are gliomas and may arise from glial cells, such as astrocytes and oligodendrocytes, or neural stem cells [4].

The WHO classification system for primary brain tumours combines tumour nomenclature with a grading system, such that the histological tumour subtype is correlated with the histological grade of the tumour. The TNM system is not used in the prognostication of CNS malignancies.

Astrocytic tumours

Low-grade astrocytomas are most commonly seen in children and young adults and tend to be relatively well defined or circumscribed. Duplications and/or mutations in the *BRAF* gene are seen.

Pilocytic astrocytomas (WHO grade I)

- Cells with 'hair-like' (piloid) processes.
- Usually occur in children and young adults.
- They are most commonly seen in the cerebellar hemispheres and midline areas such as the third ventricle and spinal cord.
- Rarely fully resectable but, if resected, may be cured.

Diffuse astrocytoma (WHO grade II)

- Most commonly seen in young adults.
- Many progress to malignant astrocytoma.

Anaplastic astrocytoma (WHO grade III)

- Exhibit higher cellularity, more marked nuclear atypia, and hyperchromasia, as well as mitoses.
- No endothelial proliferation or necrosis.

Glioblastoma (WHO grade IV)

- Pleomorphic tumours with high levels of mitotic activity and necrosis.
- Variants include giant cell glioblastoma, small cell glioblastoma, gliosarcoma, and glioblastoma with oligodendroglial component.
- Mutations in the isocitrate dehydrogenase 1 (*IDH1*) and *TP53* gene are common in these tumours. There is an association between *IDH1* gene alterations and a more favourable prognosis [5].

(continued)

- Glioblastoma may arise *de novo* (primary GBM), usually in older patients, or evolve from a low-grade glioma (secondary GBM), typically in younger patients. The observed molecular abnormalities differ in these two settings. EGFR amplification, *PTEN* mutations, and MDM2 overexpression are seen in primary GBMs, whereas secondary GBMs more commonly display *p53* mutations.

Oligodendroglial and oligoastrocytic tumours

Oligodendroglial tumour cells have round nuclei with perinuclear halos (a 'fried egg' appearance). Some have areas resembling astrocytomas and are designated oligoastrocytomas.

The WHO grading system describes grade II oligodendrogliomas and grade III anaplastic oligodendrogliomas.

- Both are characterized by increased cellularity, pleomorphism, high mitotic rate, and microvascular proliferation.
- Anaplastic oligoastrocytomas with necrosis are classified as glioblastoma with oligodendroglioma component (GBM-O—grade IV).

Oligodendroglial tumours commonly exhibit *IDH* gene mutations and the combined loss of the short arm of chromosome 1 (1p) and the long arm of chromosome 19 (19q). This is more common in oligodendrogliomas, as opposed to oligoastrocytomas or mixed tumours.

In general, the prognosis of oligodendrogliomas is better than that of diffuse astrocytic gliomas, particularly in those tumours with 1p/19q loss. Additionally, patients with oligodendrogliomas displaying 1p/19q loss derive a survival benefit from adjuvant chemotherapy given before or after radiotherapy, whereas those with tumours without the deletion do not [6].

Following recovery from surgery, he remained fit and of good PS, with no residual neurological deficit. Prior to proceeding to definitive treatment, a comprehensive assessment of patient fitness, co-morbidities, and neurological function was undertaken, along with routine blood tests to confirm satisfactory renal and liver function, prior to embarking on cytotoxic chemotherapy. He proceeded to a radical course of radiotherapy 60 Gy in 30 fractions over 6 weeks, with concurrent oral temozolomide (TMZ) chemotherapy. He tolerated treatment well and proceeded to 6 months of treatment with adjuvant TMZ chemotherapy, starting 1 month following the completion of chemoradiation.

✪ Learning point Management of GBM

- Tissue diagnosis and the first definitive treatment are usually undertaken at the same operation, ideally maximal debulking surgery.
- Assessment of patient fitness is vital before embarking upon radical treatment. Older age and poor PS have consistently been shown to be associated with shorter survival in GBM [7].
- The Stupp trial [9] excluded patients over the age of 70 and showed no benefit for concurrent chemoradiation in patients aged 61–70, regardless of PS.
- There is evidence of a modest survival benefit, compared with best supportive care, for radiotherapy alone in patients over 70 [10]. There is evidence to suggest hypofractionated, short-course radiotherapy may be equally as effective as higher doses of radiotherapy, in terms of survival benefit in the elderly [11].
- Standard UK practice has been to offer palliative radiotherapy, e.g. 30 Gy in six fractions treating three times a week for 2 weeks, to the following groups:
  o patients over 70 years of age with PS 0–2
  o patients with persistent neurological deficit (with the exception of persistent visual field defect—these patients may benefit from radical chemoradiation)
  o patients under 70 who are unlikely to tolerate radical chemoradiation

- Patients of PS 3–4 or those with significant neurological deficit or rapidly progressive disease are unlikely to benefit from palliative radiotherapy and should be offered best supportive care, which includes the use of steroids to manage symptoms arising from raised ICP.
- The gold standard treatment following debulking or biopsy is concurrent radiotherapy and chemotherapy with oral TMZ [8,9]
- Patients receive EBRT 60 Gy in 30 fractions over 6 weeks. TMZ is given concurrently at a dose of 75 mg/m^2 daily throughout radiotherapy treatment (including weekends).
- One month following completion of chemoradiation, patients proceed to 6 months of adjuvant TMZ, dosed at 200 mg/m^2 given on days 1–5 of a 28-day cycle (first cycle often dosed at 150 mg/m^2, with dose escalation if no significant thrombocytopenia)

✅ Evidence base Stupp trial: radiotherapy versus chemoradiotherapy with temozolamide [9]

- A total of 573 patients aged 18–70 years with newly diagnosed GBM, PS 0–2.
- Randomized between standard radiotherapy (60 Gy in 30 fractions) or standard radiotherapy plus concomitant daily TMZ chemotherapy followed by adjuvant TMZ.
- Patients received prophylactic co-trimoxazole or inhaled pentamidine as *Pneumocystis jirovecii* pneumonia (PCP) prophylaxis during chemoradiation.
- Combination treatment resulted in a statistically significant increase in OS (27% versus 11% at 2 years, and 10% versus 2% at 5 years), median survival benefit 2.5 months (Figure 20.2) from 5-year analysis [12]).
- Median OS 14.6 months versus 12.1 months.
- HR for death 0.63 with combination treatment.
- Methyl guanine methyl transferase (MGMT) promoter methylation shown to be a prognostic factor for improved survival as well as a predictor of benefit from chemotherapy.

Source: data from Stupp R *et al.*, Radiotherapy plus Concomitant and Adjuvant Temozolomide for Glioblastoma, *New England Journal of Medicine*, Volume 352, Number 10, pp. 987–96, Copyright © 2005 Massachusetts Medical Society. All rights reserved.

⊕ Clinical tip Patients likely to benefit from chemoradiation

- PS 0–1.
- ≤70 years.
- No residual neurological deficit (excluding seizures and visual field defects).

⊕ Clinical tip Common TMZ toxicities

- Nausea.
- Thrombocytopenia.
- Lymphopenia—patients are prescribed prophylactic co-trimoxazole during chemoradiation, as there have been recorded cases of PCP.
- Blood counts should be monitored on a weekly basis during chemoradiation, and TMZ must be omitted in the presence of a neutrophil count of <1.5 × 10^9/L or platelet count of <75 × 10^9/L. If the patient is clinically well, radiotherapy should be continued.

⊕ Clinical tip Common side effects of radical brain radiotherapy

- Fatigue.
- Local hair loss (usually permanent).
- Nausea.
- Headache.
- Increased risk of seizures.
- In longer-term survivors, cognitive impairment and early cataract formation.

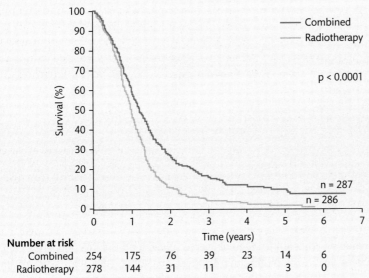

Figure 20.2 Kaplan–Meier estimates of OS by treatment group—combined radiotherapy and TMZ versus radiotherapy alone. Reprinted from *The Lancet Oncology*, Volume 10, Issue 5, Stupp R *et al.*, Effects of radiotherapy with concomitant and adjuvant temozolomide versus radiotherapy alone on survival in glioblastoma in a randomised phase III study: 5-year analysis of the EORTC-NCIC trial, pp. 459–66, Copyright © 2009 with permission from Elsevier, <http://www.sciencedirect.com/science/journal/14702045>.

✪ Learning point Radiotherapy planning in GBM

Radiotherapy planning is undertaken primarily using information from the preoperative MRI images, but post-operative MRI is being used increasingly to inform radiotherapy planning, as this gives additional information regarding residual areas of enhancement following surgery. It also provides a new baseline image for comparison to future post-chemoradiation imaging. Co-registration of planning CT images with preoperative T1-weighted contrast-enhanced axial MRI images is helpful for delineating the target volume. A gross tumour volume (GTV) is reconstructed on the planning CT images, which includes the original extent of the enhancing tumour. A margin of 2.5 cm is added to the GTV in all directions to form the clinical target volume (CTV), which should include ideally all visible oedema and is designed to cover the microscopic extent of the disease. The CTV should be trimmed back from natural barriers, such as the skull, and should normally be trimmed off the midline, as spread of the tumour to the opposite hemisphere would be unusual. In certain circumstances, there may be concern about tumour spreading across the corpus callosum, for example, in which case the 2.5 cm extent of the CTV can extend to cover the midline. A further margin is added to the CTV to create the planning target volume (PTV), commonly 0.5 cm. The size of the CTV to PTV margin may vary between radiotherapy centres, according to local set-up error measurements.

✪ Learning point Prognostic factors in GBM

Prognostic factors affecting the OS and response to treatment include age, neurological function, PS, and the extent of the initial surgical resection.

The impact of these clinical factors on outcome was illustrated in a study of 832 patients with GBM, in which the outcome was analysed using recursive partitioning analysis (RPA) [13]. Four prognostic groups were identified, based upon the age at presentation, tumour location, Karnofsky PS, and extent of surgery. Median survival varied from 37 weeks, with 2-year survival of 4%, in the high-risk group (patients aged 65 or over with Karnofsky PS <80 who had biopsy, rather than debulking) to 132 weeks, with 65% 2-year survival, in the lowest-risk group (patients up to 40 years of age with a frontal tumour).

A similar analysis in older adults, aged over 70, identified four prognostic subgroups, based on the age, extent of surgery (biopsy versus resection), and PS; median survival ranged from 2.3 months in subgroup IV (biopsy only, Karnofsky PS <70) to 9.3 months in subgroup I (surgical resection, age <75.5) [14].

⊕ Clinical tip MGMT as a prognostic marker

The enzyme MGMT is responsible for repair of DNA damage induced by alkylating agents such as TMZ. The MGMT gene may be silenced, in some tumours, by methylation of its promoter during tumour development, rendering these tumours more susceptible to the effects of TMZ. MGMT promoter methylation appears to be associated with improved survival in patients receiving TMZ [15].

In view of the apparent prognostic value of the MGMT promoter methylation status, testing for the presence of methylation is now routine in clinical trials for GBM for stratification purposes. Current guidance does not recommend routine testing outside trials, due to a lack of standardization of any specific testing method for clinical practice and as treatments for patients without MGMT promoter methylation are not yet established [16].

He remained clinically and radiologically stable for 4 months, following completion of treatment, before presenting via Accident and Emergency with seizures. Imaging revealed likely recurrence of the disease, with significant oedema and mass effect. His case was re-discussed in the neuro-oncology MDT meeting where the conclusion was that there had been progression of disease and that the changes were not due to the treatment (pseudoprogression - see clinical tip). It was felt that further debulking surgery was unlikely to improve his symptoms and therefore was not recommended. He was managed symptomatically with high-dose dexamethasone, and his seizures were controlled on levetiracetam. He was discharged home, once his seizures were controlled, and was seen in the oncology outpatient clinic to discuss further treatment options.

✪ Learning point (Acute Oncology) Management of seizures in GBM

Whilst patients with GBM are at increased risk of seizures, there is no evidence for the use of prophylactic anti-epileptic drugs (AEDs) in such patients.

Patients presenting with seizures should be commenced on an AED. However, if they subsequently proceed to optimal debulking surgery, AED can often be tapered down and discontinued in the post-operative period. Patients experiencing seizures >72 hours after surgery, or with seizures in the absence of planned surgery, should be commenced on long-term AED [17].

First-generation AEDs, e.g. phenytoin, carbamazepine, and phenobarbital, should be avoided, due to their hepatic enzyme-inducing properties which can interfere with other medications, including chemotherapy (but not TMZ). Additionally, phenytoin increases the hepatic metabolism of dexamethasone, meaning patients on both drugs may require higher doses of steroid (an increase of up to 50%) to control their symptoms.

In general, third-generation AEDs, such as levetiracetam, lamotrigine, or pregabalin, are preferred in patients with GBM and seizures [16]. If possible, monotherapy should be pursued, aiming to increase the dose of a single agent up to the maximum recommended dose, if necessary, in order to achieve seizure control, without resorting to polypharmacy with its attendant risks of drug–drug interactions and side effects [17].

⊕ Clinical tip Pseudoprogression

Pseudoprogression is defined as an increase in the size and enhancement of GBM lesions on imaging, following treatment, which subsequently decrease in size or stabilize without further treatment [18]. Following completion of chemoradiation, a proportion of patients exhibit clinical and radiological deterioration. If this is due to disease progression, this heralds a poor outcome, and proceeding to adjuvant TMZ chemotherapy would not be in the patient's best interests. The presence of pseudoprogression can produce an identical clinical and radiological picture but may be a predictive factor for a better prognosis [19].

There are no reliable means of distinguishing between the two. A change in the radiological criteria for restaging GBM after treatment attempts to address the issue [20], and future directions of study include the use of novel imaging techniques in an attempt to identify distinguishing features of pseudoprogression.

---

❻ Expert comment

A fundamental teaching in oncology is to do no harm and to withdraw a potentially toxic treatment if it is not proving beneficial. As a treatment-supervising clinician, it is therefore especially important to be wary of the phenomenon of pseudoprogression, which may, in itself, be a marker of good prognosis. In one of the largest series of radiological pseudoprogression analysed to date [19], Brandes *et al.* found that pseudoprogression occurred in 91% of patients with MGMT methylation, as opposed to only 41% in the unmethylated group, implying that patients who are more sensitive to chemotherapy (and more likely to have a better prognosis) are more likely to have pseudoprogression. The series had a selection bias because pseudoprogression was defined retrospectively on the basis of a prolonged period of response. However, these data counsel strongly against withdrawing patients from treatment too prematurely on the basis of radiological imaging alone, not just because the imaging findings may be false, but also because treatment interruption might ultimately prejudice patients with a better prognosis who paradoxically would benefit very much from longer treatment. Certainly, it is wise to continue follow-up for 3 months and repeat the imaging in patients where treatment is withdrawn, despite the fact that true disease progression is frequently diagnosed.

> ⭐ **Learning point** Role of further surgery
>
> The indications for repeat debulking at relapse are not firmly established. There is some evidence for a modest survival benefit from re-operation in selected patients, although much of these data predate the TMZ era [21,22]. The median survival for patients undergoing surgery for recurrent GBM ranges from 14 to 36 weeks.
>
> Factors that may suggest a favourable outcome from repeat debulking include:
>
> - good PS
> - young age
> - longer interval since the original surgery
> - limited extent of the second surgical resection
>
> Insertion of carmustine-impregnated polymer wafers into the tumour bed at repeat debulking may prolong survival, following re-operation for local recurrence [23]. However, this treatment is not NICE-approved in recurrent disease.

> ⭐ **Learning point** Carmustine implants
>
> Insertion of carmustine-impregnated 'wafers' into the surgical cavity at the time of debulking is NICE-approved for patients in whom at least 90% of the tumour has been resected. This is largely based on a RCT of 240 patients with grades 3 and 4 gliomas where patients received carmustine implants or placebo at operation, before undergoing radical radiotherapy (55–60 Gy in 30–33 fractions) without concurrent or adjuvant chemotherapy. In a retrospectively identified subgroup of 111 patients with GBM, in whom at least 90% of the tumour had been resected, a median OS benefit of 2.15 months was observed in the group who received carmustine implants versus those who received placebo implants [24]. In spite of NICE approval, this technology is not widely used in clinical practice in the UK. Potential complications of carmustine wafer insertion include an increased risk of post-operative infection, seizures, problems with wound healing, and exacerbation of post-operative oedema.

He consented to second-line chemotherapy with PCV (procarbazine, CCNU, and vincristine) and received two cycles, before worsening seizure control prompted a repeat MRI scan. This confirmed progressive disease, and chemotherapy was discontinued. As he remained of reasonable PS, he was offered third-line treatment with irinotecan plus bevacizumab; however, this was poorly tolerated and was discontinued after one cycle, as his PS deteriorated. The decision was made to stop active treatment and manage him with best supportive care.

Discussion

This case highlights the practical issues arising in the diagnosis and management of GBM and its complications. Standard treatment, following debulking surgery or biopsy in suitable patients, is radical radiotherapy with concomitant oral TMZ chemotherapy, followed by adjuvant TMZ. After completion of adjuvant TMZ, patients should undergo a repeat MRI of the brain to serve as a new baseline. Clinical follow-up should be undertaken on a 3-monthly basis, including documentation of the presence/evolution of neurological symptoms or seizures. In the absence of progressive symptoms, routine MRI should take place 6-monthly.

Timing of post-chemoradiation imaging in GBM varies between treatment centres. A major complicating factor in deciding on a standardized post-treatment imaging schedule is the phenomenon of pseudoprogression, which can develop on imaging performed between 4 weeks and 6 months following completion of chemoradiation. Some centres undertake repeat MRI imaging at 4 weeks post-chemoradiation, prior to adjuvant chemotherapy, whilst others proceed directly from chemoradiation to adjuvant chemotherapy 4 weeks later, without prior imaging, preferring to repeat imaging after completion of three cycles of adjuvant TMZ, proceeding with a total of six cycles of TMZ if appearances are stable or improved. The issue with these approaches is that apparent radiological progression within this time frame could be caused by pseudoprogression, which is, in fact, indicative of tumour response and yet is indistinguishable from true progression of disease.

An alternative approach is to proceed with six cycles of adjuvant chemotherapy before repeating imaging, or to perform an MRI scan after three cycles to document radiological appearances but continue with treatment, even if changes suggestive of progressive disease are seen.

An additional complication arises in the case of clinical deterioration, following completion of chemoradiation. This has previously been attributed to progression of disease and, when supported by evidence of radiological progression, is sometimes used as a justification for discontinuing or withholding adjuvant chemotherapy. However, there is evidence to suggest that pseudoprogression can also cause transient clinical decline as well as radiological progression [25].

In summary, whilst there are no reliable means of definitively making a diagnosis of pseudoprogression, clinicians should adopt a pragmatic approach to the use of adjuvant chemotherapy and timing of follow-up imaging in patients with GBM. Practical guidelines have been published to aid the scheduling of imaging and interpretation of radiological and clinical features in patients with suspected pseudoprogression [26].

The management of truly progressive GBM is challenging, and further active treatment has not been proven to prolong survival. In patients who remain fit enough for systemic therapy, options are limited. Efforts to improve chemotherapy for GBM have not, as yet, had a meaningful effect on survival. For patients progressing after first-line treatment, there is no established chemotherapy regimen available, and patients are best treated within investigational clinical protocols [16]. Outside of a trial setting, if there has been a reasonable interval (6–12 months) between completion of adjuvant TMZ and progression, rechallenge with TMZ chemotherapy is an option.

PCV chemotherapy is a commonly used second-line regimen (procarbazine, lomustine (CCNU), and vincristine). Vincristine 1.5 mg/m^2 IV and lomustine 100 mg/m^2 PO are given on day 1, and oral procarbazine 100 mg/m^2 is administered on days 1–10 of a 6-week cycle.

There is phase II evidence for the tolerability and activity of bevacizumab ± irinotecan in relapsed GBM [27]. The impact of this treatment regimen on survival is unclear.

The role of bevacizumab in first-line treatment of GBM has been addressed within the phase III AVAglio trial. In this randomized, double-blind, placebo-controlled study, patients with newly diagnosed GBM were randomized to receive standard radiotherapy plus concomitant and adjuvant TMZ, plus either bevacizumab or placebo until progression. Interim results showed a 4.4 month improvement in median PFS (10.6 months versus 6.2 months) in patients who received bevacizumab. There was no statistically significant difference in OS at interim analysis [28]. In phase II studies, bevacizumab reduced steroid requirements and has been associated with imaging evidence of tumour response, but the effect on life expectancy remains unknown [27,29]. The use of bevacizumab in GBM has given rise to the phenomenon of 'pseudoresponse', an apparent radiological improvement following treatment, which may be related to changes in vascular permeability, resulting in a reduction in peri-tumoural oedema, but not tumour shrinkage.

Current phase III trials in GBM are focussing on methods of optimizing debulking surgery, the use of IFN-alpha, in combination with TMZ, in newly diagnosed GBM in patients without MGMT promoter methylation, and exploration of optimal management of elderly patients with GBM [30].

A final word from the expert

The diagnosis of glioblastoma confers nearly as poor an outlook today as it did half a century ago. Whilst the basic treatments of maximal debulking surgery followed by radiotherapy (if PS allows), remain, a role for chemotherapy is now clear, and biological markers for determining who might benefit more from chemotherapy are established, although not yet readily available in the UK. Sadly, in an era where molecular treatments and targeted therapies abound in the treatment of other solid tumours, the evidence for the use of these in the treatment of glioblastoma have been disappointing, culminating in the recent inconclusive results from the AVAglio (adjuvant bevacizumab) study.

Population-based data confirm that the incidence of high-grade glioma is increasing and is greatest in patients aged 65 and older. Age is a key prognostic factor in the management of glioblastoma, and survival decreases for each decade of life over 50 years. It seems therefore that, at present, efforts would be better focussed on achieving a consensus approach to the management of malignant glioma in the older patient, rather than in large expensive international randomized controlled studies evaluating new treatments or modalities. In this setting, centralizing MGMT testing in a handful of reference laboratories in the UK, so that results are available rapidly and relatively inexpensively, would at least allow clinicians to stratify treatments appropriately, which would serve to improve patient outcomes, whilst avoiding toxicity from unnecessary treatment.

References

1. Batchelor T, DeAngelis LM. Medical management of cerebral metastases. *Neurosurgery Clinics of North America* 1996; **7**(3): 435–46.
2. Ryken TC, McDermott M, Robinson PD *et al.* The role of steroids in the management of brain metastases: a systematic review and evidence-based clinical practice guideline. *Journal of Neuro-Oncology* 2010; **96**(1): 103–24.
3. Pichlmeier U, Bink A, Schackert G, Stummer W; ALA Glioma Study Group. Resection and survival in glioblastoma multiforme: an RTOG recursive partitioning analysis of ALA study patients. *Neuro-Oncology* 2008; **10**(6): 1025–34.
4. Louis DN. Molecular pathology of malignant gliomas. *Annual Reviews of Pathology: Mechanisms of Disease* 2006; **1**: 97–117.

5. Hartmann C, Hentschel B, Wick W *et al.* Patients with IDH1 wild type anaplastic astro-cytomas exhibit worse prognosis than IDH1-mutated glioblastomas, and IDH1 mutation status accounts for the unfavorable prognostic effect of higher age: implications for clas-sification of gliomas. *Acta Neuropathologica* 2010; **120**(6): 707–18.

6. Van den Bent M, Brandes AA, Taphoorn MJ *et al.* Adjuvant procarbazine, lomustine, and vincristine chemotherapy in newly diagnosed anaplastic oligodendroglioma: long-term follow-up of EORTC brain tumor group study 26951. *Journal of Clinical Oncology* 2013; **31**(3): 344–50.

7. Buckner JC. Factors influencing survival in high-grade gliomas. *Seminars in Oncology* 2003; **30**(6 Suppl 19): 10–14.

8. Wick W, Platten M, Meisner C *et al.*; NOA-08 Study Group of Neuro-oncology Working Group (NOA) of German Cancer Society. Temozolomide chemotherapy alone versus radiotherapy alone for malignant astrocytoma in the elderly: the NOA-08 randomised, phase 3 trial. *The Lancet Oncology* 2012; **13**(7): 707–15

9. Stupp R, Mason WP, van den Bent MJ *et al.*; European Organisation for Research and Treatment of Cancer Brain Tumor and Radiotherapy Groups; National Cancer Institute of Canada Clinical Trials Group. Radiotherapy plus concomitant and adjuvant temozolo-mide for glioblastoma. *The New England Journal of Medicine* 2005; **352**(10): 987–96.

10. Keime-Guibert F, Chinot O, Taillandier L *et al.*; Association of French-Speaking Neuro-Oncologists. Radiotherapy for glioblastoma in the elderly. *The New England Journal of Medicine* 2007; **356**(15): 1527–35.

11. Roa W, Brasher PM, Bauman G *et al.* Abbreviated course of radiation therapy in older patients with glioblastoma multiforme: a prospective randomized clinical trial. *Journal of Clinical Oncology* 2004; **22**(9): 1583–8.

12. Stupp R, Hegi ME, Mason WP *et al.*; European Organisation for Research and Treatment of Cancer Brain Tumour and Radiation Oncology Groups; National Cancer Institute of Canada Clinical Trials Group. Effects of radiotherapy with concomitant and adjuvant temozolomide versus radiotherapy alone on survival in glioblastoma in a randomised phase III study: 5-year analysis of the EORTC-NCIC trial. *The Lancet Oncology* 2009; **10**(5): 459–66.

13. Lamborn KR, Chang SM, Prados MD. Prognostic factors for survival of patients with glioblastoma: recursive-partitioning analysis. *Neuro-Oncology* 2004; **6**(3): 227–35.

14. Scott JG, Bauchet L, Fraum TJ *et al.* Recursive partitioning analysis of prognostic factors for glioblastoma patients aged 70 years or older. *Cancer* 2012; **118**(22): 5595–600.

15. Hegi ME, Diserens AC, Gorlia T *et al.* MGMT gene silencing and benefit from temozolo-mide in glioblastoma. *The New England Journal of Medicine* 2005; **352**(10): 997–1003.

16. Stupp R, Tonn JC, Brada M, Pentheroudakis G; ESMO Guidelines Working Group. High-grade malignant glioma: ESMO Clinical Practice Guidelines for diagnosis, treatment and follow-up. *Annals of Oncology* 2010; **21**(Suppl 5): v190–3.

17. Weller M, Stupp R, Wick W. Epilepsy meets cancer: when, why, and what to do about it? *The Lancet Oncology* 2012; **13**(9): e375–82.

18. Brandsma D, Stalpers L, Taal W, Sminia P, van den Bent MJ. Clinical features, mecha-nisms, and management of pseudoprogression in malignant gliomas. *The Lancet Oncology* 2008; **9**(5): 453–61.

19. Brandes AA, Franceschi E, Tosoni A *et al.* MGMT promoter methylation status can pre-dict the incidence and outcome of pseudoprogression after concomitant radiochemother-apy in newly diagnosed glioblastoma patients. *Journal of Clinical Oncology* 2008; **26**(13): 2192–7.

20. Wen PY, Macdonald DR, Reardon DA *et al.* Updated response assessment criteria for high-grade gliomas: response assessment in neuro-oncology working group. *Journal of Clinical Oncology* 2010; **28**(11): 1963–72.

21. Dirks P, Bernstein M, Muller PJ, Tucker WS. The value of reoperation for recurrent glio-blastoma. *Canadian Journal of Surgery* 1993; **36**(3): 271–5.

22. Barker FG 2nd, Chang SM, Gutin PH *et al.* Survival and functional status after resection of recurrent glioblastoma multiforme. *Neurosurgery* 1998; **42**(4): 709–20.

23. Westphal M, Ram Z, Riddle V, Hilt D, Bortey E; Executive Committee of the Gliadel Study Group. Gliadel wafer in initial surgery for malignant glioma: long-term follow-up of a multicenter controlled trial. *Acta Neurochirurgica* 2006; **148**(3): 269–75.

24. Westphal M, Hilt DC, Bortey E *et al.* A phase 3 trial of local chemotherapy with biodegradable carmustine (BCNU) wafers (Gliadel wafers) in patients with primary malignant glioma. *Neuro-Oncology* 2003; **5**(2): 79–88.

25. Topkan E, Topuk S, Oymak E, Parlak C, Pehlivan B. Pseudoprogression in patients with glioblastoma multiforme after concurrent radiotherapy and temozolomide. *American Journal of Clinical Oncology* 2012; **35**(3): 284–9.

26. Sanghera P, Rampling R, Haylock B *et al.* The concepts, diagnosis and management of early imaging changes after therapy for glioblastomas. *Clinical Oncology* 2012; **24**(3): 216–27.

27. Friedman HS, Prados MD, Wen PY *et al.* Bevacizumab alone and in combination with irinotecan in recurrent glioblastoma. *Journal of Clinical Oncology* 2009; **27**(28): 4733–40.

28. Chinot O, Wick W, Mason W *et al.* Phase III trial of bevacizumab added to standard radiotherapy and temozolomide for newly diagnosed glioblastoma: mature progression-free survival and preliminary overall survival results in AVAglio. *Neuro-Oncology* 2012; **14**(Suppl 6): vi101–5.

29. Kreisl TN, Kim L, Moore K *et al.* Phase II trial of single-agent bevacizumab followed by bevacizumab plus irinotecan at tumor progression in recurrent glioblastoma. *Journal of Clinical Oncology* 2009; **27**(5): 740–5.

30. National Cancer Institute (NCI). *PDQ (Physician Data Query)—NCI's comprehensive cancer database.* Available at: <http://www.cancer.gov/cancertopics/pdq>. Accessed 6 May 2013.

21 Thyroid cancer and radioiodine therapy

David K Woolf

Expert commentary Nicola Dallas

Case history

A 38-year-old female presented to her GP with a 6-week history of a lump in the neck which had not noticeably changed in size or consistency over this time. It was slightly uncomfortable, but not painful, and was not associated with any other symptoms. The patient was otherwise fit and well, with no other significant medical history. She was not taking any regular medications and was allergic to penicillin causing a rash. She had no significant family history and was married, with a 2-year-old daughter. They lived in a two-bedroom flat, and she worked as a primary school teacher.

Examination revealed a diffuse mass to the left of the midline, which moved on swallowing and was felt to be consistent with a thyroid lump. The patient was clinically euthyroid, and there was no local lymphadenopathy or other clinical signs detected on systemic review. Routine blood tests, including thyroid function tests, were reported as normal.

A referral was made to the 'lump in neck clinic' at the local hospital. The patient was reviewed 2 weeks later in clinic, and an ultrasound (USS) of the neck and an FNA of the suspicious mass arranged. The results were reviewed in the MDT meeting, which included a consultant thyroid surgeon, radiologist, pathologist, endocrinologist, clinical oncologist, and specialist nurse. The USS had demonstrated a 2.5 cm predominately solid and hyperechoic mass with microcalcification in the left side of the thyroid gland. The associated lymph nodes within the neck were reported as normal. An FNA of the thyroid mass was classified as being Thy4, therefore suspicious for papillary carcinoma. The MDT recommended a total thyroidectomy without neck dissection. Details of the suspected diagnosis, operation, and associated risks were explained to the patient and her husband. The likelihood of needing radioactive iodine treatment after the operation was also introduced.

✪ Learning point Classification of thyroid cancer and prognostic factors

Thyroid cancer makes up over 95% of all cancers of the endocrine system and is becoming more common, with a 2.3-fold increase over the past 30 years. It is three times more common in females, with the peak incidence 1–2 decades earlier than in men.

Papillary cancer is the commonest histological subtype of thyroid cancer, accounting for 79% of thyroid malignancies. Less common tumour types include: follicular (13%), Hurthle (2%), medullary (4%), and anaplastic (2%) cancers [1].

The 5-year survival rate for the disease in women is 97.4%, and the most important prognostic indicators are histology, with papillary being the most favourable. Other favourable factors include smaller tumour size and earlier stage, lack of distant metastasis, female gender, and being under the age of 45.

> ⓱ **Expert comment**
>
> Whilst the incidence of thyroid cancer is increasing, this is likely to be related to improved imaging techniques and the use of neck ultrasonography. In addition, 16% of CT and MRI scans identify incidental thyroid nodules, 10% of which will turn out to be malignant. Approximately 90% of thyroid cancers are low-risk small papillary cancers which may never progress to cause symptoms or death. This explains the fact that, whilst the incidence is increasing, the death rate remains the same. There is therefore a concern that low-risk tumours are being overtreated [2].

Two weeks later, the patient was admitted for surgery. The surgery was completed successfully, with the recurrent laryngeal nerve being identified and preserved, as were the parathyroid glands and the external branch of the superior laryngeal nerves. A post-operative laryngeal cord check was normal. Routine post-operative blood tests, including serum calcium levels, were normal, so the patient was commenced on liothyronine sodium (T3) at a dose of 20 micrograms three times a day and discharged, with a follow-up appointment 2 weeks later.

> ➕ **Clinical tip** Complications associated with thyroidectomy
>
> - Infection.
> - Bleeding.
> - Anaesthetic risks.
> - Pain at the operation site.
> - Scarring.
> - Need for temporary surgical drains.
> - Vocal cord paralysis following damage to the recurrent laryngeal nerve.
> - Hypothyroidism requiring lifelong thyroxine replacement.
> - Temporary or permanent hypoparathyroidism resulting from trauma to, or removal of, the parathyroid glands at the time of surgery.

> ✅ **Evidence base** Extent of surgery affects survival for papillary thyroid cancer [5]
>
> - Retrospective review of 52 173 patients undergoing thyroid surgery for papillary cancer between 1985 and 1998.
> - Those with tumours ≥1 cm having a lobectomy, rather than a total thyroidectomy, had a 15% higher risk of recurrence and 31% higher risk of death.
> - There was no difference between lobectomy and total thyroidectomy for tumours <1 cm.
>
> *Source*: data from Bilimoria KY *et al.*, Extent of Surgery Affects Survival for Papillary Thyroid Cancer, *Annals of Surgery*, Volume 246, Number 3, pp. 375–84, Copyright © 2007 by Lippincott Williams & Wilkins.

> ⭐ **Learning point** Surgery in thyroid cancer
>
> There is significant controversy with regard to the extent of both the thyroidectomy and the nodal dissection that should be performed. The consensus is that low-risk node-negative papillary and follicular carcinomas which are <1 cm should be offered a lobectomy, rather than a total thyroidectomy. Those with a follicular tumour between 1 and 4 cm may be considered for a lobectomy, rather than total thyroidectomy, if they are otherwise low risk, at the discretion of the MDT and after discussion with the patient [3].
>
> The intention of surgery is to:
>
> - remove the primary disease
> - minimize treatment-induced morbidity
> - allow accurate histological diagnosis and staging
> - facilitate the appropriate use of radioactive iodine
> - allow long-term surveillance with serum thyroglobulin (Tg) and whole-body scans, as appropriate,
> - reduce the chances of disease recurrence and spread [4].
>
> Retrospective data have shown that patients with tumours >1 cm have a better outcome with a total thyroidectomy versus a lobectomy. This difference is particularly noticeable in patients with tumours >3 cm [5]. Other factors, including tumour histology, age, and sex, also need to be considered when making this decision.

> ⭐ **Learning point** Neck dissection in thyroid cancer
>
> Another surgical conundrum is when to offer a patient a neck dissection. The latest UK guidelines [3] suggest that patients who have papillary carcinoma are 'high risk' if any of the following are present:
>
> - male gender
> - age >45 years
> - tumour over 4 cm
> - extracapsular? spread,
> - extrathyroid disease.
>
> These patients should be offered a level VI node dissection (pre- and paratracheal lymph nodes). A selective lateral neck dissection (IIa–Vb) should be offered when disease is found in the lateral neck on preoperative imaging/biopsy or during surgery.

MDT review of the pathology revealed a multifocal papillary thyroid cancer, with the maximal size being 26 mm, no extension beyond the capsule or into extrathyroid tissues, and no lymphovascular invasion. A decision was therefore made to proceed to radioactive iodine ablation.

The patient was admitted to the ward. Her baseline bloods were all within the normal range. The consultant clinical oncologist, with an ARSAC (Administration of Radioactive Substances Advisory Committee) licence, authorized a prescription of radioiodine, a capsule with a dose of 3.7 GBq of iodine-131. On day 2, she experienced an episode of vomiting. The radiation protection supervisor (RPS) was notified immediately, and an emergency decontamination procedure put into place. The patient's symptoms were then successfully managed with regular cyclizine.

> ✪ **Learning point** Radioactive iodine treatment
>
> **Rationale**
>
> - To ablate the remaining thyroid cells.
> - To increase the chance of cure.
> - To facilitate improved monitoring with the use of serum Tg.
>
> **Preparation**
>
> - Patients should be on a low-iodine diet for 2 weeks prior to treatment (avoiding, e.g. glacé cherries, fish, kelp, and seafood, and reducing dairy products).
> - Adequate hydration should be maintained.
> - T3 replacement should be withdrawn 2 weeks prior to treatment.
> - Thyroid function tests must be undertaken prior to treatment to ensure the TSH is adequately raised (>30 mIU/L), and a serum Tg to act as a baseline measurement.
> - Female patients must have a routine pregnancy test on the day of admission.
>
> **Treatment**
>
> - Patients are admitted to a lead-lined side room where a medical physics team member administers the treatment capsule.
> - Visitors are not permitted to avoid the risk of unnecessary radiation exposure.
> - Staff are able to attend to the patient but must do so briefly and avoid contact with bodily fluids.
> - High fluid intake and frequent showers are encouraged to increase the speed of excretion and removal of the radioactive iodine.
> - Daily radiation readings are taken, in order to establish when it is safe for the patient to be discharged. The average length of stay is 3 days.
> - On the day of discharge, a whole-body post-ablation uptake scan is conducted.
>
> **Side effects**
>
> - Dry mouth.
> - Altered taste.
> - Sialadenitis.
> - Neck discomfort or swelling.
> - Small increased risk of miscarriage over the next year.
> - Pregnancy should be avoided for 6–12 months after completion of RAI therapy.
> - Small risk of secondary malignancies.

> ✚ **Clinical tip** Use of radioactive iodine ablation (RAI)
>
> *RAI is recommended for:*
>
> - known distant or lymph node metastasis
> - any gross extrathyroid extension
> - primary tumour size of ≥2 cm.
>
> *RAI is not recommended for:*
>
> - unifocal cancer <1 cm without high-risk factors
> - multifocal cancers where all foci are <1 cm without high-risk factors.
>
> **High-risk factors**
>
> - Histological subtypes: tall cell, columnar, insular and solid variant of follicular, and Hurthle cell variants of differentiated thyroid cancer.
> - Intrathyroid vascular invasion.
> - Multifocal disease (gross or microscopic).

> ✚ **Clinical tip** ARSAC
>
> In order to administer a radioactive medicinal product in the UK, such as iodine-131, a doctor is required to hold a certificate issued by ARSAC. This is under the legal jurisdiction of Section 2 of the Medicines (Administration of Radioactive Substances) Regulations 1978.

> ❝ **Expert comment**
>
> Patients often tolerate thyroid hormone replacement withdrawal quite well, particularly for the first RAI where there may still be some endogenous hormone production. However, in patients who do not tolerate this, recombinant human TSH (rhTSH) can be used. Thyroid hormone replacement is continued, and the rhTSH administered as an IM injection on the 2 days prior to RAI. This has not been shown to adversely affect the efficacy of treatment [6].

✚ Clinical tip Discharge instructions

Following discharge, the patient must be instructed to:

- avoid circumstances which place them in prolonged (half an hour or more) close contact with others, e.g. public transport, cinema, theatre
- reduce time spent in close proximity to family members
- sleep in a separate room
- avoid sexual activity
- take time away from work.

The exact period for which restrictions need to be observed, following discharge, depends on the radiation levels measured and are explained by the medical physics team.

✪ Learning point (Acute Oncology) **The unwell patient having radioiodine treatment**

If a leakage of fluid occurs from the patient, e.g. vomiting or a spill of urine

- A decontamination kit should be deployed. It contains appropriate protective equipment, absorbent material for spills, and warning signs.
- Staff should wear personal dosimeters (preferably with real-time displays), whilst dealing with these situations.
- The responsible RPS should be notified immediately.
- The responsible clinician should be notified.
- The spilt fluid should be contained, using the decontamination kit, without allowing further contamination throughout the area.
- Pregnant members of staff should not be involved in this process.
- Safety of the patient and staff remains a priority.

If a patient becomes unwell having received RAI

- The patient's health is a priority and must be dealt with appropriately, whilst considering radiation protection.
- The RPS and responsible clinician should be informed.
- Protective equipment and a dosimeter should be worn by all staff involved in the patient's care, and pregnant staff should not be involved.
- If cardiopulmonary resuscitation is needed, then this should be administered using only the required number of staff. Patients can be transferred into a high dependency/intensive care environment, but a side room should be used.
- Emergency surgery can also be performed, but care should be taken to minimize the operating time, and dosimeters should again be worn.
- If any blood work is required, this may also be radioactive, and procedures for transferring this to the laboratory, as well as analysis, should be discussed with the RPS.
- Once the incident is over, dosimeters should be reviewed to assess the risk to staff. Iodine may be administered, if needed, which will reduce the risk of iodine-131 accumulation in the thyroid.
- Any equipment used should also be monitored to allow safe decontamination, as appropriate.
- If a patient dies, whilst receiving RAI, this should be discussed with the RPS, as monitoring of the body will be required to facilitate safe handling.

The patient was discharged home 2 days later, once her radiation levels were acceptable. A whole-body post-ablation uptake scan was performed, and she was restarted on liothyronine sodium (T3) 20 micrograms tds.

✔ Evidence base Retrospective review of the role of RAI and EBRT in papillary thyroid cancer [7]

- A total of 842 patients diagnosed between 1960 and 1997, with a mean follow-up of 9.2 years.
- The 10-year cause-specific survival by stage: stage I 99.8%, stage II 91.8%, stage III 77.4%. stage IV 37.1%.
- Poor prognostic factors were: age >45, post-operative gross disease, distant metastasis at presentation, lack of RAI.
- For patients without residual or metastatic disease: RAI improved locoregional control (RR = 0.29) and metastatic failure (RR = 0.2), but not cause-specific survival.
- EBRT was particularly useful in those with gross post-operative disease (10-year locoregional control 56% versus 24% without EBRT).

Source: data from *International Journal of Radiation Oncology*Biology*Physics*, Volume 52, Issue 3, Chow SM *et al.*, Papillary thyroid carcinoma: prognostic factors and the role of radioiodine and external radiotherapy, *Radiation Oncology Biology*, pp. 784–95, Copyright © 2002 Elsevier Inc. All rights reserved.

At the follow-up appointment, 6 weeks later, the post-ablation uptake scan was reviewed and reported as demonstrating uptake in the thyroid bed, with no evidence of metastatic disease (Figure 21.1). The patient was well and asymptomatic.

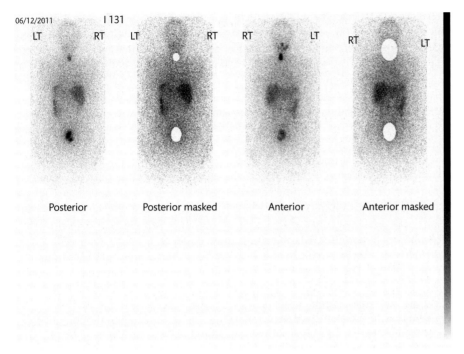

Figure 21.1 Whole-body iodine-131 post-ablation uptake scan after treatment with 3.7 GBq of iodine-131. Increased activity is projected over the thyroid bed, consistent with residual thyroid tissue at this site. The uptake seen in the salivary glands, liver, bowel, and urinary bladder is physiological. No metastatic disease is demonstrated.

A diagnostic whole-body iodine uptake scan was requested for 5 months after the RAI ablation. T3 withdrawal for 2 weeks prior to the scan is once again required. This scan was reported as normal, and the patient was converted to 150 micrograms of levothyroxine (T4) once a day and told to discontinue her three-times-a-day liothyronine sodium (T3).

The proposed follow-up regimen was explained, with 6-monthly clinic appointments for the first 2 years, and annually thereafter. Prior to each visit, routine blood tests, including thyroid function tests, calcium, and serum Tg, are performed. Clinical review included history and examination, paying particular attention to the neck and thyroid status.

Discussion

This case demonstrates a very common presentation of thyroid cancer and highlights a number of treatment decisions and management dilemmas that must be made throughout a patient's journey.

Once a diagnosis of thyroid cancer or suspected thyroid cancer has been made, based on imaging and the results of an FNA, including a Thy classification, surgery can be planned. As said previously, the extent of surgery remains controversial. In our patient with a 2.5 cm papillary carcinoma, a total thyroidectomy was performed; she was not offered a neck dissection, in keeping with her 'low-risk' preoperative disease status.

Following MDT discussion, the patient was offered, and proceeded to have, RAI. The use of iodine-131 remains controversial. Studies have either shown a lower relapse rate with RAI ablation or failed to show a benefit [8]. Patients with poor prognostic features are thought to have the most to gain from ablation therapy, in terms of improvement in relapse-free survival. The most recent European Society for Medical Oncology (ESMO) guidelines provide a useful guide of indications for thyroid remnant ablation [9]. The primary group of patients where no recommendations are made are the 1–2 cm tumours where the decision will rest with the treating clinicians and MDT in discussion with the patient.

The other area of uncertainty focusses on the use of thyrotropin alfa (recombinant human thyrotropin; rhTSH). Ordinarily, thyroid hormone replacement is withdrawn prior to the administration of RAI, in order to stimulate the uptake of the therapeutic iodine. Thyroxine (T4) treatment needs to be stopped 4 weeks prior to the administration of RAI, and liothyronine sodium (T3) 2 weeks prior. This induces hypothyroidism which, in some patients, is poorly tolerated, affecting their QoL significantly during this period. Alternatively, rhTSH stimulates the thyroid gland to take up the radioactive iodine without the need to stop hormone replacement and induce hypothyroidism. The HiLo study [6] looked at this question by randomizing patients between thyroid hormone withdrawal and thyrotropin alfa. The conclusion was that the use of thyrotropin alfa did not compromise the efficacy of treatment but showed a non-significant benefit, in terms of adverse effects.

> **❝ Expert comment**
>
> Once a decision to proceed to RAI ablation has been made, there exist two significant areas of uncertainty regarding its administration. The first is the required dose of RAI to successfully achieve ablation. The standard UK dose is considered to be 3.7 GBq (100 mCi), although, in Europe and the US, there is a tendency to use a reduced dose. This has the advantage of a reduced inpatient stay and isolation, reduced side effects, including a lower radiation dose, and reduced theoretical risk of a secondary malignancy. The HiLo study [6] randomized patients between a high dose of 3.7 GBq and a low dose of 1.1 GBq RAI ablation therapy and found no statistical difference between the two arms when measured at 6–9 months post-ablation. Follow-up of this cohort of patients continues.

> **✔ Evidence base** HiLo: high-dose, compared to low-dose, RAI therapy [6]
>
> - Low-dose RAI (1.1 Gbq) versus high-dose RAI (3.7 Gbq) for thyroid ablation.
> - Thyrotropin alfa pre-ablation versus thyroid hormone withdrawal.
> - Randomized non-inferiority factorial allocation of 438 patients to one of these four groups.
> - T1–3N0–1M0 differentiated thyroid cancer.
> - Ablation success of 85.0% in low dose versus 88.9% in high dose.
> - Ablation success of 87.1% in the thyrotropin alfa group versus 86.7% in thyroid hormone withdrawal group.
> - Statistically, all treatments non-inferior.
> - Adverse effects of 21% in low dose versus 33% in high dose ($p = 0.007$).
> - Adverse effects of 23% in the thyrotropin alfa group versus 30% in thyroid hormone withdrawal group ($p = 0.11$).
>
> *Source*: data from Mallick U et al., Ablation with low-dose radioiodine and thyrotropin alfa in thyroid cancer, *New England Journal of Medicine*, Volume 366, Number 18, pp. 1674–85, Copyright © 2012 Massachusetts Medical Society. All rights reserved.

✪ Learning point Long-term follow-up

Following successful completion of initial therapy, the patient is entered into a follow-up protocol. The aim of this is to monitor for any recurrence and detect it early, whilst managing any long-term symptoms or side effects induced by treatment.

Blood tests are reviewed at each visit, and, in particular, the dose of levothyroxine (T4) is adjusted to ensure that TSH is well suppressed (below 0.1 mIU/L). This reduces the stimulatory effects of TSH on any remaining thyroid tissue. Regular monitoring of serum Tg levels are also undertaken, as, provided surgery and ablation therapy has been successful, this will allow early indication of disease recurrence, as they should remain undetectable.

➕ Clinical tip Avoid contrast-enhanced scans

- Most contrast agents contain iodine.
- These should be avoided, if at all possible, as the large quantity of iodine means iodine-131 cannot be used to full effect for up to 3 months.

❝ Expert comment

When converting a patient from T3 hormone replacement to once-a-day thyroxine, a dose of 150 micrograms is a sensible starting point. Thyroid function tests should then be monitored 6- to 8-weekly, until TSH suppression is achieved. This will result inevitably in a slightly high free T4 in the mid to late twenties which is acceptable, as long as it is tolerated clinically by the patient. It is important to write to the patient's GP to explain the need for this apparent over-replacement of thyroid hormone; otherwise, there is a tendency for the dose of thyroxine to be reduced in the community. In low-risk patients who are unable to tolerate complete TSH suppression, a TSH between 0.1 mIU/L and 0.5 mIU/L is acceptable.

✪ Learning point Thyroglobulin (Tg)

- Thyroglobulin (Tg) is a glycosylated protein produced by the thyroid gland and plays a role in the production of thyroid hormones.
- It can be used as a tumour marker in differentiated thyroid cancer and has been the cornerstone of post-operative surveillance for decades [10].
- If all thyroid tissue has been removed by surgery and RAI, then finding a detectable level of Tg is highly specific for tumour recurrence.
- It is not a useful marker in the preoperative diagnostic setting.
- It can take many weeks after surgery for Tg levels to become suppressed or undetectable.
- Tg measurements can be complicated by anti-Tg antibodies giving a false negative reading. This issue can be addressed by testing for the antibodies, which are present in about 15% of the population.
- Provided Tg levels become very low or undetectable post-surgery, it is a sensitive test for disease relapse and should therefore be measured during routine follow-up.
- Tg sensitivity for recurrent disease is up to 65%, with a specificity of 86% [11], and increasing levels noted on serial tests has a positive predictive value of almost 100% [10].

In the event of a relapse, it is important to stage the disease accurately, in particular with a diagnostic whole-body iodine uptake scan and a non-contrast-enhanced CT scan. Depending on the site of relapse, the option of curative treatment with further surgery, RAI, and/or EBRT should be considered. If advanced metastatic or non-curative disease is present, then repeated treatments with RAI can be used to control the disease, with careful monitoring of the effects on the bone marrow. With this treatment, survival can be prolonged. However, if the disease does not concentrate iodine, then other systemic therapies, such as chemotherapy and TKIs, have, in selected cases, been shown to have activity.

❝ Expert comment

Whilst the majority of patients who are diagnosed with differentiated thyroid cancer can be cured, some will present with advanced metastatic disease and some will go on to develop iodine-refractory disease. Cytotoxic chemotherapy has been a limited option in the past, with doxorubicin consistently being shown to be the most active agent, with response rates of up to 22% at significant cost in terms of toxicity. More recently, TKIs have been shown to have activity, often better tolerated with, in some series, up to a third of patients achieving stable disease [12].

A final word from the expert

The incidence of differentiated thyroid cancer is increasing, with the vast majority of cases being of low risk, carrying an excellent prognosis. Here, the role of the multidisciplinary approach to case management is illustrated. The combination of surgery and RAI is certainly indicated for tumours larger than, or equal to, 2 cm in maximal diameter, but the challenge is not to overtreat the population with low-risk tumours who will live for many decades, with the consequences of treatment requiring lifelong hormone replacement and monitoring.

References

1. Sipos JA, Mazzaferri EL. Thyroid cancer epidemiology and prognostic variables. *Clinical Oncology* 2010; **22**(6): 395–404.
2. Brito JP, Morris JC, Montori VM. Thyroid cancer: zealous imaging has increased detection and treatment of low risk tumours. *BMJ* 2013; **347**: f4706.
3. British Thyroid Association, Royal College of Physicians. *Guidelines for the management of thyroid cancer*, 2nd edn. Report of the Thyroid Cancer Guidelines Update Group. London: Royal College of Physicians, 2007.
4. American Thyroid Association (ATA) Guidelines Taskforce on Thyroid Nodules and Differentiated Thyroid Cancer, Cooper DS, Doherty GM *et al.* Revised American Thyroid Association management guidelines for patients with thyroid nodules and differentiated thyroid cancer. *Thyroid* 2009; **19**(11): 1167–214.
5. Bilimoria KY, Bentrem DJ, Ko CY *et al.* Extent of surgery affects survival for papillary thyroid cancer. *Annals of Surgery* 2007; **246**(3): 375–84.
6. Mallick U, Harmer C, Yap B *et al.* Ablation with low-dose radioiodine and thyrotropin alfa in thyroid cancer. *The New England Journal of Medicine* 2012; **366**(18): 1674–85.
7. Chow SM, Law SCK, Mendenhall WM *et al.* Papillary thyroid carcinoma: prognostic factors and the role of radioiodine and external radiotherapy. *International Journal Radiation Oncology "Biology" Physics* 2002; **52**: 784–95.
8. Clarke SEM. Radioiodine therapy in differentiated thyroid cancer: a nuclear medicine perspective. *Clinical Oncology* 2010; **22**(6): 430–7.
9. Pacini F, Castagna MG, Brilli L, Pentheroudakis G; ESMO Guidelines Working Group. Thyroid cancer: ESMO Clinical Practice Guidelines for diagnosis, treatment and follow-up. *Annals of Oncology* 2012; **23**(Suppl 7): vii110–19.
10. Durante C, Conante G, Filetti S. Differentiated thyroid carcinoma: defining new paradigms for postoperative management. *Endocrine-Related Cancer* 2013; **20**(4): 141–54.
11. Schlumberger M, Hitzel A, Toubert ME *et al.* Comparison of seven serum thyroglobulin assays in the follow-up of papillary and follicular thyroid cancer patients. *The Journal of Clinical Endocrinology & Metabolism* 2007; **92**(7): 2487–95.
12. Chougnet C, Brassard M, Leboulleux S, Baudin E, Schlumberger M. Molecular targeted therapies for patients with refractory thyroid cancer. *Clinical Oncology* 2010; **22**(6): 448–55.

22 Neuroendocrine tumours and treatment complications

Angela Lamarca

 Expert commentary Juan W Valle

Case history

A 36-year-old man initially presented with fatigue and weight loss. Multiple investigations were performed to determine the aetiology of the non-specific presentation, and a CT scan demonstrated a potentially resectable lesion in the tail of the pancreas. Following MDT discussion, surgical management, with a distal pancreatectomy and splenectomy, was discussed with the patient. At the time of surgery, however, unresectable liver metastases were found, and a palliative partial resection of the

---

✪ Learning point Clinical presentation and diagnosis

Most functional NETs are diagnosed as a consequence of symptoms associated with excess hormone secretion (Table 22.1). Non-functional NETs may present with symptoms relating to the primary tumour (e.g. bowel obstruction, weight loss, bleeding, or fatigue).

Table 22.1 Subtypes of functional NETs

NET subtype	Most frequent location	Secreted hormone (biomarker)	Symptoms
Carcinoid tumour	Small bowel	Serotonin (blood and urine 5-hydroxyindoleacetic acid, 5-HIAA)	Flushing, diarrhoea, wheezing, valvular heart disease
Insulinoma	Pancreas	Insulin (serum insulin level)	Hypoglycaemia
Gastrinoma	Pancreas	Gastrin (serum gastrin)	Gastric or duodenal ulcer
Glucagonoma	Pancreas	Glucagon (serum glucagon)	Necrolytic migratory erythema, diabetes
Somatostatinoma	Pancreas	Somatostatin (serum somatostatin)	Steatorrhoea, gallstones
VIPoma	Pancreas	Vasoactive intestinal polypeptide (serum VIP)	Watery diarrhoea, hypochlorhydria, hypokalaemia
Phaeochromocytoma and paraganglioma	Adrenal gland and lymph nodes	Catecholamines (norepinephrine and/or epinephrine) (24-hour urinary metanephrines and catecholamines)	Hypertension, headache

---

⊗ Learning point Classification of NETs

NETs arise from neuroendocrine cells, which are widely distributed throughout the body and produce hormones to regulate normal physiological function. They most commonly arise in the intestine. These gastroenteropancreatic (GEP) NETs vary considerably in their hormone functionality, the clinical presentation, and their biological behaviour.

GEP-NETs can be classified into several groups, according to the location, symptoms, hormone secretion, and pathology characteristics (Figure 22.1):

- functional NETs (40%)—secrete inappropriate amounts of glycopeptide hormones and active amines
- non-functional NETs (60%)—which do not secrete hormones.

This classification has a direct impact on patient management. Tumour functionality is defined by the existence of symptoms and serological data (see serum biomarkers).

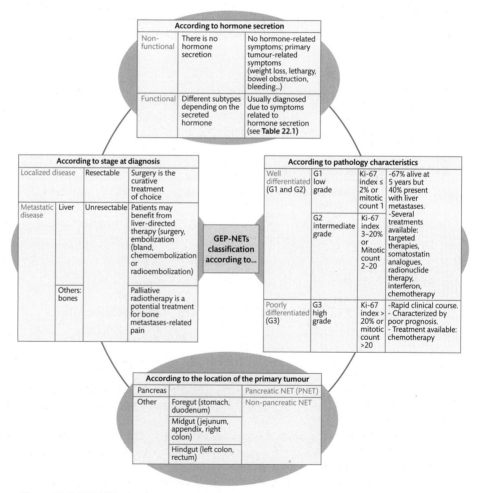

Figure 22.1 GEP-NETs classification according to the location, hormone secretion, stage, and pathology.

❝ Expert comment

Another factor to consider is the presence or absence of disease progression.

If a patient's tumour is very indolent (e.g. well-differentiated tumours with low Ki-67), with no evidence of disease progression of metastatic disease, a period of 'active monitoring' without therapy may be appropriate.

pancreatic mass was performed. Histologically, this was a well-differentiated pancreatic NET (PNET), grade 2 (with a proliferation index of 5%, as measured by Ki-67).

A post-operative octreotide scan showed uptake in the liver (in keeping with the known metastatic disease) and at the resection site (in keeping with post-operative inflammation). The local multi-disciplinary team (MDT) therefore recommended two treatments with indium-labelled octreotide, completed at 6 and 8 months after surgery. The patient achieved a partial response to therapy. The liver lesions became resectable, based on imaging, and a left lateral partial hepatectomy was performed.

➕ **Clinical tip** Mitotic count

The WHO/European Neuroendocrine Tumor Society (ENETS) guidelines specify that cell counting is to be performed on 40–50 high power fields, and 2000 cells should be counted to determine the Ki-67 index [1]. However, instead of the Ki-67 index, mitotic count (/10 high power fields) can also be employed.

✱ **Learning point** Management of liver metastases

Patients with liver metastases may become symptomatic from hormone hypersecretion, rather than from tumour bulk. Symptoms of hormonal excess can often be well controlled with systemic therapy such as somatostatin analogues. However, liver-directed therapies may be considered when the symptoms are resistant to somatostatin analogues or other systemic therapies, i.e. targeted therapies or chemotherapy, such as:

- surgery for potentially resectable liver metastases in the absence of diffuse bilobar involvement, compromised liver function, or inoperable extra-hepatic metastases
- hepatic arterial embolization in patients with hepatic-predominant metastatic cancer. Embolization of the hepatic artery can be performed by different techniques and aims to target tumour cells, which derive their blood supply from the hepatic artery, and not healthy hepatocytes which are supplied by the portal vein (PV):
  ○ bland embolization: infusion of gel foam powder into the hepatic artery through an angiography catheter
  ○ chemo-embolization: infusion of gel foam powder into the hepatic artery, in conjunction with chemotherapy
  ○ radioembolization: radioactive isotopes (e.g. yttrium-90) tagged to glass or resin microspheres and delivered selectively to the tumour via the hepatic artery
- ablation, using radiofrequency, microwaves, or now less commonly cryoablation, may be performed percutaneously or laparoscopically and may be applicable only to small lesions (up to 3 cm).

➕ **Clinical tip** Staging investigations

All patients should undergo a biopsy, a full-body CT scan, an octreotide scan, chromogranin A (CgA), urine 5-HIAA (midgut or unknown primary tumours), and fasting gut peptides (particularly PNETs) for diagnosis and staging assessment. In any biopsy recognized as having NET-like morphological features, the proliferative activity (Ki-67) should be determined. Additional investigations, depending on the presentation of the patient, may include MRI of the liver, bone scan, PET scan, echocardiogram, and meta-iodobenzylguanidine (MIBG) scan.

Three-monthly follow-up CT scans showed no evidence of disease, until 1 year later when he developed new liver metastases. The patient then received systemic chemotherapy with streptozocin, combined with 5-FU over 6 months, which stabilized the tumour growth for the following 7 years.

After this period, he developed progressive disease and was commenced on interferon-alpha (IFN) (3 MU, s/c by self-injection three times a week), which achieved stabilization of the disease on follow-up scans.

A year later, the patient was referred to the specialist NET team for discussion of further treatment options. On review, the patient was of PS 0, with symptoms of mild fatigue only. Blood tests were unremarkable, and a urinary 5-HIAA measurement

❝ Expert comment

Although this patient received radionuclide therapy at this point for his advanced disease, the sequence of this and subsequent systemic therapies is largely interchangeable. However, curative surgery is the treatment of choice in the presence of localized disease (including resectable metastatic disease).

✪ **Learning point** Biomarkers

Both tissue and serum/urine biomarkers may be used for diagnosis, monitoring the response to treatment, and surveillance for recurrence of patients with resected NETs (Table 22.1).

Tissue biomarkers

- Neuroendocrine differentiation markers CgA and synaptophysin can be demonstrated by IHC on paraffin-embedded tissue.

Serum/urine biomarkers

- *Serum CgA* is currently the most widespread serum biomarker for the diagnosis of GEP-NETs, with a diagnostic sensitivity of 60%. Levels tend to correlate with tumour volume, and therefore it is particularly useful for monitoring the response to treatment.
- *5-HIAA* (the metabolite of 5-hydroxytryptamine, or serotonin) is the most useful test for the diagnosis of carcinoid syndrome, with a sensitivity of over 70% and a specificity of close to 100%. Measurement, with 24-hour urine collections, requires appropriate dietary modifications. False positive elevations are caused by the intake of certain foods or drugs that contain the precursor of 5-HIAA (i.e. bananas, pineapple, tomatoes, plums, eggplant, kiwi, nuts).
- *Serum 5-HIAA* (recently introduced) has a good correlation with 24-hour urinary levels [2] and is more patient-friendly.

✪ **Learning point** Radiological investigations in NETs

- *Cross-sectional imaging* by CT and MRI is extensively used for the identification of patients with resectable disease and for reassessment after therapy.
- *Octreotide scanning*, employing the radioactive tracer[111]In-D-Phe-octreotide, is highly sensitive for detecting tissue with somatostatin receptors. It is the standard tool for the diagnosis, localization, staging, and screening of patients eligible for treatment with octreotide-based radionuclide therapy.
- *MIBG scintigraphy*, with ^{123}I-MIBG, a noradrenaline analogue, is the investigation of choice for phaeochromocytomas or paragangliomas. It may also be useful in selecting GEP-NET patients eligible for ^{131}I-MIBG therapy.
- *PET* is useful due to the existence of a very active amino acid transporter and hormone receptors in NET cells. These tumours demonstrate a high affinity for [68]Gallium or ^{18}F-DOPA which are used in PET. Poorly differentiated NETs tend to show high activity with radiopharmaceuticals such as ^{18}F-FDG.

✪ **Learning point** Systemic treatment

Patients with metastases often have disseminated disease involving the liver, lymph nodes, bones, or lungs as the commonest sites. In such cases, systemic therapy may be indicated.

1. *Somatostatin analogues*

   Endogenous somatostatin is a very short-acting 14-amino acid peptide that acts by binding to somatostatin receptors and inhibiting the secretion of a broad range of hormones. Somatostatin analogues, such as octreotide and lanreotide, are valuable for the management of tumours that express somatostatin receptors (octreotide scan 'positive') as they reduce tumour-related hormone secretion and associated symptoms. Somatostatin analogues are highly effective in controlling the symptoms associated with carcinoid tumours, VIPomas, and glucagonomas. Efficacy is less predictable for symptomatic insulinomas.

   Long-acting depot (monthly injection) preparations of octreotide (IM) and lanreotide (deep s/c) are available to avoid daily injections and are considered a standard approach for symptomatic treatment of advanced NETs. Both are usually well tolerated, and side effects are generally mild (nausea, bloating, abdominal discomfort, steatorrhoea, and gallstones). Although symptom control has historically been the principal aim of these treatments, there is emerging evidence that somatostatin analogues also control tumour progression [3,4].

2. *Systemic radionuclide therapy*
   Targeted radiotherapy, using radiolabelled somatostatin analogues, can be used for patients with avid tracer uptake on their octreotide scan. The most frequently used radionuclides include yttrium (^{90}Y) and lutetium (^{177}Lu) [5,6]. Usually, more than a single dose of treatment is needed; the most frequent side effects are renal impairment, pancytopenia, and myelodysplastic syndrome. MIBG is a compound resembling norepinephrine which, until the advent of yttrium and lutetium, was the only radionuclide option. For selected patients, where uptake is preferential with ^{123}I-MIBG, rather than octreotide, ^{131}I-MIBG therapy may be considered.

3. *Interferon (IFN)*
   IFN has the ability to stimulate T-cell function, controlling the secretion of tumour products, and therefore has been employed for the treatment of NETs in patients with carcinoid syndrome. In addition, IFN can inhibit tumour growth by activation of the T-cell response against the tumour and inhibition of angiogenesis. IFN has been shown to reduce symptoms related to hormone secretion in 40–50% of patients and result in a partial response rate of 10%, with disease stabilization seen in 20–40% of patients [7].

4. *Systemic chemotherapy*
   Chemotherapy is the standard treatment of choice in patients with high-grade (G3) tumours; most of whom are diagnosed with advanced/metastatic disease. The choice is usually a platinum/etoposide combination for patients with a very high Ki-67 (e.g. over 55%) [8] or with streptozocin, fluoropyrimidine or temozolomide-based combinations in patients with Ki-67 values of 20–55%.

   Chemotherapy is also used in patients with well-differentiated (G1-2) pancreatic NETs, particularly in the presence of a high tumour burden, progressive disease or higher Ki-67 (e.g. closer to 20%).

   Chemotherapy has a minor role in patients with well-differentiated intestinal NETs as studies have shown poor responses to treatment. However, for selected cases, it may be an appropriate option.

Table 22.2 Chemotherapy in NETs

Chemotherapy	Type of trial	NET type	Number of patients	Response rate (%)	Median PFS (months)	Median OS (months)	References
Chlorozotocin versus streptozocin and FU versus doxorubicin and streptozocin	Phase III	Pancreatic	33/33/36	30/45/69	17/14/18	18/16.8/26.4	Moertel et al. [9]
Temozolomide and capecitabine	Retrospective analysis	Pancreatic	30	70	18	NR	Strosberg et al. [10]
Streptozocin, doxorubicin, and FU	Retrospective analysis	Pancreatic	84	39	18	37	Kouvaraki et al. [11]
Dacarbazine	Phase II	Non-pancreatic	56	16	–	20	Bukowski et al. [12]
FU and doxorubicin versus streptozocin and FU	Phases II/III	Non-pancreatic	88/88	15.9/16	4.5/5.3	15.7/24.3	Sun et al. [13]

Clinical tip Chemotherapy for GEP-NETs

For patients with high-grade NETs, combination chemotherapy with etoposide and a platinum agent are usually recommended.

For patients with well-differentiated (especially G2) tumours, one of the most effective drugs is streptozocin, and its combination with FU is widely used. Retrospective analysis of a combination of temozolomide and capecitabine has also been reported recently; this has not yet been validated in a prospective phase III study.

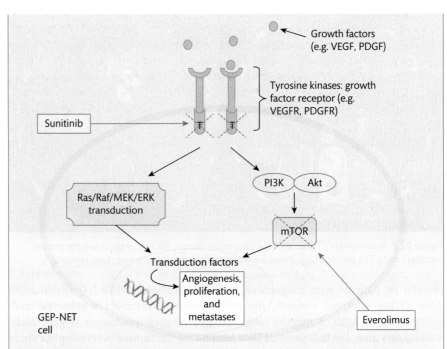

Figure 22.3 Pathway inhibition and anti-tumour effect due to the anti-targeted therapies: sunitinib and everolimus.

Table 22.3 Clinical trials employing targeted therapies for GEP-NETs

Target therapy	NET type	Trial type	Number of patients	Response rate (%)	Median PFS (months)	Reference
Sunitinib	PNETs	Phase II	66	17	7.7	Kulke et al. [15]
	Non-PNETs		41	2	10.2	
Everolimus versus placebo	Non-PNETs	Phase III (RADIANT 2 study)	216/213	2/2	16.4/11.3	Pavel et al. [16]
Sunitinib versus placebo	PNETs	Phase III	86/85	9/0	11.4/5.5	Raymond et al. [14]
Everolimus versus placebo	PNETs	Phase III (RADIANT 3 study)	207/203	5/2	11/4.6	Yao et al. [17]
Everolimus versus placebo	Non-pancreatic, non-functional	Phase III (RADIANT 4 study)	Ongoing			

Source: data from Raymond E et al., Sunitinib malate for the treatment of pancreatic neuroendocrine tumors, *New England Journal Medicine*, Volume 364, Issue 6, pp. 501–513, Copyright © 2011 Massachusetts Medical Society. All rights reserved.

⊕ Clinical tip Sunitinib

- Dose: 37.5 mg od; one cycle = 28 days of treatment.
- Dose reduction may be considered if significant side effects appear during the treatment.
- Common side effects include: hypertension, renal toxicity (proteinuria), arterial thromboembolism, myocardial toxicity (left ventricular dysfunction, clinical heart failure), thyroid dysfunction, bleeding, myelosuppression, hand–foot skin reaction, hepatotoxicity, and muscle wasting.

⊕ Clinical tip Everolimus

- Dose: 10 mg od; one cycle = 28 days of treatment.
- Dose reduction may be considered if significant side effects appear.
- Common side effects include stomatitis, rash, fatigue, hyperglycaemia, and diarrhoea. Cases of everolimus-related pneumonitis have been described, and viral infections (such as viral hepatitis) may be reactivated.

⊘ Evidence base Phase III trial of sunitinib in metastatic PNETs [14]

- Continuous administration of sunitinib (37.5 mg daily) was compared to placebo.
- A total of 171 patients with progressive (within 12 months) metastatic PNETs.
- The median PFS was significantly longer with sunitinib (11.4 months versus 5.5 months).
- Hand–foot skin reaction and hypertension were the commonest side effects.

At this point, following the newly published results of the RADIANT 3 trial [17] (Table 22.3), treatment with everolimus (10 mg od) was commenced. At the start of treatment, the patient was of ECOG PS 2 and experiencing episodic GI bleeding from the primary pancreatic tumour. Repeated embolization controlled the bleeding, and treatment with everolimus was continued, without significant side effects. The patient remains on everolimus therapy to date, with stable disease on imaging, and improved PS (ECOG PS 1) and CgA (471 ng/mL). Treatment is planned until disease progression.

⊘ **Evidence base** Phase III, everolimus in PNETs: RADIANT 3 [17]

- Everolimus monotherapy (10 mg daily) was compared to best supportive care alone.
- Phase III trial of 410 patients with progressive (within 12 months) metastatic PNETs.
- Everolimus was associated with a significant prolongation in median PFS (11.0 months versus 4.6 months), compared to the placebo group.
- The treatment was mostly well tolerated, with grades 1–2 side effects (stomatitis, rash, diarrhoea, and tiredness). Severe stomatitis and hyperglycaemia were shown in <10% of the patients.

Source: data from Yao JC et al., Everolimus for advanced pancreatic neuroendocrine tumors, *New England Journal Medicine*, Volume 364, Issue 6, pp. 514–523, Copyright ©2011 Massachusetts Medical Society. All rights reserved.

Discussion

This case exemplifies the presentation of well-differentiated PNETs. Gastro-entero-pancreatic (GEP)-NETs are a different entity, with a different epidemiology and prognosis to GI adenocarcinomas. The median age at diagnosis is in the fifth decade. NETs can develop in the context of various syndromes, entailing a hereditary predisposition, such as multiple endocrine neoplasia type 1 (MEN-1) or VHL disease. In this case, the age at diagnosis may be 15 years younger.

GEP-NETs are relatively rare, although the incidence has been rising during the last years. Due to their indolent nature (particularly with G1 and G2 tumours), the prevalence is higher, particularly with the improvement in the treatment options; they are now the second most prevalent GI malignancy, after colorectal adenocarcinoma.

According to the Surveillance, Epidemiology, and End Results (SEER) Program in the US, a significant increase in the annual age-adjusted incidence of NETs from 1973 (1.09/100 000) to 2004 (5.25/100 000) was observed [18]. Forty-nine per cent of GEP-NETs are diagnosed at localized stages, whereas 27% display metastatic disease at presentation. The prognosis of NETs depends on many factors, including the primary tumour site (rectal sites have the best prognosis, and pancreatic sites the worst), the disease stage, the histopathological grade and proliferative index, and the resectability of the tumour (even in advanced disease). Overall, the median survival for patients with distant metastases from GEP-NETs varies between 2 and 5 years, depending on the series.

Several guidelines have been developed by the most important NET expert societies, such as ENETS (European Neuroendocrine Tumour Society) UKI NETS (UK and Ireland Neuroendocrine Tumour Society), NANETS (North American Neuroendocrine Tumor Society), and ESMO (European Society of Medical Oncology) summarizing the management of the NETs, according to the most up-to-date data [19–24]. It is recommended that one of these guidelines is used by treating clinicians; usually dependent on the geographical region, as these usually reflect the available treatment options licensed and funded for therapy.

❝ Expert comment

Following a diagnosis of NET, it is important to take a detailed family history, including a history of tumours as well as of hypercalcaemia or renal calculi (indicative of parathyroid tumours, part of MEN-1 syndrome).

The treatment of choice for a patient who has a localized GEP-NET tumour is surgery. The extent of resection depends on the site of origin, size of the primary tumour and extent of local invasiveness. Primary tumour resection in the case of small bowel NET is sometimes considered. These tumours are often associated with desmoplasia and fibrosis, which can result in intermittent small bowel obstruction and, in some cases, bowel ischaemia. Resection of the primary tumour, even in the presence of distant metastases (especially for primary tumours from the small bowel), may be recommended to reduce the potential for bowel obstruction, bleeding, or abdominal pain.

To date, there is no evidence available supporting adjuvant therapy after resection, and limited evidence to make recommendations for follow-up after resection. CT scans or MRI of the abdomen and pelvis, with biochemical follow-up, e.g. fasting gut peptides (for pancreatic tumours), urine/serum 5-HIAA (for midgut tumours), and serum CgA, are usually performed.

After demonstrating initial activity in PNETs in phase II trials, two large randomized placebo-controlled trials have been completed separately with everolimus (RADIANT 3) [2] and sunitinib [14], in patients with progressive PNETs. These two phase III trials independently demonstrated a significant improvement in PFS. To date, there are no current data to determine if particular patient subgroups benefit from one or the other treatment and the best way of scheduling the drugs, with respect to each other or other therapies, at disease progression.

⊕ Expert comment

Patients should be encouraged to participate in clinical trials to help address a number of unanswered questions:

- identification of biomarkers (e.g. blood test, imaging, or tissue marker) which may predict the benefit of an individual therapy
- identification of optimal sequence of therapies
- activity in earlier stage of the disease (e.g. as adjuvant therapy after curative surgery)
- efficacy outside the indication (e.g. non-GEP-NET primary tumours such as lung NETs)
- assessment of novel emerging therapies, based on ongoing molecular biology work.

In contrast, the evidence for everolimus and sunitinib in non-PNETs is less well established. One phase III trial showed no clear benefit for everolimus (RADIANT 2) [16], and an ongoing randomized trial (RADIANT 4) has completed recruitment of patients with non-PNETs and non-functional NETs to clarify the benefit of therapy with everolimus, compared to placebo, in this setting. No randomized trial has been completed for sunitinib in non-PNETs (the SUNLAND study ((NCT01731925) is currently ongoing for patients with progressive functional midgut NETs).

A final word from the expert

NETs are fascinating, in terms of their behaviour and the emerging novel treatment options, based on a better understanding of their molecular biology. Given the increasing incidence and relative high prevalence of patients with these tumours, clinicians need to be aware of the importance of their identification, accurate diagnosis, and staging. In order to achieve the best patient outcomes, patients should be managed by neuroendocrine specialists. Moreover, patients (as in our case) should be encouraged to participate in research aimed at improving our understanding of NETs, ultimately improving patient outcomes and survival.

References

1. Rindi G, Arnold R, Bosman FT *et al.* Nomenclature and classification of neuroendocrine neoplasms of the digestive system. In: Bosman TF, Carneiro F, Hruban RH, Theise ND, eds. *WHO classification of tumours of the digestive system*, 4th edn. Lyon: International Agency for Research on cancer (IARC), 2010; p. 13.

2. Tellez MR, Mamikunian G, O'Dorisio TM, Vinik AI, Woltering EA. A single fasting plasma 5-HIAA value correlates with 24-hour urinary 5-HIAA values and other biomarkers in midgut neuroendocrine tumors (NETs). *Pancreas* 2013; **42**(3): 405–10.

3. Rinke A, Muller HH, Schade-Brittinger C *et al.* Placebo-controlled, double-blind, prospective, randomized study on the effect of octreotide LAR in the control of tumor growth in patients with metastatic neuroendocrine midgut tumors: a report from the PROMID Study Group. *Journal of Clinical Oncology* 2009; **27**(28): 4656–63.

4. Caplin M, Pavel M, Ćwikła J *et al.* Lanreotide in Metastatic Enteropancreatic Neuroendocrine Tumors *N Engl J Med* 2014;371:224-33. http://www.ncbi.nlm.nih.gov/pubmed/25014687.

5. Schillaci O, Corleto VD, Annibale B, Scopinaro F, Delle FG. Single photon emission computed tomography procedure improves accuracy of somatostatin receptor scintigraphy in gastro-entero pancreatic tumours. *Italian Journal of Gastroenterology and Hepatology* 1999; **31**(Suppl 2): S186–9.

6. Gibril F, Reynolds JC, Doppman JL *et al.* Somatostatin receptor scintigraphy: its sensitivity compared with that of other imaging methods in detecting primary and metastatic gastrinomas. A prospective study. *Annals of Internal Medicine* 1996; **125**(1): 26–34.

7. Faiss S, Pape UF, Bohmig M *et al.* Prospective, randomized, multicenter trial on the antiproliferative effect of lanreotide, interferon alfa, and their combination for therapy of metastatic neuroendocrine gastroenteropancreatic tumors—the International Lanreotide and Interferon Alfa Study Group. *Journal of Clinical Oncology* 2003; **21**(14): 2689–96.

8. Mitry E, Baudin E, Ducreux M *et al.* Treatment of poorly differentiated neuroendocrine tumours with etoposide and cisplatin. *British Journal of Cancer* 1999; **81**(8): 1351–5.

9. Moertel CG, Lefkopoulo M, Lipsitz S, Hahn RG, Klaassen D. Streptozocin-doxorubicin, streptozocin-fluorouracil or chlorozotocin in the treatment of advanced islet-cell carcinoma. *The New England Journal of Medicine* 1992; **326**(8): 519–23.

10. Strosberg JR, Fine RL, Choi J *et al.* First-line chemotherapy with capecitabine and temozolomide in patients with metastatic pancreatic endocrine carcinomas. *Cancer* 2011; **117**(2): 268–75.

11. Kouvaraki MA, Ajani JA, Hoff P *et al.* Fluorouracil, doxorubicin, and streptozocin in the treatment of patients with locally advanced and metastatic pancreatic endocrine carcinomas. *Journal of Clinical Oncology* 2004; **22**(23): 4762–71.

12. Bukowski RM, Tangen CM, Peterson RF *et al.* Phase II trial of dimethyltriazenoimidazole carboxamide in patients with metastatic carcinoid. A Southwest Oncology Group study. *Cancer* 1994; **73**(5): 1505–8.

13. Sun W, Lipsitz S, Catalano P, Mailliard JA, Haller DG. Phase II/III study of doxorubicin with fluorouracil compared with streptozocin with fluorouracil or dacarbazine in the treatment of advanced carcinoid tumors: Eastern Cooperative Oncology Group Study E1281. *Journal of Clinical Oncology* 2005; **23**(22): 4897–904.

14. Raymond E, Dahan L, Raoul JL *et al.* Sunitinib malate for the treatment of pancreatic neuroendocrine tumors. *The New England Journal of Medicine* 2011; **364**(6): 501–13.

15. Kulke MH, Lenz HJ, Meropol NJ *et al.* Activity of sunitinib in patients with advanced neuroendocrine tumors. *Journal of Clinical Oncology* 2008; **26**(20): 3403–10.

16. Pavel ME, Hainsworth JD, Baudin E *et al.* Everolimus plus octreotide long-acting repeatable for the treatment of advanced neuroendocrine tumours associated with carcinoid syndrome (RADIANT-2): a randomised, placebo-controlled, phase 3 study. *The Lancet* 2011; **378**(9808): 2005–12.

17. Yao JC, Shah MH, Ito T *et al.* Everolimus for advanced pancreatic neuroendocrine tumors. *The New England Journal of Medicine* 2011; **364**(6): 514–23.

18. Yao JC, Hassan M, Phan A *et al.* One hundred years after 'carcinoid': epidemiology of and prognostic factors for neuroendocrine tumors in 35,825 cases in the United States. *Journal of Clinical Oncology* 2008; **26**(18): 3063–72.

19. Salazar R, Wiedenmann B, Rindi G, Ruszniewski P. ENETS 2011 Consensus Guidelines for the Management of Patients with Digestive Neuroendocrine Tumors: an update. *Neuroendocrinology* 2012; **95**(2): 71–3.

20. Ramage JK, Ahmed A, Ardill J *et al.* Guidelines for the management of gastroenteropancreatic neuroendocrine (including carcinoid) tumours (NETs). *Gut* 2012; **61**(1): 6–32.

21. Anthony LB, Strosberg JR, Klimstra DS *et al.* The NANETS consensus guidelines for the diagnosis and management of gastrointestinal neuroendocrine tumors (nets): well-differentiated nets of the distal colon and rectum. *Pancreas* 2010; **39**(6): 767–74.

22. Boudreaux JP, Klimstra DS, Hassan MM *et al.* The NANETS consensus guideline for the diagnosis and management of neuroendocrine tumors: well-differentiated neuroendocrine tumors of the Jejunum, Ileum, Appendix, and Cecum. *Pancreas* 2010; **39**(6): 753–66.

23. Kulke MH, Anthony LB, Bushnell DL *et al.* NANETS treatment guidelines: well-differentiated neuroendocrine tumors of the stomach and pancreas. *Pancreas* 2010; **39**(6): 735–52.

24. Oberg K, Knigge U, Kwekkeboom D, Perren A. Neuroendocrine gastro-entero-pancreatic tumors: ESMO Clinical Practice Guidelines for diagnosis, treatment and follow-up. *Annals of Oncology* 2012; **23**(Suppl 7): vii124–30.

23 HIV-associated malignancies

Kate Smith

ⓘ **Expert commentary** Mark Bower

Case history

A 36-year-old Nigerian man presented to his local emergency department (ED) with a 4-month history of fevers, nights sweats, and breathlessness. He had a past medical history of appropriately treated pulmonary *Mycobacterium tuberculosis* infection. He volunteered no other past medical history and took no regular medication. He had lived in the UK for 10 years and had not travelled outside the country during this time. He was married with two children.

On arrival, he was febrile (temperature 40°C), tachycardic, and hypotensive (BP 90/70 mmHg). The ED doctor noted extensive cervical, axillary, and inguinal lymphadenopathy, hepatosplenomegaly, and reduced air entry at both lung bases. Multiple discrete purple nodules, 2–4 cm in size, were evident over the dorsum of both feet and over his chest (Figure 23.1). Examination of his mouth demonstrated a solitary flat purple lesion on his hard palate.

Routine blood tests revealed anaemia, leucocytosis, thrombocytopenia, renal dysfunction, and an elevated CRP (Table 23.1). A peripheral blood film showed anisocytosis and poikilocytosis, with no malignant cells. A chest radiograph revealed bilateral pleural effusions. He was fluid-resuscitated and started on broad-spectrum antibiotics with piperacillin and tazobactam.

The general medical registrar was concerned the clinical findings were in keeping with a haematological malignancy and that the skin lesions were characteristic of Kaposi's sarcoma (KS). The patient was therefore consented for an HIV test, which confirmed HIV-1 positivity, and his management taken over by the specialist HIV team.

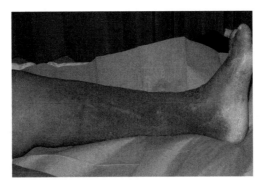

Figure 23.1 Typical Kaposi's sarcoma lesions.

Additional blood tests demonstrated a wild-type HIV-1 virus (no resistance mutations present). Other test results are shown in Table 23.1. He had evidence of cleared previous hepatitis B infection (hepatitis B core antibody positive, hepatitis B surface antigen negative). Plasma human herpesvirus-8 (HHV-8) levels were elevated at 250 000 copies/mL. Multiple blood cultures, urine cultures, and sputum cultures demonstrated no bacterial, fungal/ or mycobacterial infection.

Table 23.1 Key blood test results on admission

Haematology	Biochemistry	Virology	Immunology
Hb 10.6 g/dL	Na 134 mmol/L	HIV-1 viral load 250 000 copies/mL	HIV-1 antibody positive
WCC 17×10^9/L	K 4.2 mmol/L	HIV genotypic resistance assay: wild-type virus	Lymphocyte subsets: CD4 count 350 cells/mm^3
Platelets 75×10^9/L	Urea 6.8 mmol/L	HHV-8 viral load 250 000 copies/mL	Hepatitis A IgG negative
INR 1.1	Creatinine 160 μmol/L	EBV viral load 0 copies/mL	Hepatitis B core antibody positive
	ALT 54 IU/L	CMV viral load 0 copies/mL	Hepatitis B surface antigen negative
	ALP 80 IU/L	VZV viral load 0 copies/mL	Hepatitis C IgG negative
	Bilirubin 35 μmol/L	Cryptococcal antigen negative	Syphilis EIA negative
	CRP 75 mg/L		*Toxoplasma gondii* IgG negative

Bone marrow aspirate and trephine showed changes consistent with HIV with a hypercellular marrow and plasmacytosis; there was no evidence of haematological malignancy or opportunistic infection.

A CT scan of his neck, chest, abdomen, and pelvis (NCAP) demonstrated lymphadenopathy within the thorax, abdomen, and pelvis, with bilateral pleural effusions and hepatosplenomegaly.

⊕ Learning point Acquired immune deficiency syndrome (AIDS)-defining malignancies

AIDS-defining malignancies are often caused by oncogenic viruses. The three AIDS-defining malignancies are [1]:

- KS (caused by HHV-8)
- high-grade B-cell NHL (associated with EBV and HHV-8)
- invasive cervical cancer (caused by HPV).

⊕ Learning point Immunosuppression and link to cancer

- Environmental and genetic risk factors common to the general population attenuate immunosuppression-associated cancer pathogenesis [2,3].
- Oncogenic viruses are implicated, particularly HPV, EBV, HHV-8, and hepatitis B (HBV) and hepatitis C virus (HCV) [4].
- The degree of immunosuppression correlates with the risk of malignancy. In transplant recipients, more intensive immunosuppression is associated with a greater risk of malignancy and a more aggressive tumour phenotype [5].
- For HIV-positive patients, the risk of AIDS-defining malignancies increases, as the CD4 count falls; this is not the case for all non-AIDS-defining malignancies [1].
- In HIV-positive patients, traditional risk factors for malignancy, such as smoking and viral hepatitis, are more common [6].

Inguinal lymph node excision biopsy was performed under ultrasound guidance. Histology was consistent with multicentric Castleman disease (MCD), with large plasmablasts within the mantle zone of B-cell follicles which stained positively for the HHV-8-associated latent nuclear antigen-1 (LANA-1) and expressed high levels of IgMλ restricted cytoplasmic immunoglobulin.

The patient was discussed in the lymphoma and HIV MDT meetings. It was recommended that he start highly active antiretroviral therapy (HAART), in combination with rituximab and etoposide for his MCD. Consequently, he started combination antiretroviral therapy with the nucleoside reverse transcriptase inhibitors (NRTIs) abacavir and lamivudine, in combination with the non-nucleoside reverse transcriptase inhibitor (NNRTI) efavirenz. His chemotherapy treatment was overseen by a specialist oncology team and consisted of weekly rituximab 375 mg/m^2 and etoposide 100 mg/m^2 for 4 weeks. Appropriate opportunistic infection (OI) prophylaxis was commenced with co-trimoxazole 960 mg od, aciclovir 400 mg bd, fluconazole 50 mg od, and azithromycin 1250 mg weekly.

Two weeks after commencing chemotherapy, the KS lesions over the dorsum of both feet became more pronounced, and he developed pitting oedema up to his knees. Progression of KS is a well-recognized complication of rituximab therapy. Consequently, after completion of the 4-week therapy with rituximab and etoposide for MCD, he was started on liposomal doxorubicin 20 mg/m^2 every 3 weeks for six cycles. Seven weeks after admission to hospital, he was discharged. His fevers had resolved, the KS lesions had regressed, and the KS-associated oedema significantly improved. The liposomal doxorubicin was completed as an outpatient regimen, and prophylaxis for opportunistic infection continued.

> ⊕ **Clinical tip** TIS staging of Kaposi's sarcoma and risk stratification
>
> Poor-risk disease in HIV-associated KS is an indication for systemic chemotherapy.
>
> | TIS staging of KS | Good risk (all of the following) 0 | Poor risk (any of the following) 1 |
> |---|---|---|
> | (T) Tumour | Confined to skin, lymph nodes, or minimal oral disease | • Tumour-associated oedema or ulceration
• Extensive oral KS
• GI KS
• KS in other non-nodal viscera |
> | (I) Immune status | CD4 cell count >150 cells/microlitre | CD4 cell count <150 cells/microlitre |
> | (S) Systemic illness | Karnovsky PS >70 | Karnovsky PS <70 or other HIV-related illness |
>
> Reproduced from Mark Bower et al., British HIV Association guidelines for HIV-associated malignancies 2014, HIV Medicine, Volume 15, Supplement 2, pp. 1–92, Copyright © 2014 British HIV Association, with permission from John Wiley & Sons, Inc. Included data from: Krown S. et al., Kaposi's sarcoma in the acquired immune deficiency syndrome: a proposal for uniform evaluation, response, and staging criteria. AIDS Clinical Trials Group Oncology Committee, Journal of Clinical Oncology, Volume 7, Number 9, pp. 1201–07, Copyright © 1989 by the American Society of Clinical Oncology; and Krown S. et al., AIDS-related Kaposi's sarcoma: prospective validation of the AIDS Clinical Trials Group staging classification. AIDS Clinical Trials Group Oncology Committee, Volume 15, Number 9, pp. 3085–3092, Copyright © 1989 by the American Society of Clinical Oncology.

Three months post-treatment, he remained asymptomatic. CT NCAP confirmed a significant radiological response of his multicentric Castleman's disease (MCD), and his KS lesions had further regressed. Plasma HHV-8 viral load titre was undetectable, and his HIV viral load had fallen to 200 copies/mL.

Eighteen months later, his fevers returned. He developed bilateral pleural effusions, splenomegaly, and cervical and axillary lymphadenopathy. His CRP was 50 mg/L, and plasma HHV-8 levels 200 000 copies/mm^3. CT NCAP demonstrated axillary and mediastinal lymphadenopathy, and appropriate investigations were conducted to exclude other pathology. An excision biopsy of an axillary lymph node confirmed relapsed MCD. In view of his PS of 0 at this time and the lack of organ dysfunction, he was commenced on single-agent rituximab (375 mg/m^2 for 4 weeks), with continuation of his HAART regimen, and achieved a complete response.

> ✪ **Learning point** Diagnosis of multicentric Castleman disease (MCD) in an HIV-positive patient
>
> MCD is a 'great mimic'. In immunosuppressed patients, pathologies often coexist, and the differential diagnosis is broad. A comprehensive history (including travel history), examination, and focused appropriate investigations must be obtained. The diagnosis should be made histologically, and HHV-8 DNA is almost always detectable in the blood of patients with active disease.
>
> Potential differential diagnoses include:
>
> • bacterial infections, e.g. *Streptococcus pneumoniae*
> • viral infections, e.g. *Haemophilus influenzae*
> • lymphoma
> • *Mycobacterium tuberculosis*
> • atypical disseminated mycobacterial infection
> • *Pneumocystis carinii* infection
> • fungal infection, e.g. cryptococcal infection
> • KS
> • drug fever
> • other neoplastic processes, e.g. RCC.
>
> (continued)

MCD is a relapsing–remitting disease. Once a histological diagnosis has been made, the diagnosis of an MCD 'attack' (in the absence of other aetiology) should include:

1. fever

2. at least three of the following symptoms:

- peripheral lymphadenopathy
- splenomegaly
- oedema
- pleural effusion
- ascites
- cough
- nasal obstruction
- xerostomia
- rash
- central neurological symptoms
- jaundice
- autoimmune haemolytic anaemia

3. CRP level (>20 mg/L) [7].

ⓘ Expert comment

It is thought that cytokines, in particular IL-6, are responsible for the majority of the clinical systemic features of MCD. In the case of KS-associated herpesvirus (KSHV)-associated MCD, the IL-6 may be of either a viral origin from the viral homologue vIL-6, encoded by KSHV, or human hIL-6, derived from host cells. Human hIL-6 acts via the IL-6 receptor (IL-6R) and a co-receptor gp130, leading to the stimulation of the JAK–STAT intracellular pathway. In contrast, viral vIL-6 is thought to activate the same pathway by binding only the co-receptor gp130. The importance of this finding is that the mAbs siltuximab, which targets hIL-6, and tocilizumab, which binds IL-6R, are effective therapies for MCD that is not associated with HIV or KSHV but appear to be ineffective in KSHV-associated MCD in people living with HIV.

✪ Learning point   Management of multicentric Castleman's disease (MCD)

The prognosis of MCD has improved considerably in the post-HAART era, with a 2-year OS of >80%, compared to a median OS of 14 months in the pre-HAART era [7].

- HIV-positive patients should be started on HAART.
- The standard therapy for HHV8-associated MCD in people living with HIV/AIDS is rituximab.
- Etoposide should be added for patients with a severe attack, as evidenced by poor PS or end-organ involvement.
- Anti-viral agents, e.g. valganciclovir, may have a role [7].
- Patients are at a 15-fold increased risk of NHL, compared to the HIV-positive population, as a whole—rituximab administration may reduce this risk [8].

✪ Learning point   Kaposi's sarcoma (KS)

MCD and KS are both driven by HHV-8 infection and frequently coexist. KS is a low-grade vascular tumour, characterized by red/purple papules typically on the lower legs/feet, chest, and oral mucosa. Lesions are typically painless but may become exophytic and ulcerated. Systemic involvement (typically with lung involvement) is seen in 10% of HIV/transplant-associated cases [1,9]. The diagnosis is made clinically with skin biopsy for histological confirmation.

Four variants are described:

- HIV-associated: the commonest HIV-associated malignancy [9]
- transplant-associated: the relative risk of KS is related to the duration and intensity of immunosuppression [9]

(continued)

- classic: seen particularly in people of Jewish and Mediterranean descent
- endemic: commonest in Central Africa.

Patients with classic and endemic KS often do not require treatment; single lesions can be excised, and disease often regresses spontaneously. Transplant and HIV-associated disease is often aggressive, and lymph nodes with mucosal and visceral involvement are more commonly seen.

The treatment of small lesions includes excision, cryotherapy, and photodynamic therapy; recurrence with local treatments is, however, common. Intralesional chemotherapy with vinblastine or vincristine may be used. EBRT, using a single fraction of 8–12 Gy delivered to an extended field, may be successful in patients with a few lesions in a limited area [1].

All HIV-positive patients should be started on HAART, and good virological control is often sufficient to control early disease. In transplant-associated KS, reducing or switching immunosuppressants may lead to resolution. In advanced KS, liposomal anthracyclines are the treatment of choice, with either liposome-encapsulated daunorubicin (40 mg/m^2 every 2 weeks) or pegylated liposomal doxorubicin (20 mg/m^2 every 3 weeks) demonstrating equivalence [10]. In anthracycline-refractory disease, paclitaxel (100 mg/m^2 every 2 weeks) may be considered [1].

Two years after relapse of his MCD, his night sweats and temperatures returned, in association with significant anorexia and weight loss. Plasma HHV-8 levels were not elevated, and CT NCAP and ^{18}F-FDG-PET-CT demonstrated widespread cervical, axillary, and inguinal lymphadenopathy, with splenomegaly. Cervical lymph node excision biopsy was consistent with extra-cavity primary effusion lymphoma (PEL). Histology demonstrated large malignant cells, with round irregular nuclei and variable morphology. These stained positively for the plasma cell-specific antigen CD138/syndecan-1 and for the HHV-8-associated antigen LANA-1, with negative staining for CD20. Bone marrow biopsy and lumbar puncture demonstrated no marrow or CNS involvement.

✪ Learning point The outcome of diffuse large B cell lymphoma (DLBCL) according to the International Prognostic Index (IPI) score in HIV-positive patients [11]

PEL typically has a poor prognosis, with a median OS of 11 months in extra-cavity disease and 4 months in cavity PEL. Most HIV-associated non-Hodgkin's lymphoma (NHL) have better outcomes, and the IPI is a useful tool to predict outcome and guide treatment.

IPI adverse factors: age >60, LDH > ULN, stages III–IV disease, ECOG PS ≥2, extranodal sites ≥2.

Risk group	Number of adverse factors	3-year OS (%)
Low	0–1	64
Low intermediate	2	64
High intermediate	3	50
High	4–5	13

Source: data from Lim, Soon-Thye *et al.*, Prognostic factors in HIV-related diffuse large-cell lymphoma: before versus after highly active antiretroviral therapy, *Journal of Clinical Oncology*, Volume 23, Number 33, pp. 8477–8482, Copyright © 2005 by American Society of Clinical Oncology.

He was started on CHOP chemotherapy every 21 days (cyclophosphamide 750 mg/m^2, doxorubicin 50 mg/m^2, vincristine 1.4 mg/m^2, and prednisolone 40 mg/m^2 (days 1–5)), with G-CSF support for a total of six cycles, in combination with full prophylaxis against opportunistic infections, and the efavirenz switched to raltegravir. He achieved an excellent partial response to treatment, and his symptoms resolved fully.

❻ Expert comment

Knowledge of the metabolism of cytotoxic chemotherapy agents and antiretrovirals is essential for the management of these patients. Table 23.2 and Table 23.3 show the main hepatic enzymes involved in the metabolism of CHOP and the induction and inhibition of these enzymes by antiretrovirals.

Table 23.2 Some potential interactions with CHOP

	Drug	Catabolism
C	Alkylating agents (e.g. cyclophosphamide)	CYP2B6, CYP2C9, 2C19, CYP3A4, 3A5
H	Anthracyclines (e.g. doxorubicin)	CYP3A4, CYP2D6
O	Vinca alkaloids (e.g. vincristine)	CYP3A4
P	Glucocorticoids (e.g. prednisolone)	CYP3A4

Source: data from *The Lancet Oncology*, Volume 12, Issue 9, Michelle A. Rudek *et al.*, Use of antineoplastic agents in cancer patients with HIV/AIDS, pp. 905–912, Copyright © 2011 Elsevier Ltd. All rights reserved.

Table 23.3 Chemotherapy and antiretroviral agents

Drug	Effects
Efavirenz	↑ CYP2B6, 3A4 ↓ CYP2C9, 2C19, 3A4
Ritonavir	↑ CYP2B6 ↓ CYP2C9, 2D6, 3A4
Daraunavir	↓ CYP3A4
Atazanavir	↓ CYP3A4, UGT1A1
Raltegravir	–
Maraviroc	–

Source: data from *The Lancet Oncology,* Volume 12, Issue 9, Michelle A. Rudek *et al.*, Use of antineoplastic agents in cancer patients with HIV/AIDS, pp.905–912, Copyright © 2011 Elsevier Ltd. All rights reserved.

✪ Learning point HIV-associated lymphomas

Non-Hodgkin's lymphoma (NHL) is the second commonest HIV-associated malignancy and is an AIDS-defining illness [1]. The median survival in HIV-associated NHL in those receiving chemotherapy has increased from 2 to 13 months in the pre-HAART era to >24 months [12]. Advanced disease at diagnosis is common, although, with appropriate management, survival is the same as in immunocompetent patients when matched for IPI. Commencing non-interacting HAART and prophylaxis for OIs is essential. Patients with HIV-associated malignancies should only be managed in centres with integrated HIV and oncology services and experience with caring for these patients.

HIV-associated non-Hodgkin's lymphoma (NHL)

- NHL occurs more frequently in patients with advanced or poorly controlled HIV infection and is frequently EBV-driven; rarer subtypes are associated with HHV-8.
- DLBCL predominates, followed by Burkitt's lymphoma (BL).
- BL often presents earlier in the HIV natural history and is associated with higher CD4 counts; DLBCL often presents later and is associated with lower CD4 counts.

(continued)

- HIV-associated primary CNS lymphoma (PCL) is becoming increasingly rare. It is associated with profound immunosuppression (CD4 count typically <50 cells/mm^3) [12] and, unlike PCL, in HIV-negative patients, is always EBV-driven. Survival is very poor, typically a few weeks, compared to 2 years in immunocompetent patients.
- Plasmablastic lymphoma (PBL) and primary effusion lymphoma (PEL) are aggressive forms of NHL that occur almost uniquely in HIV-positive patients [13,14].
- EBV-driven PBL characteristically arises in the jaw and oral cavity, whilst lymph node PBL is characteristically HHV-8-associated.
- HHV-8-associated PEL may arise in body cavities as a malignant effusion; increasingly, patients present with extra-cavity disease with solid tumour masses.
- PBL and PEL typically do not express CD20; rituximab plays no role in CD20-negative disease [13].
- The optimal therapy for HIV-associated NHL has yet to be defined; CHOP-like chemotherapy is generally used first-line, alongside rituximab [15].
- HIV-positive patients with BL often present with advanced disease, and aggressive chemotherapy regimens are typically used (e.g. R-CODOX-M/R-IVAC) [12].
- All patients with CNS involvement by systemic lymphoma should receive intrathecal chemotherapy and whole-brain radiotherapy. Treatment of patients with high-risk disease, without CNS involvement (e.g. in patients with BL), should incorporate CNS-penetrating chemotherapy and intrathecal chemotherapy [1].
- The International Working Group response criteria, defined for NHL in the general population, are used to assess response to treatment [1].

HIV-associated Hodgkin's lymphoma

- Mixed cellularity and lymphocyte-depleted subtypes predominate [1].
- Standard chemotherapy with ABVD (doxorubicin, bleomycin, vinblastine, and dacarbazine) is the first-line treatment of choice, although more intensive regimens may be considered.
- Salvage chemotherapy, followed by high-dose chemotherapy and autologous stem cell transplantation, should be considered in patients who relapse [1].
- The International Prognostic Score (IPS) Hasenclever index for Hodgkin's lymphoma is applicable.
- The prognosis is now identical to that in HIV-negative patients.
- Non-interactive HAART and prophylaxis for opportunistic infections are essential.

He continued 3-monthly outpatient review in the joint haematology/HIV clinic and was maintained on the same HAART regimen. Nine months after the initial diagnosis of PEL, his night sweats and temperatures returned, and relapsed PEL was confirmed. He quickly deteriorated and requested that he receive no further chemotherapy and was transferred to a hospice where he died 3 weeks after relapse.

Table 23.4 Other HIV-associated malignancies

Cervical cancer and cervical intraepithelial neoplasia	• Typically HPV-associated • Presents at more advanced stage, compared to HIV-negative patients (prognosis typically worse) • Cervical intraepithelial neoplasia more common and more likely to recur • HIV-positive patients should be screened annually and undergo baseline colposcopic examination • Role for HPV screening not yet established [1]
Anal carcinoma	• 90% of cases associated with HPV positivity • Presence of multiple sexual partners/sexually transmitted infections, history of cervical intraepithelial neoplasia of the cervix, vagina, or vulva, cigarette smoking, and iatrogenic immunosuppression are additional risk factors • Most are squamous cell (epidermoid) • Increasingly, anal cytology and anoscopy are employed for surveillance of those at highest risk, although evidence for its routine use is lacking [1]
Germ cell tumours	• Increased risk of seminoma but not non-seminomatous germ cell tumours • The prognosis is excellent and no worse than that in immunocompetent patients [1]
Head and neck carcinomas	• KS and NHL are the commonest head and neck cancer • Nasopharyngeal carcinoma, mucosal SCC, and some salivary tumours (lymphoepithelial carcinoma and Merkel cell carcinoma) are more common and associated with worse prognosis and more aggressive disease • Generally associated with oncogenic viruses; smoking is also a significant risk factor [16]
HCC	• Hepatitis B and C co-infections are common; the exact contribution of HIV to the development of HCC is therefore unclear • HIV infection accelerates the progression of HBV infection and hastens cirrhosis in patients with chronic HCV infection [1]
Lung cancer	• Incidence of NSCLC is increasing in the HIV population, independently of traditional risk factors • Typically, such patients present at a younger age with more aggressive disease [1]

Source: data from Bower, M., et al., British HIV Association guidelines for HIV-associated malignancies 2008, HIV Medicine, Volume 9, Issue 6, pp. 336–88, Copyright © British HIV Association 2008; and Purgina, B., L. Pantanowitz and R.R. Seethala, A Review of Carcinomas Arising in the Head and Neck Region in HIV-Positive Patients, Pathology Research International, Volume 11, Volume 2011, Article ID 469150 Copyright © Bibianna Purgina et al. 2011.

Discussion

The challenges of managing HHV-8-associated KS and MCD in an HIV-positive patient, who then develops a further HHV-8-associated malignancy (NHL), are highlighted by this case study.

Following the diagnosis of HIV infection, the patient's initial management was overseen by a specialist HIV–oncology team. All patients with immunosuppression-associated malignancies should be managed in specialist centres; this is associated with a better clinical outcome [1]. Appropriate MDT discussion and close collaboration between oncologists and HIV physicians are crucial.

Acute deterioration in immunosuppressed patients may happen quickly, and identifying an aetiology may be a challenge. In MCD, cytokine and virokine production may account for systemic symptoms, with patients presenting acutely unwell and deteriorating quickly. As multi-organ dysfunction can develop quickly, early referral to the ICU is potentially lifesaving. Studies have shown that HIV-positive patients admitted to the ICU now have a similar chance of survival to hospital discharge as other medical patients, and an aggressive management approach should therefore be adopted [17].

Unless there are clear contraindications, all patients with HIV-associated malignancies should continue combination antiretroviral therapy (cART) indefinitely. When choosing appropriate antiretroviral therapy, the presence of HIV-associated resistance mutations, renal and liver dysfunction, drug interactions, e.g. with other chemotherapy agents, and patient preference should be taken into account. cART regimens may need to be modified during the course of a patient's treatment, e.g. after the development of chemotherapy-induced renal dysfunction or as a consequence of treatment-related side effects. The importance of pharmacokinetic interactions between ritonavir-boosted protease inhibitors and hepatically metabolized cytotoxic chemotherapy cannot be overestimated. The concomitant administration of drugs that block CYP 3A4 and 2B6 with chemotherapy agents that are metabolized by these enzymes will result in severe chemotherapy toxicity and usually prolonged myelosuppression. Switching cART to a different regimen, based on NNRTI or integrase inhibitors, avoids this risk.

Many immunosuppression-associated malignancies are potentially preventable through screening and appropriate vaccination. The British HIV-Association (BHIVA) has issued clear guidelines for the screening of HIV-positive patients, e.g. for cervical and anal cancers. Early diagnosis and treatment of immunosuppression-associated malignancy is associated with better long-term outcomes; better still is the prevention of malignancy in the first place.

> ✪ **Learning point** Reducing the cancer risk in HIV-positive patients
>
> - Cancer risk and CD4 counts are associated in AIDS-defining malignancies; early diagnosis and treatment of HIV infection are therefore essential.
> - All patients should be screened for hepatitis B and C infections and vaccinated against hepatitis B.
> - All women should undergo a baseline colposcopic examination and annual smear tests; all women with abnormal smears should be referred for colposcopy.
> - Men who have sex with men should be considered for anoscopic examination and cytology for anal intraepithelial neoplasia.
> - Appropriate advice regarding smoking cessation and alcohol consumption should be offered [1].

A final word from the expert

Advances in the survival of people living with HIV who develop AIDS-defining malignancies is one of the greatest achievements of modern oncology. A decade ago, the 5-year survival of MCD was 15%; now it is 90%. Similarly, the prognosis for people with AIDS-related NHL is the same as for NHL in the HIV-negative population. Indeed, for most malignancies, the OS is the same, regardless of the HIV status. This can only be achieved by close collaboration between experienced oncologists and HIV physicians, and by careful attention to opportunistic infection prophylaxis and pharmacological interactions between cytotoxics and antiretrovirals.

References

1. Bower M, Collins S, Cottrill C *et al.*; AIDS Malignancy Subcommittee. British HIV Association guidelines for HIV-associated malignancies 2008. *HIV Medicine* 2008; **9**(6): 336–88.

2. Vajdic CM, van Leeuwen MT. Cancer incidence and risk factors after solid organ transplantation. *International Journal of Cancer* 2009; **125**(8): 1747–54.

3. Zafar SY, Howell DN, Gockerman JP. Malignancy after solid organ transplantation: an overview. *The Oncologist* 2008; **13**(7): 769–78.

4. Gutierrez-Dalmau A, Campistol JM. Immunosuppressive therapy and malignancy in organ transplant recipients: a systematic review. *Drugs* 2007; **67**(8): 1167–98.

5. Dantal J, Hourmant M, Cantarovich D *et al.* Effect of long-term immunosuppression in kidney-graft recipients on cancer incidence: randomised comparison of two cyclosporin regimens. *The Lancet* 1998; **351**(9103): 623–8.

6. Clifford GM, Polesel J, Rickenbach M *et al.* Cancer risk in the Swiss HIV Cohort Study: associations with immunodeficiency, smoking, and highly active antiretroviral therapy. *Journal of the National Cancer Institute* 2005; **97**(6): 425–32.

7. Bower M. How I treat HIV-associated multicentric Castleman disease. *Blood* 2010; **116**(22): 4415–21.

8. Gerard L, Michot JM, Burcheri S *et al.* Rituximab decreases the risk of lymphoma in patients with HIV-associated multicentric Castleman disease. *Blood* 2012; **119**(10): 2228–33.

9. Antman K, Chang Y. Kaposi's sarcoma. *The New England Journal of Medicine* 2000; **342**(14): 1027–38.

10. Cooley T, Henry D, Tonda M, Sun S, O'Connell M, Rackoff W. A randomized, double-blind study of pegylated liposomal doxorubicin for the treatment of AIDS-related Kaposi's sarcoma. *The Oncologist* 2007; **12**(1): 114–23.

11. Sehn LH, Berry B, Chhanabhai M *et al.* The revised International Prognostic Index (R-IPI) is a better predictor of outcome than the standard IPI for patients with diffuse large B-cell lymphoma treated with R-CHOP. *Blood* 2007; **109**(5): 1857–61.

12. Stebbing J, Marvin V, Bower M. The evidence-based treatment of AIDS-related non-Hodgkin's lymphoma. *Cancer Treatment Reviews* 2004; **30**(3): 249–53.

13. Chen YB, Rahemtullah A, Hochberg E. Primary effusion lymphoma. *The Oncologist* 2007; **12**(5): 569–76.

14. Castillo JJ, Reagan JL. Plasmablastic lymphoma: a systematic review. *The Scientific World Journal* 2011; **11**: 687–96.

15. Ezzat H, Filipenko D, Vickars L *et al.* Improved survival in HIV-associated diffuse large B-cell lymphoma with the addition of rituximab to chemotherapy in patients receiving highly active antiretroviral therapy. *HIV Clinical Trials* 2007; **8**(3): 132–44.

16. Purgina B, Pantanowitz L, Seethala RR. A Review of Carcinomas Arising in the Head and Neck Region in HIV-Positive Patients. *Pathology Research International* 2011; **2011**: 469150.

17. Casalino E, Mendoza-Sassi G, Wolff M *et al.* Predictors of short- and long-term survival in HIV-infected patients admitted to the ICU. *Chest* 1998; **113**(2): 421–9.

24 Late cardiovascular complications of cancer treatment

Fatima El-Khouly

Expert commentary Chris Plummer

Case history

A 55-year-old woman was initially treated for ER+, PR+, HER2+ invasive ductal carcinoma of the left breast, staged T2N2M0, with a wide local excision and axillary lymphadenectomy, six cycles of FEC-T chemotherapy, and adjuvant radiotherapy to the left breast and supraclavicular fossa (40 Gy in 15 fractions). She then completed 1 year of adjuvant trastuzumab and 5 years of tamoxifen.

Five years later, she re-presented to her GP with fatigue, shortness of breath, and reduced exercise tolerance. On clinical examination, she had moderate bilateral peripheral pitting oedema to the mid calf and a raised jugular venous pressure. Her pulse rate was 100 bpm, with a BP of 165/90 mmHg. The remaining examination was normal.

> ⊙ **Learning point** Adjuvant chemotherapy regimens
>
> The mainstay of adjuvant chemotherapy in breast cancer includes anthracycline-based regimens where guidance on specific regimens have been taken from data produced from the Early Breast Cancer Trialists' Collaborative Group (EBCTCG) [2]. Local policies determine whether doxorubicin or epirubicin are used.
>
> **Options**
>
> | High-risk patients | Low-risk patients |
> |---|---|
> | FEC × 6 | AC × 4 |
> | Day 1, IV bolus repeated every 21 days | IV bolus repeated every 21 days |
> | 5-FU 500 mg/m^2 | Doxorubicin 60 mg/m^2 |
> | Epirubicin 75 mg/m^2 | Cyclophosphamide 600 mg/m^2 |
> | Cyclophosphamide 500 mg/m^2 | |
> | | |
> | FEC × 3, followed by Taxotere® × 3 | CMF × 6 |
> | Day 1, cycles 1–3, repeated every 21 days | Cyclophosphamide* 100 mg/m^2 (max 150 mg) PO |
> | 5-FU 500 mg/m^2 | daily days 1–14 |
> | Epirubicin 100 mg/m^2 | Methotrexate 40 mg/m^2 IV bolus days 1 and 8 |
> | Cyclophosphamide 500 mg/m^2 | 5-FU 600 mg/m^2 IV bolus days 1 and 8 |
> | Day 1, cycles 4–6 | Repeat every 28 days |
> | Docetaxel 100 mg/m^2 | Give folinic acid 15 mg orally 24 and 36 hours after |
> | | methotrexate |
> | | |
> | The use of taxanes in node-positive early breast cancer is approved by NICE, based on 5 and 10 years' outcome of BCIRG 001 trial [3] | Improvement outcomes of AC × 4 and CMF × 6 are equivalent, but toxicity is different. |
>
> *If necessary, can give cyclophosphamide IV in this regime (instead of orally) in a dose of 600 mg/m^2 on days 1 and 8.
> Source: data from *The Lancet*, Volume 379, Issue 9814, Early Breast Cancer Trialists' Collaborative Group (EBCTCG), Comparisons between different polychemotherapy regimens for early breast cancer: meta-analyses of long-term outcome among 100,000 women in 123 randomised trials, pp. 432–44, Copyright © 2012 Elsevier Ltd; and *Lancet Oncology*, Volume 14, Issue 1, Mackey JR *et al.*, Adjuvant docetxel, doxorubicin and cyclophosphamide in node-positive breast cancer: 10-year follow-up of the phase 3 randomised BCIRG 001 trial, pp. 72–80, Copyright © 2013 Elsevier Ltd. All rights reserved.

> ✪ **Learning point** HER2 and trastuzumab
>
> - Approximately 20% of breast cancers exhibit an overexpression of HER2 [4].
> - HER2 gene amplification in breast cancer is both a biomarker for adverse prognosis and a target for treatment [4–6].
> - Two main methods are employed in clinical laboratories for detecting HER2: IHC techniques, using antibodies to measure proteins, and *in situ* hybridization (ISH) methods, using nucleic acid probes to measure HER2 gene amplification [7–9].
> - National and international guidelines recommend that, for breast cancers with equivocal IHC, HER2 testing by ISH is mandatory [9].
> - FISH evaluation for HER2 gene amplification has the greatest evidence base and is most commonly used.
> - Other ISH methods include chromogenic and silver techniques, whilst evaluation of different technologies to target DNA/RNA and proteins are in progress.
> - ER2 is one of four plasma membrane-bound receptor tyrosine kinases of the EGFR family (EGFR/ErbB).
> - Heterodimerization of HER2 can occur with any of the other three receptors, resulting in autophosphorylation of tyrosine residues within cytoplasmic domains of receptors, thus initiating a number of signalling pathways which promote cell proliferation and oppose apoptosis.
> - Trastuzumab is a humanized mAb directed against the HER2 protein.
> - Patients with HER2-positive early breast cancer treated with adjuvant trastuzumab have shown significant improvement in both DFS and OS outcomes, compared to those not given trastuzumab (50% relative reduction risk of recurrence) [10].

A transthoracic echocardiogram revealed a dilated left ventricle with severely impaired left ventricular systolic function fraction (LVEF 30%; normal range ≥55%). An ECG showed sinus tachycardia. FBC and renal and liver function tests were normal. She was reviewed by a cardiologist who confirmed her diagnosis of heart failure with New York Heart Association (NYHA) class III symptoms. She was started on furosemide 40 mg daily and ramipril 1.25 mg bd. She lost 4 kg over the following 2 weeks, and, within 6 weeks, her exercise tolerance had improved.

> ✪ **Learning point** Risk of developing congestive heart failure (early and delayed onset)
>
> The risk of heart failure after anthracycline chemotherapy increases with the total lifetime dose and also the peak plasma concentration, with lower rates of toxicity seen after longer infusions than bolus administration. The risk of cardiovascular toxicity can be reduced by liposomal encapsulation of the drug. The recommended maximum cumulative doses vary between anthracyclines, depending on the efficacy and cardiovascular risk [11,12]:
>
> | Anthracycline | Accumulative dose associated with cardiotoxicity | Recommended maximum dose (MHRA) |
> |---|---|---|
> | Doxorubicin | 400–700 mg/m^2 | 450–500 mg/m^2 |
> | Epirubicin | 550–900 mg/m^2 | 900 mg/m^2 |
> | Liposomal doxorubicin (pegylated forms available) | 550 mg/m^2 | 450 mg/m^2 |
>
> It is important to recognize that doses below these limits can result in cardiomyopathy and that cardiac toxicity is often evident only after long-term follow-up.
>
> *Source*: data from Medicines and Healthcare products Regulatory Agency (MHRA), © Crown Copyright 2014, available from <http://www.mhra.gov.uk/Safetyinformation/Medicinesinformation/SPCandPILs/index.htm>; and *Pharmacology and Therapeutics*, Volume 125, Issue 2, Raschi E *et al.*, Anticancer drugs and cardiotoxicity: Insights and perspectives in the era of targeted therapy, pp. 196–218, Copyright © 2009 Elsevier Inc. All rights reserved.

The patient's only cardiovascular risk factor was untreated hypertension. There were no documented echocardiograms prior to starting chemotherapy, but her scan prior to commencing trastuzumab showed a LVEF of 64%. During her trastuzumab treatment, she was persistently hypertensive, with systolic BPs >155 mmHg, and an echocardiogram carried out midway through treatment had shown a drop in the LVEF to 50%. Her trastuzumab was continued, in accordance with NICE guidance, and 3-monthly echocardiograms measured the LVEF between 50% and 55%. She had no breaks in treatment, and an end-of-treatment echocardiogram was not performed.

> **Clinical tip** Trastuzumab
>
> - This should not be given concurrently with anthracyclines, because of the high risk of cardiac toxicity, but can be given with taxanes.
> - The HERA trial (median 8 years follow-up) has shown that 2 years of trastuzumab has an unfavourable benefit–risk ratio, compared with 1 year of treatment (increased cardiac events) [6].
> - There are no data to support 6 months' treatment versus 1 year; therefore, guidelines on adjuvant trastuzumab remains 1 year (it can be given until disease progression in the metastatic setting).
> - LVEF should be monitored every 3 months, whilst on treatment (echocardiography is preferred to nuclear ventriculography, because of the additional structural and functional information provided and the absence of ionizing radiation).

> **Clinical tip** Considering cardiac risk factors
>
> - A full medical history is needed—has the patient been exposed to previous anthracyclines, e.g. treatment for a previous contralateral breast cancer?
> - Any known cardiovascular risk factors.
> - Baseline LVEF.
> - Previous irradiation to the mediastinum.
> - Increasing age.

Discussion

The advances in third-generation chemotherapy for adjuvant management of breast cancer (FEC-T) have shown improved OS rates and decreased recurrence. Most trials have focussed on the efficacy of cancer treatment, rather than the late effects of treatment. Cardiac toxicity is a well-known side effect of several cytotoxic drugs, especially the anthracyclines, and encompasses a number of side effects, including impairment in either myocardial contraction (systolic dysfunction) or relaxation (diastolic dysfunction), changes in BP, myocardial ischaemia, or arrhythmias. The development of cardiac toxicity can lead to long-term morbidity.

> **Learning point** Mechanisms of cardiac toxicity [13]
>
> Understanding the mechanisms of cardiovascular toxicity in cancer treatment is a field of active research. Many hypotheses have been proposed, but the data supporting them are limited—it may be that different mechanisms are important in different clinical scenarios.
>
> **Anthracyclines [14]**
>
> *Oxidative stress hypothesis*
>
> - One-electron reduction of doxorubicin to form doxorubicin semiquinone radical by a reduced flavoenzyme, e.g. NADPH-cytochrome P450 reductase.
> - Semiquinone radical complexes with iron to form an anthracycline–iron free radical complex.
> - This complex then reduces oxygen to produce superoxide.
> - Cardiac cells are then subjected to oxidative stress (low levels of antioxidant enzymes in the heart).
> - The formation of oxidative free radical can initiate apoptosis of cardiac myocytes.
>
> *Metabolite theory*
>
> - Inhibition of cardiac lipid peroxidation by doxorubicin and hydrogen peroxide.
> - Metabolite doxorubicinol mediates iron release and negatively affects the function of apoprotein as a regulatory protein.
>
> (continued)

Influence on calcium homeostasis

- Oxidative stress can make changes to mitochondrial calcium transport, leading to tissue injury, cell death, and impaired cardiac contraction.
- The precise role of anthracyclines in changes to calcium regulation and its subsequent implications for cardiotoxicity are unclear.

Role of immune system

- A study in hypertensive rats demonstrated an increase in antigen-presenting cells after treatment with doxorubicin. Interestingly, pretreatment with dexrazoxane reduced this increase, suggesting an immunogenic reaction following oxidative stress [15].

Taxanes [13,14]

- In early clinical trials, paclitaxel was associated with a 30% incidence of asymptomatic sinus bradycardia, without any clinical consequences.
- To enhance drug solubility, paclitaxel is formulated in a cremophor EL vehicle.
- It has therefore been suggested that the vehicle, and not the cytotoxic drug itself, is responsible for the cardiac effects through histamine release.
- The cardiac toxicity of doxorubicin is increased by concurrent paclitaxel administration.
- This appears to be caused by paclitaxel reducing doxorubicin hepatic elimination, and therefore leading to increased plasma concentration of doxorubicin.
- Docetaxel shows no increase in cardiac toxicity when combined with doxorubicin.

5-FU

- The pathophysiological mechanism of 5-FU-induced cardiotoxicity is unknown.
- Multiple hypotheses have been postulated.
- Currently, the most plausible is direct toxicity to the myocardium.

Trastuzumab [11,17]

- The incidence of cardiomyopathy with concurrent trastuzumab and anthracycline treatment is up to 28%, and is not recommended.
- When used as a single agent, before anthracyclines or 90 days after the completion of anthracycline chemotherapy, the incidence of asymptomatic falls in the LVEF is approximately 7%, with <1% of patients experiencing severe heart failure symptoms.
- The mechanism of trastuzumab cardiac toxicity is thought to be reduced cardiac myocyte contractility, rather than cell loss.
- For this reason, left ventricular dysfunction is usually reversible.
- Risk factors for cardiac dysfunction include age older than 50 years, lower LVEF before treatment, structural heart disease, previous anthracycline use (cumulative doses >300 mg/m^2), and timing of trastuzumab initiation in patients previously treated with anthracyclines.

Bevacizumab [14]

- Bevacizumab is a humanized mAb directed against VEGF.
- It is associated with hypertension, with antihypertensive drug treatment required in about 10%.
- Serious adverse events (grades 4–5 toxicity) due to hypertension are rare (<1%).
- Heart failure associated with bevacizumab is rare (<1%) and is associated with prior anthracycline treatment.

Many other agents have been linked to cardiovascular toxicity, although the data supporting these links are much weaker than for those shown above. These risks should be carefully assessed, with the other risks of chemotherapy, against their potential benefits for each individual patient.

⊗ **Learning point** Late effects of anthracyclines

- Cardiac toxicity usually develops late after completion of anthracycline-based chemotherapy.
- Anthracycline cardiomyopathy presents with reduced LVEF and/or signs and symptoms of heart failure [18]:
  - common:
    - dyspnoea
    - fatigue
    - peripheral oedema
    - raised jugular venous pressure
    - gallop rhythm
  - late features:
    - pulmonary oedema
    - pleural effusion
    - cardiomegaly
    - hepatomegaly
    - ascites.
- The risk of congestive heart failure is increased by:
  - increasing total cumulative dose of anthracycline
  - radiation therapy to the mediastinal area.

⊕ **Expert comment**

Heart failure may be much more common after anthracycline chemotherapy than was previously thought—the incidence appears to increase with the duration of follow-up. The cumulative incidence of congestive heart failure, 30 years after receiving ≥250 mg/m^2 of anthracycline for childhood cancer, is estimated at approximately 8%, with a similar proportion having asymptomatic left ventricular systolic dysfunction [19]. In women aged 66–70 years undergoing adjuvant treatment for early breast cancer with an anthracycline-containing regimen, there was an absolute 9.7% increase in heart failure events after 10 years, compared to women not receiving chemotherapy [20].

⊗ **Learning point** Chemotherapy-related cardiac dysfunction [21,22]

	Type I (myocardial damage)	Type II (myocardial dysfunction)
Characteristic agent	Doxorubicin	Trastuzumab
Clinical course	May stabilize; underlying damage appears to be permanent and irreversible	High likelihood of recovery (to or near baseline cardiac status) in 2–4 months (reversible)
Dose effect	Cumulative, dose-related	Not dose-related
Mechanism	Free radical formation—oxidative stress/damage	Blocked ErbB2 signalling
Ultrastructure	Vacuoles; myofibrillar disarray and dropout; necrosis (changes resolve over time)	No apparent ultrastructural abnormalities
Non-invasive cardiac testing (echocardiogram or nuclear studies, e.g. MUGA)	Decreased ejection fraction Global reduction in wall motion	Decreased ejection fraction Global reduction in wall motion
Effect of re-challenge	High probability of recurrent progressive dysfunction May result in intractable heart failure and death	Increasing evidence for the relative safety of re-challenge (additional data needed)
Effect of late sequential stress	High likelihood of sequential stress-related cardiac dysfunction	Low likelihood of sequential stress-related cardiac dysfunction

Source: data from Ewer MS and Lippman SM, Type II chemotherapy-related cardiac dysfunction: Time to recognize a new entity, *Journal of Clinical Oncology*, Volume 23, Number 19, pp. 2900–2, Copyright © 2005 by American Society of Clinical Oncology; and Ewer MS *et al.*, Reversibility of trastuzumab-related cardiotoxicity: New insights based on clinical course and response to medical treatment, *Journal of Clinical Oncology*, Volume 23, Number 31, pp. 7820–6, Copyright © 2005 by American Society of Clinical Oncology.

In this clinical case, the patient had several risk factors for developing cardiac dysfunction: untreated hypertension, both anthracycline chemotherapy and trastuzumab therapy, as well as irradiation to the left breast leading to potential radiation effects. This clinical presentation is rare, however, but heart failure after anthracycline chemotherapy becomes more common with increasing duration of follow-up. The cardiac toxicity caused by trastuzumab is usually reversible, if identified early by routine echocardiography. This allows appropriate treatment to be given, before there has been significant cardiac enlargement.

This patient's history demonstrates that her LVEF had fallen by 14 points from before trastuzumab to after the sixth cycle. Her treatment continued without a break, and cardiac management was not optimized. Both UK and US guidelines indicate the suspension of trastuzumab if the LVEF falls by >10 points to below 50%, whereby repeat echocardiogram and commencement of angiotensin-converting enzyme (ACE) inhibitors are recommended.

⊕ **Clinical tip** Managing falls in LVEF whilst on trastuzumab

Current NICE guidance [23] recommends that:

- assessments of cardiac function should be repeated every 3 months, whilst a patient is receiving trastuzumab therapy
- trastuzumab treatment should be suspended if the LVEF drops by 10 percentage (ejection) points or more from baseline and to below 50%
- the decision to restart trastuzumab should be based on further cardiac assessment, as well as a fully informed discussion of the risks and benefits between the patient and their clinician.

Current National Cancer Research Institute (NCRI) guidance [24] recommends:

- *echocardiography prior to anthracycline chemotherapy*
  o patients with an LVEF below the lower limit or normal (<55% on echocardiography)
    - start an ACE inhibitor, and refer to a cardiologist
    - consideration of a non-anthracycline regimen
- *echocardiography prior to trastuzumab treatment*
  o patients with an LVEF below the lower limit or normal (<55% on echocardiography)
    - start an ACE inhibitor, and refer to a cardiologist
    - defer trastuzumab (if LVEF remains ≥40% and returns to normal, it may be possible to start trastuzumab, but risks and benefits should be considered)
- *echocardiography during trastuzumab treatment*
  o patients with an LVEF above the lower limit or normal (≥55% on echocardiography):
    - continue trastuzumab—repeat echocardiography in 4 months
  o patients with an LVEF below the lower limit or normal (<55% on echocardiography) but >40% and/or a 10-point LVEF fall from baseline:
    - start an ACE inhibitor, and refer to a cardiologist
    - continue trastuzumab—repeat echocardiography in 6–8 weeks
  o patients with an LVEF ≤40% and/or signs or symptoms of heart failure:
    - start an ACE inhibitor, and refer to a cardiologist
    - stop trastuzumab—repeat echocardiography within 6 weeks (if LVEF returns to normal, it may be possible to start trastuzumab, but risks and benefits should be considered).

> ⊕ **Clinical tip** Drug management of fall in LVEF on trastuzumab
>
> Current NCRI guidance recommends a more proactive approach to cardiovascular management during trastuzumab treatment [24]:
>
> - symptomatic heart failure
>   - trastuzumab should be interrupted; the patient should be commenced on an ACE inhibitor (and furosemide if there is evidence of fluid retention) and referred to a cardiologist
> - asymptomatic fall in LVEF
>   - if the LVEF falls to ≤40%, then trastuzumab should be interrupted; the patients should be started on an ACE inhibitor and referred to a cardiologist
>   - the LVEF should be measured within 6 weeks or as clinically indicated
>   - trastuzumab may be restarted if the LVEF recovers to the normal range (≥55%)
>   - if the LVEF falls by 10 points or more but remains above 40%, an ACE inhibitor should be started, but trastuzumab may be continued.
>
> ACE inhibitors are initiated if a fall in the LVEF is identified, whether or not the patient has heart failure symptoms. If significant cardiac toxicity is identified, then patients should be reviewed by a cardiologist before continuing treatment. These principles are applicable to the treatment of other malignancies. There are currently no licensed cardioprotective agents, but there is some evidence that hypertensive patients, already on beta-blockers, ACE inhibitors, and aspirin, may benefit from both an anti-cancer effect as well as cardiac protection.

> ✪ **Learning point** Other cardiovascular protection considerations
>
> - *Dexrazoxane* [11]
>   - An iron chelator, binding to intracellular iron, thus affecting the anthyracycline–iron complex, aimed to prevent free radical formation.
>   - Two phase III trials showed that 15% of patients treated with dexrazoxane developed cardiac side effects versus 31% of patients on placebo (HR 2.63; p <0.001).
>   - Based on pharmacokinetic studies, there is a theoretical possibility that dexrazoxane administered with epirubicin will reduce exposure and hence the efficacy of epirubicin.
>   - Since July 2011, following two reports of a non-statistically significant excess of secondary malignancies in dexrazoxane-treated patients, its use has been restricted to adults with advanced or metastatic breast cancer who have previously received a minimum cumulative dose of 300 mg/m^2 of doxorubicin or 540 mg/m2 of epirubicin.
> - *Lipid-lowering agents* [25]
>   - Mice models have shown Probucol, a lipid-lowering agent and an antioxidant, to lower the cardiotoxic effects of anthracycline.
>   - Feleszko *et al.* showed both a potentiation of anti-tumour activity and a cardioprotective effect by the cholesterol-lowering HMG-coenzyme A reductase inhibitor lovastatin in mice treated with doxorubicin.
> - *Changes in formulation* [26–28]
>   - Liposomes are preferentially being taken up by tissues with phagocytic reticuloendothelial cells and with a sinusoidal capillary system, like the liver and spleen, rather than cardiac or skeletal muscle.
>   - Liposomal anthracycline formulations have been shown to have lower cardiac toxicity.
> - *Changes in administration*
>   - Bolus administration of anthracyclines has been shown to have a significantly higher incidence of early and late anthracycline cardiac toxicity than prolonged infusion [29].

Another factor that could have been relevant in this patient's case is the role of adjuvant radiotherapy to the left breast in contributing towards cardiotoxicity. Several mechanisms of injury can occur following radiation to the mediastinal region, and, although caution would have been taken to avoid the cardiac field, it cannot be excluded completely. However, the commonest presentation of radiation-induced cardiac toxicity is with coronary artery disease, which does not appear to have been the cause of this woman's heart failure.

25 Cancer of unknown primary

Anna C Olsson-Brown

ⓘ **Expert commentary** Madhumita Bhattacharyya

Case history

A 65-year-old woman presented to her GP with a 3-month history of abdominal bloating and distension, similar to her long-standing symptoms of irritable bowel syndrome (IBS). Baseline investigations revealed an elevated CA125 only, so the patient was referred under the 2-week rule to the gynaecologists for further clinical review. On presentation, the patient was systemically well. Her past medical history included IBS and rheumatic valve disease, which had developed because of rheumatic fever in childhood. The patient was not on any regular medication and had no known allergies. Her family history was positive for malignancy; her sister and father had had breast and lung cancer, respectively. There was no family history of gynaecological or colorectal malignancy. Her sister had tested negative for a *BRCA1/2* mutation.

At presentation, the patient had an ECOG performance status (PS) of 1 and appeared clinically well, with an absence of jaundice, pallor, lymphadenopathy, or digital clubbing. On abdominal examination, there was evidence of mild distension and palpable, non-tender hepatomegaly. Breast examination was unremarkable. There was no evidence of ascites. There were no palpable adnexal masses, and vaginal examination was unremarkable. Cardiovascular examination revealed a pansystolic murmur.

The patient's pelvic ultrasound was unremarkable, with no evidence of ovarian or endometrial pathology. Baseline blood tests were repeated and again were unremarkable, except for a raised CA125 of 2138 U/mL and mildly deranged liver function, with AST of 66 IU/L and ALP of 114 IU/L. Levels of CEA were within the normal range.

A CT CAP was arranged. This showed multiple hypodense lesions in both lobes of the liver, with a little irregularity of the liver outline, in keeping with multiple hepatic metastases. Unfortunately, the scan did not identify an obvious primary source. Mammography was performed to exclude a breast primary; this was unremarkable. Following discussion with the acute oncology service (AOS), it was felt that, in the absence of any other symptoms, an endoscopy was not necessary. In the presence of unresectable disease, it was also decided that a PET-CT would not contribute further to the diagnostic work-up.

> ⊕ **Clinical tip** Assessment of Performance status
>
> PS activities of daily living (ADLs) to infer the physiological reserve and fitness for anti-cancer treatment.
>
> The WHO (ECOG) performance score provides sufficient distinction for the management of patients in oncological practice [1]. A score of ≤2 is normally acceptable for therapy. Performance status may also be assessed using the Karnofsky score [2].

> ⊕ **Clinical tip** Role of endoscopy
>
> Endoscopic investigations are low-yield in the absence of specific symptoms [3,4]. Targeted endoscopy in patients with an appropriate clinical indication is endorsed. It is not recommended to perform endoscopies, unless a GI malignancy is suspected radiologically or if the patient has symptoms to warrant it [5].

✪ **Learning point** Investigations based on metastatic distribution

Clinical information regarding the pattern of metastases from different tumour types can help focus the choice of investigations performed initially to increase the chance of locating the primary source (Table 25.1).

Table 25.1 Investigations based on metastatic distribution [4,6]

Site of lesion	Additional investigations that could be considered
Supraclavicular/axillary lymphadenopathy	Mammogram ± breast MRI PSA (M)
Mediastinal lymphadenopathy	Mammogram ± breast MRI AFP, HCG PSA (M) Testicular USS (M)
Pleural disease	Mammogram ± breast MRI CA125 (F), testicular USS (M)
Peritoneal disease/malignant ascites	CA125 (F)
Retroperitoneal lesion	Beta-HCG (M), AFP (M), testicular USS (M)
Liver	Ca19-9, AFP, mammogram ± breast MRI, endoscopy
Inguinal lymphadenopathy	Proctoscopy, CA125 (F), PSA (M)
Bone	Isotope bone scan, PSA

MRI, magnetic resonance imaging; PSA, prostate-specific antigen; AFP, alpha fetoprotein; USS, ulrasound; M, male; F, female.
Source: data from Pavilidis N. and Pentheroudakis G., Cancer of unknown primary site, *The Lancet*, Volume 379, Issue 9824, pp. 1428–1435, Copyright © 2012 and National Comprehensive Cancer Network, *NCCN Clinical Practice Guidelines ion Oncology: Occult Primary*, Copyright © 2013, available from <http://www.nccn.org>.

✪ **Learning point** PET-CT in CUP

Radioactive glucose (^{18}F-FDG) is used to identify metabolically active cells, including, but not limited to, malignant cells. PET scans are read alongside concurrent CT images, so that anatomic information can be amalgamated with metabolic information. Research suggests that PET/CT in CUP has intermediate specificity and high sensitivity [6,7]; PET/CT is more successful in identifying a primary site than either CT or MRI (20–40% versus 20–27%, respectively). In a meta-analysis, it was concluded that PET/CT is able to detect a primary origin in 37% of malignancies; however, prospective information is required to validate this [8].

PET/CT is recommended in isolated cervical adenopathy for confirmation of a radiotherapy field and confirming a single metastatic site with potentially curative intent [9]. PET/CT use in widespread metastases is limited, because determining the primary site from metastasis is complex. It may prove valuable if the histopathological investigation is suggestive of the origin but not confirmatory. At present, however, PET/CT does not form part of routine investigations in the assessment of patients presenting with a CUP, but it may become increasingly used in the future [7,9].

The AOS recommended an ultrasound-guided biopsy of a liver metastasis. In light of the elevated CA125, the patient's case was discussed with the results at the gynaecological MDT meeting. Histological review revealed morphological changes consistent with a poorly differentiated carcinoma. The IHC profile favoured a metastatic, poorly differentiated carcinoma, as opposed to a hepatic primary. Positive staining with CA125 and WT-1 raised the possibility of a gynaecological origin, but the IHC pattern was insufficient to be conclusive

⭐ **Learning point** IHC

Identification of a tumour type using IHC is split into three phases:

1. A basic IHC panel of stains is performed to identify the cell lineage of the tumour, i.e. carcinoma, lymphoma, sarcoma, or melanoma.
2. Subtypes of carcinoma should then be defined, e.g. adenocarcinoma, germ cell tumour, HCC, RCC, thyroid, neuroendocrine, or squamous cell.
3. If the tumour is classified as an adenocarcinoma, then IHC may help identify the site of origin [10,11]. The differential pattern of IHC staining for a panel of antibodies may indicate the site of origin (Figure 25.1).

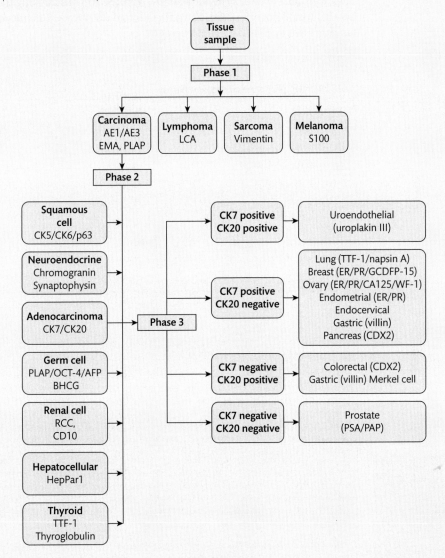

Figure 25.1 **Algorithm for IHC staining in relation to determining the primary origin of a metastatic tumour. IHC in the diagnosis of CUP [6,7,10–12]** AE1/AE3, broad-spectrum cytokeratins; EMA, epithelial membrane antigen; PLAP, placenta-like alanine phosphatase; CK5, cytokeratin 5; CK6, cytokeratin 6; OCT-4, octamer-binding transcription factor 4; AFP, alpha fetoprotein; BHCG, B-human chorionic gonadotropin; RCC, renal cell carcinoma; CD10, neprilysin; HepPar1, hepatocyte-specific antigen; TTF-1, thyroid transcription factor 1; ER, oestrogen receptor; PR, progesterone receptor; GCDFP-15, gross cystic disease fluid protein 15; CA125, cancer antigen 125; WT-1, Wilms' tumor-1; PSA, prostate-specific antigen; PAP, prostatic acid phosphatase.

Source: data from National Comprehensive Cancer Network 2013; Kim KW *et al.* 2013; Greco FA *et al.* 2012; Varadhachary GR *et al.* 2004; and Pavlidis N and Pentheroudakis G 2010.

(Table 25.2). It was also felt that the presentation was unusual for ovarian cancer, given the widespread hepatic metastases in the absence of serosal or peritoneal disease. The medical oncology team present at the meeting recommended that the patient be treated as a CUP.

When the patient met with the medical oncology team, they sensitively explained that she had an incurable, unresectable metastatic malignancy of unknown origin. They were able to offer systemic therapy, with the aim of shrinking the tumour bulk, but this would not offer cure. The patient found this a very difficult concept to grasp but was keen to consider chemotherapy.

Table 25.2 IHC properties of the liver biopsy

Positive	Negative
Pancytokeratin	Mucin
Cytokeratin (CK) 19 (weakly positive)	CK5, CK7, CK20
CA125 (focal, weak staining)	S100
WT-1 (patchy, weak staining)	Melan A
MOC 31	CDX2
	GCDFP
	TTF-1
	ER
	HepPar1

⭐ Learning point Definition of CUP

The diagnosis of CUP is made in a confirmed metastatic malignancy, for which a primary site of origin cannot be identified, following standard diagnostic investigations [7]. It is a common diagnosis, accounting for 3–5% of all malignancies diagnosed per annum [13,14] and equating to 10 000 cases in the UK annually [15,16], and is the fourth commonest cause of cancer-related deaths [12]. CUP affects males and females equally, and the average age of presentation is 60 years [17].

CUP comprises a heterogeneous collection of malignancies which display different natural histories and biological characteristics [14], often following an aggressive biological and clinical course [12]. The majority of CUP presentations are considered unfavourable, and this is reflected in poor outcomes with limited life expectancy, illustrated by a median survival of 6–12 months, with a 1-year survival of <1 in five patients [18]. Between 30% and 50% of all CUP patients present with three or more metastatic sites [19].

The majority of CUP patients present with vague, non-specific symptoms such as lethargy, anorexia, weight loss, and night sweats. Emergency presentation with intestinal obstruction, pathological fracture, or metastatic spinal cord compression (MSCC) is not uncommon, with CUP accounting for 10% of MSCC presentations [17,20].

Review of the data from post-mortem examinations suggest that the commonest primary sites include the lung (27%), pancreas (24%), liver or bile duct (8%), kidney or adrenal glands (8%), colorectal (7%), genital system (7%), and stomach (6%) [4].

⓰ Expert comment

Females with adenocarcinoma confined to axillary lymphadenopathy should be managed by the breast team, and referral to the MDT is appropriate. Standard breast investigations, such as mammography and ultrasound, should be performed, and a dynamic contrast-enhanced MRI considered if no breast primary tumour identified.

✪ **Learning point** The pathogenesis of CUP

Historically, CUP malignancies were thought to originate from different primary sites and were linked by their ability to metastasize early and aggressively, with regression or dormancy of the primary malignancy, an uncharacteristic pattern of disease, and chemoresistance [4,6,12]. It remains unclear whether they belong together purely as a consequence of their exclusion from primary origin groups or whether they are, in fact, a clinical entity in their own right with a unifying pathological basis [7]. Whilst there has been extensive research to identify a unique biological behaviour or genetic signature to demark CUP as a discrete group, no specific factor has been identified [7,12]. Recent investigations of genetic profiling, angiogenesis, hypoxic mechanisms, and signalling have failed to identify a CUP-specific signature [13].

However, with a primary origin only identified in 30% of cases, the most successful outcomes, at present, are in patients who receive site-specific chemotherapy directed at a primary, with empirical therapy offering limited benefit [21].

Pathological classification of CUP presentations illustrated that 60% are moderately differentiated carcinomas, 29% poorly differentiated adenocarcinomas or undifferentiated carcinomas, 5% SCCs, 5% poorly differentiated malignant neoplasms, and 1% neuroendocrine malignancies of unknown origin [6,12].

✪ **Learning point** Prognostic characteristics of CUP, based on histology and site of presentation

CUP can be divided into different prognostic groups, based on the likely chance of being able to offer curative treatment.

1. *Favourable CUP (approximately 20% of cases)* [22]

   These cases may be treated radically with curative intent:
   - presentation with axillary lymph node involvement only
   - SCC with cervical nodes only
   - isolated inguinal lymphadenopathy
   - small potentially resectable metastasis

   In addition, the following presentations may be treatable:
   - poorly differentiated adenocarcinoma with a midline distribution
   - women with papillary adenocarcinoma of the peritoneal cavity
   - neuroendocrine malignancy
   - males with elevated PSA levels and blastic bone lesions

2. *Unfavourable CUP (approximately 80% of cases) for which curative treatment is unlikely* [23,24]
   - Adenocarcinoma metastatic to the liver or other organs.
   - Non-papillary malignant ascites of adenocarcinomatous origin.
   - Multiple cerebral metastases of either adenocarcinomatous or squamous origin.
   - Multiple lung or pleural metastases of adenocarcinomatous origin.
   - Widespread cutaneous metastases.

Other prognostic variables have been identified for CUP which can also help predict the outcome. These include:

1. *Independent factors associated with favourable outcomes:*
   - female gender
   - good PS
   - absence of systemic symptoms
   - a low number of metastatic sites
   - functional bone marrow
   - normal LDH, ALP, CEA, and albumin

2. *Independent factors associated with poor outcomes* [3,18,25]:
   - male gender
   - multiple sites of metastatic disease, particularly in the liver
   - adenocarcinomatous subtype
   - poor PS
   - bone or pleural metastases

Empirical chemotherapy with epirubicin, cisplatin, and capecitabine (ECX) was commenced. This regimen was chosen, as it is commonly used in unknown primary cancers and has activity in oesophageal, gastric, breast, gynaecological, and urothelial malignancies. The patient received three cycles of ECX in total. Over the course of her treatment, her CA125 continued to rise. A restaging scan at the end of three cycles showed progression of the hepatic disease, but no new sites of disease.

Despite disease progression, the patient remained PS 1 and so was offered second-line gemcitabine/paclitaxel treatment. The patient had to stop paclitaxel after one dose, due to severe back and leg pain which started during infusion of the drug. The symptoms were thought to be related to an allergic reaction to paclitaxel. They did not improve with slowing down the rate of the paclitaxel infusion, so docetaxel was substituted into the regimen for cycle 2.

Following six cycles of gemcitabine and taxane chemotherapy, the patient's CA125 level had returned to normal limits (Figure 25.2), and an end-of-treatment CT CAP showed a 50% reduction in hepatic metastasis, with no other sites of malignancy (Figure 25.3).

❻ Expert comment

Both these cytotoxic drugs show activity in ovarian cancer. Gemcitabine is also active in hepatobiliary malignancy. Given the progression on ECX, it was decided to use drugs active in ovarian cancer on the basis of the raised CA125. This case is unusual, as often the CUP population is too unwell to have several lines of anti-cancer therapy.

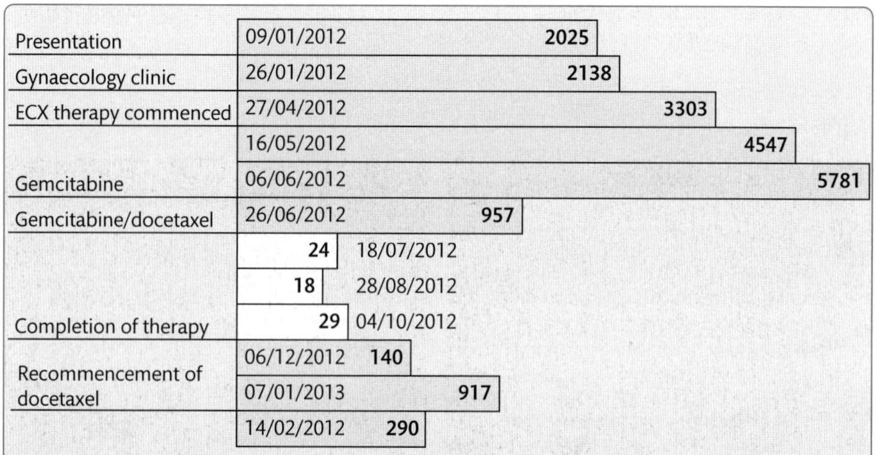

Figure 25.2　CA125 levels over the course of treatment.

	Date	CA125
Presentation	09/01/2012	2025
Gynaecology clinic	26/01/2012	2138
ECX therapy commenced	27/04/2012	3303
	16/05/2012	4547
Gemcitabine	06/06/2012	5781
Gemcitabine/docetaxel	26/06/2012	957
	18/07/2012	24
	28/08/2012	18
Completion of therapy	04/10/2012	29
	06/12/2012	140
Recommencement of docetaxel	07/01/2013	917
	14/02/2012	290

❻ Expert comment

Historically, the only treatment option in CUP malignancies was empirical chemotherapy, with approximately 70% of primary sites remaining elusive. If a primary site can be determined, site-specific chemotherapy can be delivered with improved outcomes.

★ Learning point Chemotherapy in CUP

Poorly differentiated adenocarcinomas and undifferentiated carcinomas appear to respond to platinum-based chemotherapy, traditionally cisplatin or carboplatin. In the majority of cases, platinum agents are used in combination with various additional agents, including gemcitabine, paclitaxel, docetaxel, 5-FU/capecitabine, and etoposide, depending on the metastatic distribution. Single-agent treatment is an option for patients who would not tolerate the toxicity of a multiple-treatment therapy. Recently, newer biological agents have been trialled in the empirical setting. In a phase II trial, results with bevacizumab and erlotinib, in combination with carboplatin/paclitaxel, were encouraging, but further research is required [12,26].

Trials have suggested that CUP malignancies of determined primary do not reflect the response of the associated originally diagnosed primary of equivalent stage [12]. However, whilst the site-specific treatments may show less affinity for malignancies which present as CUP, the likelihood is that the response will be better than for empirical chemotherapy which is currently relatively ineffective (Table 25.3) [27].

(continued)

Table 25.3 Treatment of favourable presentation CUP [6,12]

Pathological diagnosis	Chemotherapy regime
Poorly differentiated carcinoma with midline nodal disease	Treated as extragonadal germ cell malignancy with platinum-based chemotherapy
Peritoneal serous papillary adenocarcinoma	Treated as stages III–IV ovarian malignancy with platinum-based chemotherapy ± surgery
Isolated axillary lymph node involvement	Treated as stages II–III breast cancer with surgery plus adjuvant chemoradiotherapy ± hormonal therapy
SCC with cervical nodes only	Treated as locally advanced head and neck malignancy with surgery plus radiotherapy (plus chemotherapy in N2/N3 disease)
Isolated inguinal lymphadenopathy	Treated as lymphoma with nodal dissection ± radiotherapy ± chemotherapy
Neuroendocrine malignancies	Treated as SCLC with platinum ± etoposide chemotherapy
Blastic bone metastasis	Treated as prostate cancer with hormonal therapy ± chemotherapy

Source: data from National Institute for Health and Clinical Excellence (NICE), *Diagnosis and management of metastatic malignant disease of unknown primary origin*, Copyright © NICE 2010, available from <https://www.ncbi.nlm.nih.gov/books/NBK82159/pdf/TOC.pdf> and Pavlidis N and Pentheroudakis G, Cancer of unknown primary site: 20 questions to be answered, *Annals of Oncology*, Volume 21, Issue Supplement 7, pp. vii303–vii307, Copyright © The Author 2010. Published by Oxford University Press on behalf of the European Society for Medical Oncology. All rights reserved.

❝ Expert comment

Curative surgery should be considered where patients have squamous carcinoma confined to the inguinal nodes and patients referred to an appropriate surgeon. Superficial lymphadenectomy may be considered with post-operative radiotherapy, if there are multiple involved nodes or extracapsular spread. If a simple excision of clinically involved nodes is performed, radiotherapy is recommended.

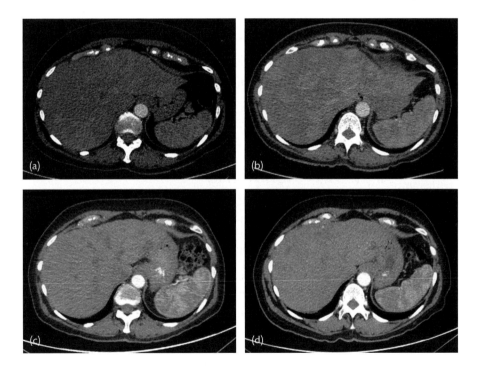

Figure 25.3 CT changes during treatment. (A) CT displaying liver metastasis at presentation, with multiple lesions throughout both lobes of the liver; (B) progression of disease following ECX chemotherapy; (C) progression of disease on single-agent gemcitabine; (D) 50% regression of hepatic metastasis following gemcitabine/docetaxel combination therapy.

At this point, the patient had received 9 months of chemotherapy, and therefore a chemotherapy holiday was recommended to try and maximize bone marrow health, before further treatment was required. However, during this chemotherapy-free period, the patient's CA125 began to rise again, and therefore further single-agent chemotherapy was reinstituted with docetaxel chemotherapy, to which she showed a further biochemical and radiological response. The patient then remained stable for 3 months, before becoming symptomatic with right upper quadrant pain and a rising CA125. A CT scan confirmed progression in her hepatic metastases, and she commenced treatment with weekly topotecan, which produced a symptomatic response and a decrease in CA125 after two cycles. She proceeded to three further cycles following which she developed heart failure leading her to discontinue chemotherapy.

Discussion

The current case identifies a well patient presenting with very non-specific symptoms and an isolated elevated CA125. The case highlights some of the diagnostic and management difficulties faced when assessing and treating patients with CUP.

The extent to which patients with CUP are investigated remains controversial. National guidelines recommend that investigations should only be undertaken if the results will directly impact on treatment, and the patient understands the indication, risk, and benefits of any treatment being offered and will accept treatment [28]. CUP patients generally have aggressive, time-limiting disease, and exhaustive investigations may not optimize the QoL or outcome. In certain cases, referral to palliative care for symptom control may be more appropriate [28]. The diagnostic process should aim to identify patients with favourable presentations in a timely manner, to optimize treatment outcomes [12,14]. CUP patients with poor PS and aggressive disease are unlikely to benefit from exhaustive investigations.

Molecular profiling may be an important diagnostic tool in the CUP work-up in the future. This process identifies the genomic profile of the tumour and may be used to determine the malignant origin. It also has the potential to help individualize therapy.

The genetic expression profile of the biopsied tissue, acquired using a reverse transcriptase polymerase chain reaction (RT-PCR) assay, is compared to a database of profiled tumour types, ranging from ten to 92 reference profiles [29]. The assay predictions are considered to be accurate in approximately 75% of cases, based on the eventual identification of the primary site from analysis of historical samples. The issue of concern is the potential incorrect identification of the primary tumour site, which will lead to the recommendation of incorrect treatments and false predictive and prognostic data [11,17,27,30]. Current guidance does not routinely advocate the routine incorporation of molecular profiling into the diagnostic pathway of patients with CUP [6,28]. In the future, however, molecular profiling may become an integral contributor to the clinicopathological picture [30,31].

⊕ Expert comment

Early oncological input in guiding investigations may identify patients at a stage where they are fit for treatment. Furthermore, unnecessary investigations may be avoided in patients who would not be treatable. The formation of CUP MDTs and keyworkers, and the introduction of AOS, working closely with palliative care services, is critical to this.

A final word from the expert

This is a rather unusual case of CUP, in that the patient remained fit for several lines of chemotherapy, despite presenting with hepatic metastases. Often, such patients present late with advanced symptomatic disease, with a PS that makes treatment difficult. Furthermore, CUP is considered to be relatively chemoresistant, and she has displayed a significant response to taxanes.

With the advent of gene expression profiling and personalized medicine in the future, it is hoped that the outcomes in CUP will be improved both by improving identification of the primary and by establishing individualized therapeutic targets.

References

1. Oken MM, Creech RH, Tormey DC *et al.* Toxicity and response criteria of the Eastern Cooperative Oncology Group. *American Journal of Clinical Oncology* 1982; **5**(6): 649–55.
2. Karnofsky DA, Burchenal JH. The clinical evaluation of chemotherapeutic agents in cancer. In: MacLeod CM, ed. *Evaluation of chemotherapeutic agents.* New York: Columbia University Press, 1949; p. 196.
3. Nishimori H, Takahashi S, Kiura K *et al.* Cancer of unknown primary site: a review of 28 cases and the efficacy of cisplatin/docetaxel therapy at a single institute in Japan. *Acta Medica Okayama* 2010; **64**(5): 285–91.
4. Pavilidis N, Pentheroudakis G. Cancer of unknown primary site. *The Lancet* 2012; **379**(9824): 1428–35.
5. National Institute for Health and Care Excellence. *Metastatic malignant disease of unknown primary origin.* 2010. Available at: <http://www.nice.org.uk/guidance/cg104>.
6. National Comprehensive Cancer Network. *NCCN clinical practice guidelines on oncology: occult primary.* 2013. Available at: <http://www.nccn.org>.
7. Kim KW, Krajewski KM, Jagannathan *et al.* Cancer of unknown primary sites: what radiologists need to know and what oncologists want to know. *American Journal of Roentgenology* 2013; **200**(3): 484–92.
8. Kwee TC, Kwee RM. Combined FDG-PET/CT for the detection of unknown primary tumours: systematic review and meta-analysis. *European Journal of Radiology* 2009; **19**(3): 731–44.
9. Seve P, Billotey C, Brussolle C *et al.* The role of 2-deoxy-2(F-18)fluoro-D-glucose positron emission tomography in disseminated carcinoma of unknown primary site. *Cancer* 2006; **109**(2): 292–9.
10. Greco FA, Oien K, Erlander M *et al.* Cancer of unknown primary: progress in the search for improved and rapid diagnosis leading towards superior patient outcomes. *Annals of Oncology* 2012; **23**(2): 298–304.
11. Varadhachary GR, Abbruzzese JL, Lenzi R. Diagnostic strategies for unknown primary cancer. *Cancer* 2004; **100**(9): 1776–85.
12. Pavlidis N, Pentheroudakis G. Cancer of unknown primary site: 20 questions to be answered. *Annals of Oncology* 2010; **21**(S7): vii303–7.
13. Kamposioras K, Pentheroudakis G, Pavlidis N. Exploring the biology of cancer of unknown primary: breakthroughs and drawbacks. *European Journal of Clinical Investigation* 2013; **43**(5): 491–500.

14. Matsubara N, Mukai, Nagai S *et al.* Review of primary of unknown cancer: cases referred to the National Cancer Centre Hospital East. *International Journal of Clinical Oncology* 2010; **15**(6): 578–82.

15. Jemal A, Siegel R, Ward E *et al.* Cancer statistics, 2009. *CA: A Cancer Journal for Clinicians* 2009; **59**(4): 225–49.

16. Office for National Statistics. *Cancer survival: England and Wales, 1991–2001, twenty major cancers by age group.* London: Office for National Statistics, 2005.

17. Randen M, Lewin F, Helde Frankling M *et al.* Cancer with unknown primary—implementation of a regional referral process and clinical practice guidelines. *Clinical Oncology* 2008; **20**(7): 564.

18. Culine S, Kramar A, Saghatchiam M *et al.* Development and validation of a prognostic model to predict length of survival in patients with carcinoma of unknown primary site. *Journal of Clinical Oncology* 2002; **20**(24): 4679–83.

19. Van de Wouw AJ, Jansen RLH, Speel EJM *et al.* The unknown biology of the unknown primary tumour: a literature review. *Annals of Oncology* 2003; **14**(2): 191–6.

20. Douglas S, Schild SE, Rades D. Metastatic spinal cord compression in patients with cancer of unknown primary. Estimating the survival prognosis with a validated score. *Strahlentherapie und Onkologie* 2012; **188**(11): 1048–51.

21. Golfinopoulos V, Pentheroudakis, Slanti G *et al.* Comparative survival with diverse chemotherapy regimes for cancer of unknown primary site: multiple-treatments meta-analysis. *Cancer Treatment Reviews* 2009; **35**(7): 570–3.

22. Pavidis N, Petrakis D, Golfinopoulos V *et al.* Long-term survivors among patients with cancer of unknown primary. *Critical reviews in Oncology/Haematology* 2012; **84**(1): 85–92.

23. Pavlidis N, Fizazi K. Cancer of unknown primary (CUP). *Critical Reviews in Oncology/Haematology* 2005; **54**(3): 243–50.

24. Koca R, Ustundag MD, Kargi E *et al.* A case with widespread cutaneous metastases of unknown primary origin: grave prognostic finding in cancer. *Dermatology Online Journal* 2005; **11**(1): 16.

25. Ayoub JP, Hess KR, Abbruzzese MC *et al.* Unknown primary tumours metastatic to the liver. *Journal of Clinical Oncology* 1998; **16**(6): 2105–12.

26. Hainsworth JD, Spigel DR, Thompson DS *et al.* Paclitaxel/carboplatin plus bevacizumab/erlotinib in the first line treatment of patients with carcinoma of unknown primary site. *The Oncologist* 2009; **14**(12): 1189–97.

27. Greco FA, Spigel DR, Yardley DA *et al.* Molecular profiling in unknown primary cancer: accuracy of tissue of origin prediction. *The Oncologist* 2010; **15**(5): 500–6.

28. National Institute for Health and Care Excellence. *Metastatic malignant disease of unknown primary origin.* 2010. Available at: < http://www.nice.org.uk/guidance/cg104>.

29. Talantov D, Baden J, Jatkoe T *et al.* A quantitative reverse transcriptase-polymerase chain reaction assay to identifiy metastatic carcinoma of tissue origin. *Journal of Molecular Diagnosistics* 2006; 8(3): 320–9.

30. Greco FA. Cancer of unknown primary or unrecognized adenexal skin primary carcinoma? Limitations of gene expression profiling diagnosis. *Journal of Clinical Oncology* 2013; **31**(11): 1479.

31. Chiang WM, Kapadia M, Laver NV *et al.* Cancer of unknown primary: from immunohistochemistry to gene expression profiling. *Journal of Clinical Oncology* 2012; **30**(29): 300–2.

INDEX

figures, diagrams and pictures are given in italics